LANGUAGE AND READING DISABILITIES

Third Edition

LANGUAGE AND READING DISABILITIES

Alan G. Kamhi

University of North Carolina at Greensboro

Hugh W. Catts

University of Kansas

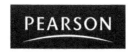

Boston   Columbus   Indianapolis   New York   San Francisco   Upper Saddle River
Amsterdam   Cape Town   Dubai   London   Madrid   Milan   Munich   Paris   Montreal   Toronto
Delhi   Mexico City   São Paulo   Sydney   Hong Kong   Seoul   Singapore   Taipei   Tokyo

Vice President and Editorial Director: Jeffery W. Johnston
Executive Editor and Publisher: Stephen D. Dragin
Editorial Assistant: Jamie Bushell
Vice President, Director of Marketing: Margaret Waples
Marketing Manager: Weslie Sellinger
Senior Managing Editor: Pamela D. Bennett
Project Manager: Pat Brown
Senior Art Director: Jayne Conte
Cover Designer: Bruce Kenselaar
Cover Art: Fotolia
Full-Service Project Management: Niraj Bhatt/Aptara®, Inc.
Composition: Aptara®, Inc.
Text Printer/Binder and Cover Printer: LSC Communications
Text Font: Times

Credits and acknowledgments for materials borrowed from other sources and reproduced, with permission, in this textbook appear on appropriate page within text.

Every effort has been made to provide accurate and current Internet information in this book. However, the Internet and information posted on it are constantly changing, so it is inevitable that some of the Internet addresses listed in this textbook will change.

Library of Congress Cataloging-in-Publication Data
Kamhi, Alan G.
    Language and reading disabilities / Alan G. Kamhi, Hugh W. Catts. — 3rd ed.
        p. cm.
    Rev. ed. of: Language and reading disabilities : Boston : Pearson/A & B. 2nd ed. 2005.
    ISBN-13: 978-0-13-707277-4
    ISBN-10: 0-13-707277-5
    1. Reading disability—United States.   2. Children—United States—Language.   3. Reading—Remedial teaching—United States.   4. English language—Composition and exercises—Study and teaching—United States.
I. Catts, Hugh W. (Hugh William),   II. Kamhi, Alan G., Language and reading disabilities.   III. Title.
    LB1050.5.L25 2012
    371.91′44—dc22

                                                                                                2011010228

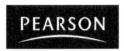

www.pearsonhighered.com

ISBN 10:   0-13-707277-5
ISBN 13: 978-0-13-707277-4

CONTENTS

PREFACE

More than 20 years have passed since the first version of this book was published in 1989. Readers who remember this book with its unique blue and pinkish-purple cover know that the title was different, *Reading Disabilities: A Developmental Language Perspective*, and the authorship order was reversed. Readers are more likely to remember the first edition of *Language and Reading Disabilities*, which was published in 1999, with Hugh as the first author. The second edition followed six years later in 2005, and this third edition will appear in 2011, six years after the second edition. The pace of advances in research and instruction in reading disabilities has obviously not slowed. Indeed, 10 years after the passing of the No Child Left Behind legislation, more attention than ever is focused on students achieving adequate levels of reading proficiency. The third edition attempts to keep pace with the rapid changes in our knowledge about language and reading disabilities.

NEW TO THIS EDITION

The most significant change in this edition is the addition of two new chapters, one on reading comprehension (Chapter 6, Kamhi) and one on spelling (Chapter 8, Apel, Masterson, & Brimo). The chapter on reading comprehension supplements the chapter by Carol Westby (Chapter 7) that has appeared in previous editions. Westby's chapter focuses on the cognitive and language aspects of comprehension. The new chapter tackles definitional issues that affect the way reading is assessed and taught. A model of comprehension is presented to help practitioners and educators develop appropriate measures of understanding and determine how to integrate strategy-based instruction with instruction that targets content and disciplinary literacy.

The chapter on spelling is a welcome addition to the book. Kenn Apel and his colleagues discuss the four-block model of spelling that he and Julie Masterson have developed and refined over the years. The model focuses on four types of knowledge (phonologic, orthographic, morphologic, and semantic) that contribute to the development of word-specific orthographic representations, or what they call "mental graphemic representations." The chapter contains numerous suggestions to help educators and practitioners assess and treat students with spelling difficulties.

Another major change in this edition is the consolidation of information on defining and classifying reading disabilities into one chapter (Chapter 3) and the addition of Suzanne Adlof as a coauthor. The two topics are obviously related, and consolidating them allowed us to add additional chapters. Suzanne also assisted us in the revision of Chapter 4 on the causal bases of reading disabilities.

With the exception of Chapter 1, every other chapter was significantly revised. Chapter 1 was updated, but the basic content stayed the same. Some of the significant changes are highlighted here:

- New section on comprehension development in Chapter 2
- New information about RTI and subgroups of poor readers in Chapter 3
- New information about auditory processing deficits and poor comprehenders in Chapter 4
- New section and information about response to instruction (RTI) and poor responders in Chapter 5

- New information about developing literate vocabulary and complex syntactic structures in Chapter 7
- Additional information about how to write genre-specific texts in Chapter 9
- New information about cognitive/linguistic skills in writing in Chapter 10

ORGANIZATION OF THIS TEXT

As mentioned earlier, the book now has 10 chapters. In Chapter 1, which discusses the convergences and divergences of language and reading, Hugh and I begin by presenting a model depicting the processes involved in both spoken and written language. Although spoken and written language share common processes, there are also important nontrivial differences between the two. A major point in the chapter is that reading, spelling, and writing are not simple derivatives of understanding and producing spoken language.

Chapter 2 focuses on the development of reading abilities. In the first part of the chapter, the importance of early exposure to literacy materials and experiences is stressed. Stage theories of reading development are then compared to more current models that emphasize the role of self-teaching mechanisms in learning to read. Although it is clear that instruction is critical to learning to read, becoming a proficient reader is largely "self-taught" and based on children's phonological, orthographic, and language knowledge. The last section of the chapter tackles the development of comprehension. It is a relatively short section because the complexity and variability of comprehension make it difficult to tell a coherent story of comprehension development.

Chapter 3 considers the difficult issues involved in defining and classifying reading disabilities. We begin by tracing the historic roots of the study of reading disabilities, focusing on how professionals came to recognize that language processes play a central role in reading disabilities. We then address the confusions surrounding terminology and provide a brief discussion of prevalence and gender issues. In the next section, we define dyslexia and other reading disabilities. The distinction between dyslexia and other language-based reading disabilities leads to a discussion of the classification of reading disabilities. We review the evidence for individual differences among children with reading disabilities and consider various attempts to subtype poor readers based on these individual differences. We suggest that children should be classified using the Simple View of Reading, which views reading comprehension as the product of word recognition and language comprehension abilities. Poor readers are classified into subgroups based on their word recognition and language or listening comprehension abilities: dyslexic (poor word recognition, good listening comprehension), specific comprehension deficit (good word recognition, poor listening comprehension), and mixed (poor word recognition and poor listening comprehension). We think that this classification system will allow practitioners to provide more appropriate intervention for children with reading disabilities.

In Chapter 4, the wealth of information about causal factors related to reading disabilities is reviewed. After discussing the impact of early literacy experiences and reading instruction, we delve into the many possible intrinsic causes of reading disabilities—genetic, neurological, visual, auditory, attentional, and language factors. Although multiple factors interact to cause reading disabilities, language deficits are central to most reading disabilities. Importantly, language deficits are both a cause and a consequence of reading disabilities.

Chapters 5, 6, and 7 are devoted to the assessment and treatment of the basic components of reading disabilities: word recognition and comprehension. In Chapter 5, Al Otaiba and her colleagues review procedures and measures used to assess phoneme awareness and discuss how to maximize the effectiveness of phoneme awareness instruction. They proceed to review issues in the assessment of word-recognition instructional activities to teach word-reading skills. As mentioned earlier, Chapters 6 and 7 focus on the assessment and treatment of comprehension problems. Chapter 8 addresses spelling.

In the last two chapters, writing disorders are addressed. In Chapter 9, Cheryl Scott discusses the writing process and what is known about how children learn to write. She also addresses the writing problems encountered by children with language and reading disabilities. This chapter lays the groundwork for Chapter 10, in which Carol Westby provides an extensive discussion of the philosophies and frameworks for assessing and facilitating written language development.

NEW! COURSESMART eTEXTBOOK AVAILABLE

CourseSmart is an exciting new choice for students looking to save money. As an alternative to purchasing the printed textbook, students can purchase an electronic version of the same content. With a CourseSmart etextbook, students can search the text, make notes online, print out reading assignments that incorporate lecture notes, and bookmark important pssages for later review. For more information, or to purchase access to the CourseSmart eTextbook, visit www.coursesmart.com.

ACKNOWLEDGMENTS

More than 20 years ago, I wrote about how the origins of this book could be traced to a hotel restaurant in Cincinnati at the 1983 ASHA convention. I related the story of how someone spelled the name on a matchbook sitting on the table (H-a-t-h-a-w-a-y). I noted that there was considerable variability in the ability of four adults to say what the word was. It's time to set the record straight. There were not four adults sitting in a hotel restaurant. It was just Hugh and me sitting in our hotel room. The matchbook was real, as was the problem Hugh had figuring out what I was spelling. He kept asking me to spell it again, but despite the repetitions and slow rate of spelling, he never got it. The story is important because it began Hugh's transition from a speech scientist at Case Western Reserve University to a language and reading specialist at the University of Kansas. Our studies in the 1980s began this transition by investigating phonological processing abilities in children and adults with language and reading disabilities. Hugh's own difficulties with phonological processing led him to develop one of the earliest prototypes of the nonword repetition task that is now commonly used to measure phonological encoding.

In that first acknowledgment, I also mentioned how we ruminated about whether the Cleveland Indians would win the pennant in our lifetimes. This was 1988, when the Indians always finished in last place or close to last. In 1998, when it came time to write the acknowledgment for the first edition of this book, I wanted to correct the fatal (not too strong a word) mistake I made by wishing for a pennant rather than a World Series. Hugh was the first author of that book, though, and had little interest in baseball or in making any amends to the baseball gods. Truth be told, a primary motivation for me in being first author of this edition was to finally atone for the mistake I made 23 years ago.

Yes, it matters what you wish for. I firmly believe that if I had written "World Series" instead of "pennant," the Indians would have won the World Series in 1997. Do you need proof that fans make a difference? Well, here's proof. In September 2010, a film of the dramatic seventh game of the 1960 World Series between the Pittsburgh Pirates and the New York Yankees was found in Bing Crosby's wine cellar near San Francisco. No film existed of this famous game because NBC destroyed all the tapes. Crosby, who was a part owner of the Pirates at the time, was nervous that he would jinx the team if he watched the game in person. Thinking that the Pirates' chances of winning would be even better if he was out of the country, he flew to Paris and listened to the game on radio while some of his employees filmed the game. Needless to say, the Pirates won the game.

So let my conscience finally be cleared: I'm sorry, Cleveland, for setting my hopes too low and wishing for a pennant and not a World Series. We should always set our goals too high rather than too low, wish for the improbable rather than the probable, and strive for what seems unattainable at the moment rather than what is clearly attainable. The likelihood of a Cleveland championship in the near future seems as improbable in November, 2010, as the likelihood of eliminating reading failure in the near future, but this should not keep Cleveland fans from continuing to support their teams, just as it should not keep us from doing all we can to help our nation's children and adolescents become more proficient readers.

Well, I feel better. The true story about the Hathaway matchbook has finally been told, and the baseball gods have hopefully been appeased. Now for the thank-yous. We would like to thank the other contributors to this book, Suzanne Adlof, Stephanie Al Otaiba, Marcia Kosanovich, Cheryl Scott, Joe Torgesen, Kenn Apel, Julie Masterson, Danielle Brimo, and Carol Westby, who took time out from their busy schedules to update their chapters. A particular thank-you goes to Carol Westby and Cheryl Scott, who have been contributing to this book since the first edition in 1989. We would also like to thank Mary Kristen Clark for her assistance in proofreading and checking references. Steve Dragin, our long-term editor at Pearson/Allyn & Bacon, deserves a special acknowledgment for encouraging (persuading) us to complete this edition in a timely manner. Thanks also to the staff at Pearson, particularly Jamie Bushell and Linda Bayma, Niraj Bhatt at Aptara, and copyeditor Karen Slaght for their excellent support in getting the book to press. We would also like to acknowledge the support we received from our respective departments at the University of North Carolina at Greensboro and the University of Kansas.

We would also like to acknowledge the reviewers of the previous edition: Martha Dunkelberger, University of Houston; Mona Greenfield, New York University; Diane Newman, Southern Connecticut State University; and Jeanne O'Sullivan, University of New Hampshire. Their reviews identified the areas that needed better coverage in this edition.

As we did in the first edition of this book, we would like to thank all the people who took the time to let us know how the information in this book helped them provide better services to children with language and learning problems. Your comments provide an important bridge between the academic world in which we primarily reside and the schools and clinics in which you work. We would like to dedicate this book to you, the teachers and clinicians who spend every day of the week trying to improve children's language and literacy skills.

Alan Kamhi

CONTRIBUTORS AND AFFILIATIONS

EDITORS

Alan G. Kamhi, Ph.D.
Department of Communication Sciences
  and Disorders
University of North Carolina at Greensboro
Greensboro, NC

Hugh W. Catts, Ph.D.
Department of Speech-Language-Hearing:
  Sciences and Disorders
University of Kansas
Lawrence, KS

CONTRIBUTORS

Suzanne M. Adlof, Ph.D.
Department of Speech-Language-Hearing:
  Sciences and Disorders
University of Kansas
Lawrence, KS

Stephanie Al Otaiba, Ph.D.
Florida Center for Reading Research
Florida State University
Tallahassee, FL

Kenn Apel, Ph.D.
School of Communication Science and
  Disorders
Florida State University
Tallahassee, FL

Danielle Brimo, M.A.
School of Communication Science and
  Disorders
Florida State University
Tallahassee, FL

Marcia L. Kosanovich, Ph.D.
Florida Center for Reading Research
Florida State University
Tallahassee, FL

Julie J. Masterson, Ph.D.
Communication Sciences and Disorders
Missouri State University
Springfield, MO

Cheryl M. Scott, Ph.D.
Department of Communication Disorders
Rush University Medical Center
Chicago, IL

Joseph K. Torgesen, Ph.D.
Florida Center for Reading Research
Florida State University
Tallahassee, FL

Carol E. Westby, Ph.D.
Research Center for Family and Community
Albuquerque, NM

Chapter *1*

Language and Reading: Convergences and Divergences

Alan G. Kamhi and Hugh W. Catts

It is now well accepted that reading is a language-based skill. This was not the case over 20 years ago when we first wrote this chapter. At that time, the idea that most reading disabilities were best viewed as a developmental language disorder was an emerging one. A developmental language perspective of reading disabilities was the major theme of our original book and continues to be the major theme of the present book. This view rests, in part, on the fact that there are numerous similarities between spoken and written language. Reading shares many of the same processes and knowledge bases as talking and listening. Reading, however, is not a simple derivative of spoken language. Although spoken language and reading have much in common in terms of the knowledge and processes they tap, there are also fundamental, nontrivial differences between the two. Knowledge of the similarities and differences between spoken language and reading is critical for understanding how children learn to read and why some children have difficulty learning to read. In this chapter, we begin by defining language and reading. This is followed by an in-depth comparison of the processes and knowledge involved in understanding spoken and written language. Other differences between spoken and written language are then discussed.

DEFINING LANGUAGE

Definitions of language are broad based and highly integrative. An example of such a definition is offered by the American Speech-Language-Hearing Association (ASHA, 1983):

> Language is a complex and dynamic system of conventional symbols that is used in various modes for thought and communication. Contemporary views of human language hold that: (a) language evolves within specific historical, social, and cultural contexts; (b) language, as rule-governed behavior, is described by at least five parameters—phonologic, morphologic, syntactic, semantic, and pragmatic; (c) language learning and use are determined by the interaction of biological, cognitive, psychosocial, and environmental factors; and (d) effective use of language for communication requires a broad understanding of human interaction including such associated factors as nonverbal cues, motivation, and sociocultural roles. (p. 44)

1

As reflected in the definition, it is generally agreed that there are five parameters of language. These parameters are described briefly in the next section.

Phonology

Phonology is the aspect of language concerned with the rules that govern the distribution and sequencing of speech sounds. It includes a description of what the sounds are and their component features (phonetics), as well as the distributional rules that govern how the sounds can be used in various word positions and the sequence rules that describe which sounds may be combined. For example, the /ʒ/ sound that occurs in the word *measure* is never used to begin an English word. Distributional rules are different in different languages. In French, for example, the /ʒ/ sound can occur in the word-initial position, as in *je* and *jouer.* An example of a sequence rule in English would be that /r/ can follow /t/ or /d/ in an initial consonant cluster (e.g., *truck, draw*), but /l/ cannot.

Semantics

Semantics is the aspect of language that governs the meaning of words and word combinations. Sometimes semantics is divided into lexical and relational semantics. *Lexical semantics* involves the meaning conveyed by individual words. Words have both intensional and extensional meanings. Intensional meanings refer to the defining characteristics or criterial features of a word. A dog is a dog because it has four legs, barks, and licks people's faces. The extension of a word is the set of objects, entities, or events to which a word might apply in the world. The set of all real or imaginary dogs that fit the intensional criteria becomes the extension of the entity *dog*.

Relational semantics refers to the relationships that exist between words. For example, in the sentence *The Panda bear is eating bamboo,* the word *bear* not only has a lexical meaning, but it also is the agent engaged in the activity of eating. *Bamboo* is referred to as the "patient" (Chafe, 1970) because its state is being changed by the action of the verb. Words are thus seen as expressing abstract relational meanings in addition to their lexical meanings.

Morphology

In addition to the content words that refer to objects, entities, and events, there is a group of words and inflections that conveys subtle meaning and serves specific grammatical and pragmatic functions. These words have been referred to as *grammatical morphemes*. Grammatical morphemes modulate meaning. Consider the sentences *Dave is playing tennis, Dave plays tennis, Dave played tennis,* and *Dave has played tennis.* The major elements of meaning are similar in each of these sentences. The first sentence describes an action currently in progress, whereas the next sentence depicts a habitual occurrence. The last two sentences describe actions that have taken place sometime in the past. What differentiates these sentences are the grammatical morphemes (inflections and auxiliary forms) that change the tense and aspect (e.g., durative or perfective) of the sentences.

Syntax

Syntax refers to the rule system that governs how words are combined into larger meaningful units of phrases, clauses, and sentences. Syntactic rules specify word order, sentence organization, and the relationships between words, word classes, and sentence constituents, such as noun phrases and verb phrases. Knowledge of syntax enables an individual to make judgments of well-formedness or grammaticality. For example, all mature English speakers would judge the sentence *The boy hit the ball* as well formed and grammatical. In contrast, the sentence *Hit the boy ball the* would be judged as ungrammatical. It should be apparent that knowledge of syntax plays an important role in understanding language.

Pragmatics

Pragmatics concerns the use of language in context. Language does not occur in a vacuum. It is used to serve a variety of communication functions, such as declaring, greeting, requesting information, and answering questions. Communicative intentions are best achieved by being sensitive to the listener's communicative needs and nonlinguistic context. Speakers must take into account what the listener knows and does not know about a topic. Pragmatics thus encompasses rules of conversation or discourse. Speakers must learn how to initiate conversations, take turns, maintain and change topics, and provide the appropriate amount of information in a clear manner. Different kinds of discourse contexts involve different sets of rules (Lund & Duchan, 1993; Schiffrin, 1994). The most frequent kinds of discourses children encounter are conversational, classroom, narrative, and event discourses.

DEFINING READING

Reading, like spoken language, is a complex cognitive activity. Gates (1949), for example, defined reading as "a complex organization of patterns of higher mental processes . . . [that] . . . can and should embrace all types of thinking, evaluating, judging, imagining, reasoning, and problem-solving" (p. 3). A view of reading that emphasizes higher-level thinking processes is a broad view of reading (Perfetti, 1986). Thinking guided by print is another way to characterize a broad view of reading. Reading ability defined in this way is associated with skill in comprehending texts. Although this is a widely accepted view of reading, particularly among practitioners, there are both practical and theoretical problems with this broad definition.

The fundamental problem with the broad view of reading is that it conflates two very different abilities—word recognition (word-level reading) and comprehension. Word recognition involves a well-defined scope of knowledge (e.g., letters, sounds, words) and processes (decoding) that can be systematically taught. Comprehension, in contrast, is not a skill with a well-defined scope of knowledge; it is a complex of higher-level mental processes that includes thinking, reasoning, imagining, and interpreting (see Kamhi, 2009a). With a broad definition of reading, a theory of reading necessarily becomes a theory of inferencing, a theory of schemata, and a theory of learning (Perfetti, 1986). The problems with the broad view of reading led Gough and his colleagues (Gough & Tunmer, 1986; Hoover & Gough, 1990) to propose the Simple View of Reading. The central claim of the Simple View is that reading consists of two components: decoding and linguistic comprehension. *Decoding* refers to word recognition processes that transform print into words. *Linguistic comprehension* (i.e., *listening comprehension*) is defined as the process by which words, sentences, and discourses are interpreted (Gough & Tunmer, 1986).

The Simple View of Reading has appealed to many researchers and practitioners. Some researchers, however, prefer restricting the definition of reading to just the decoding component (e.g., Crowder, 1982). One advantage of a narrow view of reading is that it delineates a restricted set of processes to be examined (Perfetti, 1986). Crowder (1982), who advocates a narrow view of reading, made the following analogy between the "psychology of reading" and the "psychology of braille." The psychology of braille does not include such topics as inferences and schema application. These abilities involve broad-based cognitive-linguistic processes. Crowder argued that it was superfluous to make the study of these higher level processes part of the study of braille. The study of braille is necessarily restricted to the decoding process, or how a reader decodes braille to language. By analogy, the study of reading should also be restricted to the decoding process.

Kamhi (2009a, b) recently suggested that embracing the narrow view may provide a solution to the reading crisis in the United States. The basic argument was that it is possible to eliminate reading failure if reading is defined narrowly as decoding abilities. Reading proficiency levels should reach 90 percent, at a minimum, given the numerous research-supported instructional programs that have been shown to effectively teach word-level reading (National Reading Panel [NRP], 2000; Simmons et al., 2007). As Catts (2009) pointed out, a narrow view of reading promotes a broad view of comprehension that recognizes its complexity. Not only are there different levels of understanding (e.g., literal, analytic, creative), but comprehension also depends on thinking and reasoning processes that are domain and content specific rather than domain general (cf. Kintsch, 1998). This is why the best predictor of comprehension is often familiarity with content knowledge domains (Hirsch, 2006; Willingham, 2006). A more detailed discussion of the complexity of comprehension is provided in Chapter 6.

It should be apparent that the way one defines reading will have a significant impact on how reading is measured and taught. We encourage educators to embrace a view of reading that clearly distinguishes word recognition processes from the reasoning and thinking processes involved in comprehension.

MODELS OF SPOKEN AND WRITTEN LANGUAGE COMPREHENSION

In a book about language and reading, an understanding of the similarities and differences between spoken and written language is crucial. The sections that follow compare the specific processes and knowledge involved in comprehending spoken and written language. To set the stage for these comparison, a brief overview of models of language and reading is provided.

Models of spoken and written language comprehension have often been divided into three general classes: bottom-up, top-down, and interactive. Bottom-up models view spoken and written language comprehension as a step-by-step process that begins with the initial detection of an auditory or visual stimulus. The initial input goes through a series of stages in which it is "chunked" in progressively larger and more meaningful units. Top-down models, in contrast, emphasize the importance of scripts, schemata, and inferences that allow one to make hypotheses and predictions about the information being processed. Familiarity with the content, structure, and function of the different kinds of spoken and written discourse enables the listener and the reader to be less dependent on low-level perceptual information to construct meanings.

Reliance on top-down versus bottom-up processes varies with the material being processed and the skill of the reader. Bottom-up processes are presumed to be necessary when reading isolated, decontextualized words, whereas top-down processes facilitate not only word recognition but also discourse-level comprehension. Top-down processes are especially important when reading partially illegible material, such as cursive writing.

Many language and reading theorists (Perfetti, 1985; Rumelhart, 1977; Stanovich, 1985) have advocated interactive models in which both bottom-up and top-down processes contribute to reading and language comprehension. An interactive model of reading comprehension, for example, would acknowledge that individuals must have proficient word recognition skills as well as higher-level linguistic and conceptual knowledge to be good readers. Whereas bottom-up and top-down models emphasize sequential processing, interactive models allow for parallel or simultaneous processing to occur. Later stages could thus begin before earlier stages have been completed. Although more complex than serial processing models, parallel processing models better reflect the types of processing that occur in complex tasks such as reading.

Connectionist models have also been used to explain how children learn to recognize words (e.g., Seidenberg, 1995; Seidenberg & McClelland, 1989). With this approach, the lexicon is viewed as an interactive network of connections among different layers of processing. Instead of depicting different routes (top-down or bottom-up) to access meaning, Seidenberg and McClelland (1989) propose two different layers of units, orthographic and phonological, that connect with each other and another layer of units that represents meaning. Because activation levels are input driven, word frequency has a significant impact on word recognition because the more often a particular set of units is activated together (e.g., phonological, orthographic, conceptual), the greater the strength of the pathway associated with the particular word (cf. Whitney, 1998). A detailed review of parallel processing models of spoken and written language processing is beyond the scope of this chapter. For our purposes, it is sufficient to note that simplistic serial processing models, whether bottom-up or top-down, cannot adequately capture the complex interactions that occur within and between different processing levels.

COMPREHENDING SPOKEN AND WRITTEN LANGUAGE

We have found that the model depicted in Figure 1.1 provides a useful framework for comparing the processes and knowledge involved in comprehending spoken and written language. This model, though unique, shares components with other processing models (Gough & Tunmer, 1986; Thomson, 1984). Although the components of the model will be discussed in a linear, bottom-up fashion, the model should be viewed as an interactive one that allows for parallel processing within and between levels.

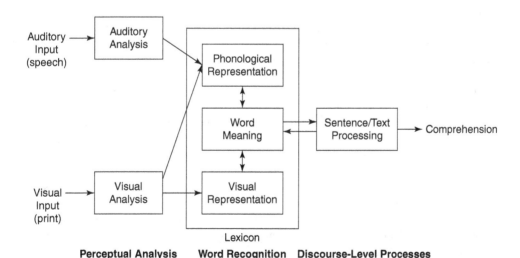

FIGURE 1.1 A Model of Spoken and Written Language Comprehension

Perceptual Analyses

The input to the perceptual analysis is speech or print. For this input to be recognized, it must be detected and analyzed. The sensory mechanisms involved in the detection of speech and print are distinctive; the ear is used to detect speech, and the eye is used to detect print. Sensory deficits involving hearing or vision place a child at risk for spoken and written language problems. Children born deaf cannot detect the speech signal through the auditory modality and, as a result, have considerable difficulty developing intelligible speech. Individuals who are blind cannot detect print through the visual modality. Braille, which relies on the tactile modality, is one way to bypass the visual deficit. An intact auditory system provides the blind another avenue to access text material by way of tape recordings.

Once the input has been detected, the segmental and suprasegmental features of spoken and written words are analyzed. In speech, the processes underlying phonetic discrimination and phonemic identification are involved. *Phonetic discrimination* refers to the ability to hear the difference between two sounds that differ acoustically and phonetically. For example, the initial *t* in the word *tap* is phonetically different from the final *t* in the word *bat*. Phonetic differences that do not affect meaning are often referred to as *allophonic variations*. If the *t* sounds in the preceding words were changed to *k* sounds, this would change the meaning of the words. *Tap* would become *cap*, and *bat* would become *back*. The phonetic differences between /t/ and /k/ are thus also phonemic differences because they change the meaning of the word. The task for the young child learning language is to determine which differences between sounds make a difference in meaning.

The language a child is learning determines which phonetic differences are phonemic. In Japanese, for example, the differences between /r/ and /l/ are allophonic. In English, however, the phonetic differences between /r/ and /l/ make a difference in meaning. In French, the front rounded vowel /y/ is phonemically different from the back rounded /u/. An American who does not make this distinction will not be able to differentiate between the words *tout* (all) and *tu* (you). These examples are meant to illustrate that learning phonemic categories requires knowledge of the language being learned. The acquisition of phonological knowledge about language necessarily involves higher-level conceptual processes. Low-level perceptual processes, such as detection and discrimination, do not lead to knowledge about phonemic categories. In light of these points, it is important to note that in most listening situations, individuals seldom have to make distinctions between minimal phoneme pairs (e.g., *p/b* in the words *pin* and *bin*) that are common stimuli on tests of discrimination. In many instances, lexical and higher-level language knowledge often eliminate the need for phonemic-level identification.

In reading, just as with speech, discrimination and identification processes are involved. In reading, *discrimination* refers to the ability to see the visual differences between letters. *Identification* requires knowledge of the correspondences between letters and phonemes. For example, the child who confuses the letters *b* and *d* in words such as *bad* and *dad* is often said to have a visual discrimination problem. It is more likely, however, that the child can perceive the visual differences between the letters *b* and *d* but has not learned that the letter *b* is associated with the phoneme /b/ and the letter *d* is associated with the phoneme /d/. In other words, the child has not learned the phoneme–letter correspondences for these two sounds.

To illustrate the difference between low-level visual discrimination ability and higher-level conceptual (identification) ability, consider the following analogy. In teaching large classes, it is common to confuse students. The first author once called a girl named Aimee, Anna. Although Aimee and Anna were both 20-something female graduate students, they could be easily differentiated by their physical characteristics, personalities, clothes, and so forth. He had no difficulty differentiating between the two students. The problem he had was associating a particular characteristic or a set of characteristics with a name. The similarity between the two names makes it more difficult to consistently use the right name with the right student. This is similar to the problem children have associating the features of a particular phoneme with the features of a particular letter. When letters and sounds are similar, as is the case for "b" and "d," it is particularly difficult to learn the correct correspondences.

These examples are meant to show that sound or letter confusions are not necessarily caused by phonetic or visual discrimination problems. With respect to spoken language, the difficulty is learning which phonetic differences make a difference in meaning. With respect to reading, the difficulty is learning which sounds are associated with which letters. In both cases, what often appear to be discrimination problems are in fact identification problems.

Word Recognition

Reading and spoken language begin to share similar knowledge domains and processes in the word recognition stage. Until this point, the processing of print and speech involves different sensory and perceptual processes. In the word recognition stage, the features identified in the previous perceptual stage are used to access the mental lexicon. The words heard or seen must activate or be associated with previously stored concepts in the individual's mental lexicon. These stored concepts in the mental lexicon represent one's vocabulary. Importantly, the content and structure of the mental lexicon is essentially the same for both reading and spoken language. The content of the lexicon includes information about the word's phonological or visual form as well as information about the word's meaning and how the word relates to other words. Consider, for example, the kind of conceptual information that might appear in the mental lexicon for the word *pencil*.

> It refers to an instrument used for writing or drawing; it is a manmade physical object, usually cylindrical in shape; and it functions by leaving a trail of graphite along a writing surface. . . .
> A pencil is one of a class of writing instruments and a close relative of the *pen, eraser,* and *sharpener.* (Just & Carpenter, 1987, p. 62)

The mental lexicon also includes syntactic and semantic information that indicates part of speech (e.g., noun, verb, or adjective) and possible syntactic and semantic roles. For example, the syntactic information about *pencil* might indicate that it is a noun that functions semantically as an instrument ("She wrote the letter with a pencil") or as a patient ("Peggy bought a pencil").

The structure of the mental lexicon has received considerable research attention during the past 30 years. Network models consisting of nodes corresponding to concepts and features have been a popular way to depict the structure of the lexicon (Collins & Loftus, 1975; Collins & Quillian, 1969). Early network models were hierarchical in nature, with the ordering in the hierarchy defined by set inclusion relations. For example, higher-order concepts such as *animal* included lower-order concepts such as *bird* and *sparrow*. Other network models have been referred to as *heterarchical,* reflecting concepts from ill-structured domains (Just & Carpenter, 1987). Although theorists might differ in their portrayal of the content and structure of the mental lexicon, they generally agree that the mental lexicon is the same for language and reading. The way in which word meanings are accessed can differ, however, in spoken language and reading.

In processing speech, word meaning is accessed through a word's phonological representation. The output of the perceptual analysis is a representation of a word's acoustic and phonetic features. These acoustic–phonetic representations of speech input are used by the listener to activate or instantiate a word's phonological representation in the lexicon. This may involve the listener in attempting to match acoustic–phonetic representations with phonological representations. Phonological representations are directly linked to a word's meaning because this information is stored together for each word in the mental lexicon.

Phonological representations of words stored in the mental lexicon can take one of several forms. Words may contain discrete phonetic and phonemic segments or syllable segments, or be represented as whole words or short phrases (e.g., "it's a" as "itsa" and "did you know" as [dIdʒəno]). Although young children's phonological representations begin to contain more discrete phonetic and phonemic information as they progress through the preschool years, the ability to access this information may not develop until age 5 or later, depending on early literacy experiences and formal instruction. Studies of young children's speech perception (e.g., Nittrouer, Manning, & Meyer, 1993) have found that there is a gradual shift in the acoustic cues used to make phonological decisions. Nittrouer and colleagues hypothesize that as children gain experience with a native language, they become more sensitive to phonetic structure. In a more recent study, Nittrouer (1996) showed that this shift is related to children's developing phonemic awareness. It seems that early exposure to reading as well as developmental changes in speech perception both contribute to young children's ability to represent speech as discrete phonemic segments.

In contrast to speech, in which there is only one way to access a word's meaning, in reading there are two ways: indirectly, by way of a phonological representation, or directly, by way of a visual representation (see Figure 1.1). Use of a visual representation to access the lexicon is variously referred to as the *direct, visual, look-and-say,* or *whole-word* approach. In accessing the lexicon in this way, the reader locates the word in the lexicon whose visual representation contains the same segmental and/or visual features as those identified in the previous perceptual analysis stage. In other words, a match is made between the perceived visual configuration and a visual representation that is part of the mental lexicon for the particular word.

Word meaning can also be accessed through a phonological representation. With this *indirect* or *phonological* approach, the reader uses knowledge of phoneme–letter correspondence rules to recode the visually perceived letters into their corresponding phonemes. Individual phonemes are then blended together to form a phonological sequence that is matched to a similar sequence in the lexicon. The phonological approach is particularly important in the development of reading. The ability to decode printed words phonologically allows children to read words they know but have never seen in print. Reading by the phonological approach also causes the child to attend to the letter sequences within words. The knowledge gained about letter sequence makes the child's visual representations more precise (see Chapter 2).

Reading by the phonological route is thus similar to speech recognition in that a word is recognized by way of its phonological representation. There is one important difference, however, in using phonological representations to access meaning in comprehending spoken and written language. To successfully use the phonological route in reading, one must have explicit awareness of the phonological structure of words, specifically, the knowledge that words consist of discrete phonemic segments (Liberman, 1983). These segments are not readily apparent to young children because the sound segments of speech are blended together in the acoustic signal. For example, the word *cat* is one acoustic event; its sound segments do not correspond exactly to its three written symbols. Although preschool children might show some phonological awareness, much explicit instruction and practice is usually required for a child to become efficient in using the phonological approach.

The recognition that there were two possible routes to word recognition led to the popularity of dual-route models of word recognition (cf. Stanovich, 1991). Although early proponents of dual-route models agreed that there were two routes to word recognition, they differed in assumptions about the various speeds of the two access mechanisms and how conflicting information was resolved. The size of the sound–letter correspondences in the phonological route also differed from model to model (e.g., sound-by-sound, syllables, word level). Discussions of the different variations of these models can be found in Coltheart, Curtis, Atkins, and Haller (1993), Patterson and Coltheart (1987), and Rayner and Pollatsek (1989).

Questions about the nature of the print-to-sound conversion have recently taken a new turn due to the increasing popularity of parallel-distributed processing models that contain no word-level representations or lexicon in the network (Share & Stanovich, 1995). Regardless of how the print-to-sound conversion takes place, there is recent evidence that this conversion is essential for the large numbers of low-frequency words that cannot be recognized on a visual basis (Share & Stanovich, 1995). In contrast, high-frequency words seem to be recognized visually with minimal phonological recoding even in the very earliest stages of reading acquisition (Reitsma, 1990). The more exposure a child has to a word, the more likely a visual approach will be used. The use of a visual versus a phonological approach to word recognition depends on the frequency of the word rather than the particular reading stage a child is in. More will be said about the development of word recognition skills in the next chapter.

Discourse-Level Processes

Up to this point, we have considered the processes involved in recognizing words. Spoken and written language, however, consists of longer discourse units, such as sentences, conversations, lectures, stories, and expository texts. Psycholinguistic studies carried out in the 1960s and 1970s (cf. Carroll, 1994; Clark & Clark, 1977) explored the role that syntactic, semantic, and world knowledge played in comprehending larger units of spoken and written discourse. By focusing on the independent contribution these different types of knowledge made toward meaning, these early studies were limited in what they could tell us about the interaction of different types of knowledge and whether different discourse types are processed the same way by listeners and readers. Despite these limitations, it is useful to consider how structural, propositional, and situation or world knowledge can be used to construct meaning.

STRUCTURAL KNOWLEDGE.   A variety of structural cues are used by listeners and readers in comprehending speech and text. These cues include word order, grammatical morphemes, and function words such as relative pronouns, conjunctions, and modals. Listeners and readers often use syntactic and morphologic cues to figure out the meaning of unknown words. Grammatical morphemes, for example, provide information about word classes. Adverbs are signaled by the inflections -*ly* and -*y*, whereas adjectives are marked by the suffixes -*able* and -*al*. Verbs are signaled by the inflections -*ed, -ing,* and -*en*. Nouns are marked by definite and indefinite articles, plural and possessive markers, and suffixes such as -*ment* and -*ness*. The reason why readers are able to make any sense at all out of a sentence like "Twas brillig and the slithy toves did gyre and gimble in the wabe" is that inflections (*y* and *s*) and syntactic markers (*the* and *did*) provide cues about grammatical form class.

Clark and Clark (1977) provide an excellent review of studies that demonstrate the influence syntactic and morphologic knowledge have on sentence comprehension. It has been shown, for example, that listeners use function words to segment sentences into constituents, classify the constituents, and construct meanings from them (e.g., Bever, 1970; Fodor & Garrett, 1967). Consider the following two sentences, one with relative pronouns and one without:

1. The pen that the author whom the editor liked used was new.
2. The pen the author the editor liked used was new.

Fodor and Garrett (1967) found that listeners had more difficulty paraphrasing sentences like (2) than sentences like (1). More recent studies have continued to attempt to prove that the initial segmentation of a sentence (i.e., parsing) is performed by a syntactic module that is not influenced by other kinds of knowledge (e.g., Frazier, 1987).

PROPOSITIONAL KNOWLEDGE.   Although structural knowledge may play an important role in understanding sentences, memory for extended discourse rarely maintains structural information. The fact that we generally store and remember the gist of what we hear or read suggests that processing resources must be devoted primarily to constructing meaningful propositions. A proposition is an *idea-unit* that consists of a predicate and its related arguments. It is generally agreed that listeners and readers use their knowledge of predicates and their inherent arguments to construct propositions. The predicate *give,* for example, requires three noun phrases or arguments: an agent to do the giving, an object to be given, and a recipient of the object. When listeners hear a sentence like *Alison gave the book to Franne,* they look for the three arguments entailed by the predicate *give.*

A simple semantic strategy suggested years ago by Bever (1970) is that listeners and readers might use content words alone to build propositions that make sense. For example, if the words *pile, raked, girl, leaves* were presented without any other syntactic information, it would be apparent that two propositions were involved: *The girl raked the leaves* and *the leaves were in a pile.* To show that listeners used content words to build propositions, researchers (e.g., Stolz, 1967) showed that semantically constrained sentences (3) were much easier to paraphrase than semantically unconstrained sentences (4).

3. The vase that the maid that the agency hired dropped broke on the floor.
4. The dog that the cat that the girl fought scolded approached the colt.

It has also been shown that propositional complexity influences processing time. Kintsch and Keenan (1973), for example, showed that sentence 5, which contains eight propositions, took significantly more time to read than sentence 6, which contained only four propositions. Note that the two sentences have about the same number of words.

5. Cleopatra's downfall lay in her foolish trust in the fickle political figures of the Roman world.
6. Romulus, the legendary founder of Rome, took the women of the Sabine by force.

Subsequent studies have examined the hierarchical networks of propositions that listeners and readers construct to link propositions within spoken discourse and text. Not surprisingly, researchers have found that the propositions listeners and readers construct are affected by many factors, such as nature of the discourse/text, knowledge of the world, processing capacity, interest level, and so forth.

WORLD KNOWLEDGE.   Structural and propositional knowledge are crucial for constructing meaning, but an individual's knowledge of the world or what has come to be called *situation model representations* also plays an important role in comprehension. Consider, for example, how world knowledge makes the sentence *Jake ate the ice cream with relish* unambiguous, whereas a similar sentence, *Jake ate the sausage with relish*, is ambiguous (Just & Carpenter, 1987). We know that relish is normally not eaten with ice cream. Such information is not specific to language; instead, it reflects general knowledge about the tastes of foods to assign with *relish*.

World knowledge can be divided into knowledge of specific content domains and knowledge of interpersonal relations. Specific content domains would include academic subjects such as history, geography, mathematics, and English literature; procedural knowledge such as how to fix a car, tie a shoelace, and play tennis; and scriptlike knowledge of familiar events. Interpersonal knowledge involves such things as knowledge of human needs, motivations, attitudes, emotions, values, behavior, personality traits, and relationships. It should be evident how these kinds of world knowledge play an important role in processing spoken and written language.

Because world knowledge can be so broad, psychologists have focused attention on the situation-specific world knowledge that listeners and readers use to construct meaning (e.g., van Dijk & Kintsch, 1983). The assumption is that as we process discourse, we construct a mental or situational model of the world as described by the discourses.

MODELS OF DISCOURSE PROCESSING.   To understand larger units of spoken and written discourse, it is necessary not only to construct representations that consider structural, propositional, and situational information, but also to relate these representations to one another. One must also use this information to make inferences about meaning and make decisions about which information should be remembered. Given the variety of knowledge types and cognitive processes involved in discourse processing, no one model can expect to capture all these facets of discourse processing. It is useful, however, to consider the kinds of models that have been proposed. Although these models deal primarily with how readers construct meaning from texts, their basic principles can be applied to spoken language discourse as well.

Kintsch and van Dijk's initial model of text comprehension proposed that multiple levels of representation were needed to construct meanings based on different kinds of knowledge (Kintsch & van Dijk, 1978; van Dijk & Kintsch, 1983). Three levels of representation correspond to the three knowledge types: structural, propositional, and knowledge of the situation/world.

This initial model of comprehension relied on schema-driven, top-down processing to build the knowledge of the world (i.e., situation model) representation. Kintsch (1988), however, felt that these notions were not adaptive to new contexts, were too inflexible, and could not account for how schemas were initially constructed. His most recent theory, called construction integration theory, acknowledges that many elements enter into the comprehension process (Kintsch, 1998). These include perceptions, concepts, ideas, images, or emotions. A crucial consideration in the theory is where these elements come from—from the world via the perceptual system or from the individual in the form of memories, knowledge, beliefs, body states, or goals. For Kintsch, the heart of the theory "is a specific mechanism that describes how elements from these two sources are combined into a stable mental product in the process of comprehension" (Kintsch, 1998, p. 4).

Kintsch goes on to provide a brief synopsis of the theory: One starts with a reader who has specific goals, a given background of knowledge and experience, and a given perceptual situation, such as printed words on a page of text. The propositional idea units created from these words are then linked to the reader's goals, knowledge, and experiences to create an interrelated network of idea units. Unlike Kintsch's earlier schema-driven models in which context was used to construct meaning, the construction of the network of idea units is viewed as an entirely bottom-up process, unguided by the larger discourse context. The initial context-insensitive construction process is followed by "a constraint-satisfaction, or integration, process that yields if all goes well, an orderly mental structure out of initial chaos" (Kintsch, 1998, p. 5). The constraint-satisfaction process involves selectively activating those elements from the network of idea-units that fit together and deactivating the rest.

If it all sounds pretty complicated, it is because complicated models and theories are needed to explain how text information is integrated with a reader's background knowledge and experiences to construct meaning. Simplistic bottom-up and top-down models are too general to explain how meaning is actually constructed, but some of the notions from these models, such as scripts and schemas, still work well for understanding how children construct meaning for certain prototype forms of discourse such as familiar events and stories. A schema is generally thought of as a structure in memory that specifies a general or expected arrangement of a body of information. Familiar events, for example, are well captured by scripts, which are a particular type of schema. Scripts contain slots for the components of an event, such as the main actions, participants, goals, and typical position of each action. Scripts make it easier to process familiar events by providing individuals with a coherent structure into which they can insert new information. Scripts also allow individuals to add necessary information that might be omitted in spoken or written discourse. For example, familiarity with a restaurant script allows listeners and readers to anticipate some mention of the menu. If no mention of the menu is made, but information about the kind of restaurant is given (e.g., Italian), one can infer the contents of the menu.

Certain types of discourse, such as stories, seem to have a consistent structure or grammar. This was recognized years ago when researchers proposed that stories had a common story grammar or schema. A story schema can be viewed as a mental framework that contains slots for each story component, such as a setting, goal, obstacle, and resolution. Story grammars represent a slightly different characterization of the knowledge of story structures. Story grammars specify the hierarchical relations among the components more directly than a story schema (Mandler & Johnson, 1977; Stein & Glenn, 1979). Story grammars attempt to specify the structural organization of stories in the same way that syntactic grammars specify the structural organization of sentences (Just & Carpenter, 1987, p. 231). The main structural components of a story are a setting and an episode. The setting introduces the characters and the context of the story. Episodes can be further divided into an initiating event, internal response, attempt, consequence, and reaction. Knowledge of the structure and function of stories, like knowledge of scripts, can facilitate comprehension of spoken and written language (Just & Carpenter, 1987; Perfetti, 1985).

OTHER METAPHORS FOR DISCOURSE AND TEXT UNDERSTANDING.   The notion that multiple sources of knowledge or representations are involved in processing discourse and text is an important one for understanding what is involved in comprehension. Other notions about comprehension, however, are important as well. Graesser and Britton (1996) have found that five metaphors capture the essence of the various ways of thinking about text comprehension. The first metaphor, *understanding is the assembly of a multileveled representation,* has already been discussed. Speech-language pathologists and other educators are familiar with at least two of the other metaphors: *understanding is the process of managing working memory* and *understanding is inference generation.* The two metaphors we may not be familiar with are *understanding is the construction of a coherent representation* and *understanding is a complex dynamical system.* To these five metaphors, we will add a sixth: *understanding is a metacognitive ability.* Although Graesser and Britton apply these metaphors to text understanding, in most cases they can be applied to spoken discourse as well. Each of these last five metaphors will be discussed briefly next.

Understanding Is the Management of Working Memory.   Most psychologists and educators are comfortable with the assumption that comprehension is managed in a limited-capacity working memory. Every educator has had firsthand experience with this metaphor. For example, when the demands of comprehension exceed the limitations of working memory, students' comprehension decreases dramatically. Students with low working memory spans often experience difficulty when comprehension components tax working memory. Poor comprehenders have also been shown to have problems suppressing irrelevant information from working memory (Gernsbacher, 1996).

Understanding Is Inference Generation.   The ability to construct meaning requires more than interpreting explicit propositions. It involves accessing relevant world knowledge and generating inferences that are needed to make sentences cohere (local coherence) and to relate text to world knowledge (global coherence). A number of different systems exist to classify inferences. In several studies comparing inferencing abilities in good and poor readers (e.g., Kucan & Beck, 1997; Laing & Kamhi, 2002; Trabasso & Magliano, 1996), inferences were classified as either predictions, associations, or explanations. A *predictive inference* speculates about events or actions that may occur based on what has already occurred in a story or text. For example, a predictive inference for the sentence *She played hard everyday* would be *She probably will be in good physical shape*. An *associative inference* is a statement that makes generalizations about characters, actions, objects, or events in a story or text. Associative inferences can also be specifications of procedures or responses to *wh*-questions. An associative inference for the sentence *He ate ice cream* would be that *He likes ice cream* or *He was hungry*. An explanatory inference provides causal connections between actions and events in a story or text. They are usually responses to "why" questions that provide explanations for a state, event, or action. For example, in a story about a child who wants a faster computer, an explanatory inference might be *He was not very happy because he wanted a new computer*. The proportion of explanatory inferences generated has been found to be significantly related to comprehension performance (e.g., Trabasso & Magliano, 1996). This is not surprising because explanatory inferences require retrieving and remembering causal information that serves to unite propositions in a story.

Inferences can also be distinguished according to whether they are derived from the content of activated world knowledge structures (e.g., scripts and schemas) or whether they are novel constructions that are needed to construct the situation model. Inferences that are generated from existing world knowledge tend to be generated "online." Graesser and Britton (1996) argue that a satisfactory model of text understanding should be able to accurately predict inferences that are quickly or automatically made during comprehension as well as those that are time consuming. Inferences generated online include those that address readers' goals, assist in establishing local or global coherence, and are highly activated from multiple information sources (e.g., Long, Seely, Oppy, & Golding, 1996). Inferences that are more time consuming may be caused by minimal world knowledge about the topic or by contradictions, anomalies, or irrelevant propositions in the text. Readers attempt to generate explanations and justifications to resolve the contradictions and anomalies. The process of generating these "elaborative inferences" is necessarily time consuming and may not be used by readers with low motivation (Graesser & Britton, 1996, p. 350).

Understanding Is the Construction of Coherent Representations.   The basic notion with this metaphor is that the more coherent the discourse or text, the easier it is to understand. A text is fully connected if every proposition is conceptually connected to one or more other propositions. Some theorists, following Kintsch (1974), believe that noun-phrase arguments are critical for connecting propositions and establishing coherence. More recent research, however, has shown that argument overlap is neither a necessary nor sufficient condition for establishing coherence;

instead, it is merely one type of connection (cf. Graesser & Britton, 1996). Other types of connections that have been considered include the connections between predicates of propositions (Turner, Britton, Andraessen, & McCutchen, 1996), causal connections and goals of story characters (van den Broek, Risden, Fletcher, & Thurlow, 1996), and the connections that tie deep metaphors to lexical items and explicit expressions (Gibbs, 1996).

Despite the challenge of identifying the specific types of connections that tie texts together, the "understanding-as-coherence" metaphor makes a large number of predictions about comprehension performance. Most of these predictions are generally intuitive. For example, a proposition has a greater likelihood of being recalled when it has more connections to other propositions in the text, and reading time increases when there is a break in coherence. However, some are counterintuitive. For example, Mannes and St. George (1996) found that there are more connections (or stronger ones) between text and world knowledge if there is a discrepancy between an outline and text content. The discrepancy causes improved problem solving, though recall for the text suffers.

Understanding Is a Complex Dynamic System. As mentioned earlier in this chapter, static, linear models of spoken and written language may be useful to identify specific processes and knowledge domains, but they do not have the flexibility to handle complex dynamic systems such as comprehension. A detailed description of a dynamic text comprehension model is beyond the scope of this chapter (cf. Graesser & Britton, 1996). It is interesting to note, however, that even researchers committed to these models recognize the difficulty involved in testing their psychological plausibility (Graesser & Britton, 1996, p. 347). Despite the difficulty in determining which dynamic model provides the best "goodness of fit," no cognitive theorist has rejected the "understanding is a complex dynamic system" metaphor.

Understanding Is a Metacognitive Ability. Metacognition refers to one's knowledge and control of one's cognitive system (Brown, 1987). Metacognitive abilities have been associated with several aspects of reading, including establishing the purpose for reading, identifying important ideas, activating prior knowledge, evaluating the text for clarity, compensating for failure to understand, and assessing one's level of comprehension (Brown, 1987). Brown added that it is not clear whether all or just certain components of these activities are metacognitive.

The ability to monitor comprehension plays an important role in both spoken and written language comprehension (e.g., Dollaghan & Kaston, 1986). When faced with a word, sentence, paragraph, or other text element that is not understood, it is necessary to do something to aid understanding, such as ask for clarification or reread the text in question. Individuals who are adept at monitoring their comprehension are more proficient processors of spoken and written language.

Summary

We have attempted in this section to provide a way of thinking about the knowledge and processes involved in understanding spoken and written language. Although the emphasis has been primarily on the similarity of knowledge and processes, some important differences in the word recognition processes were acknowledged. In our discussion of discourse comprehension processes, we tended to treat research as if it applied both to spoken and written language comprehension when, in fact, it rarely did. Our assumption here was that a model of comprehension that is sufficiently dynamic, flexible, and multifaceted would apply equally well to both spoken and written discourse. Although the six metaphors discussed were meant to illuminate the different aspects of comprehension, perhaps they made a complete muddle of comprehension for some. Graesser and Britton (1996) thought that after reading through their book on text understanding with all its different models and views of comprehension, someone might ask, "What is text understanding?" Readers of this chapter might wonder the same thing about our view of comprehension. With a slight modification to include discourse as well as text comprehension, the definition of comprehension Graesser and Britton suggest provides a good answer to the question:

> Text [and discourse] understanding is the dynamic process of constructing coherent representations and inferences at multiple levels of text and context, within the bottleneck of a limited-capacity working memory. (p. 350)

Having emphasized the similarities between spoken and written language up to this point, in the next section we consider some of the differences between the two.

DIFFERENCES BETWEEN SPOKEN AND WRITTEN LANGUAGE

Delineating the similarities and differences in the processes and knowledge involved in spoken and written language comprehension only begins to capture the complex relationship that exists between language and reading. Consider, for example, the following question posed by Gleitman and Rozin (1977, p. 2): Why is the more general and complex task of learning to speak and understand less difficult and less variable than what appears to be a trivial derivative of this (i.e., learning to read and write)? These authors proceed to point out two major differences between learning to talk and learning to read. We add a third important difference.

The first major difference is that learning to read requires explicit knowledge of the phonological aspects of speech. To become an efficient reader, one must learn the various correspondences between phonemes and letters. The knowledge that words consist of discrete phonemes is crucial for constructing phoneme–grapheme correspondence rules. Spoken language comprehension also requires analysis of utterances into smaller phonological units. But the analysis of the speech stream by the listener is carried out below the level of consciousness by evolutionarily old and highly adapted auditory perceptual processes (Lieberman, 1973). The human perceptual system is thus biologically adapted to process speech. In contrast, the human visual system is not biologically adapted to process written text. This introduces the second major difference between learning to talk and learning to read: Reading is a comparatively new and arbitrary human ability for which specific biological adaptations do not yet exist.

A third important difference is that almost all humans are reared in environments in which spoken language is the principal means of communication. Thus, not only are we biologically endowed to learn language, but we are also socialized to use spoken language to communicate. This is not true for reading. In 2008, there were 796 million illiterate adults worldwide and two-thirds of them (64%) were women (UNESCO Institute for Statistics, 2010). More than half (412 million) of these individuals live in Southern Asia and about 20% (176 million) reside in sub-Saharan Africa. These are regions with limited educational opportunities and cultures that place little value on reading.

Perera (1984) points out additional differences between spoken and written language. An understanding of these differences helps to further explain why reading is not a simple derivative of spoken language. The differences discussed in the following sections, however, in no way diminish the language bases of reading and reading disabilities.

To emphasize the contrasts between written and spoken language, Perera (1984) compared prototypical speech (conversation) to prototypical written language (literature or informative prose). She acknowledged, however, that there is a full range of spoken and written discourse types. Certain discourse types have some characteristics of written language and vice versa. For example, speeches and lectures can be planned much like writing, radio talk lacks a visual dimension and contextual support, and tape recordings arc durable.

Physical Differences

Whereas speech consists of temporally ordered sounds, writing consists of marks made on a surface (e.g., paper) in a two-dimensional space. As such, writing is relatively durable; it can be read and reread. Speech, unless it is recorded, is ephemeral. It has no existence independent of the speaker. The durability of writing gives the reader control over how fast or slow to read. Certain texts can be savored, whereas others can be skimmed. The listener, in contrast, is tied to the fleeting speech of the speaker. Missed words or sentences will be lost if clarification is not requested.

Perera (1984, p. 161) noted that readers often have the benefit of a whole range of visual cues, such as running headlines, different-size type, color, and summaries or abstracts. In addition, a device such as the footnote allows the writer to provide additional information without interrupting the main thread of the text. Such devices allow the reader to decide the level at which he or she will read. The listener, in contrast, is completely dependent on the speaker's selection of material. Note, however, that the listener could choose not to listen to the speaker's message.

Situational Differences

The most frequent type of spoken language is face-to-face communication. Conversations are often interactive exchanges between two or more individuals. Questions are followed by answers, requests by responses, and statements by acknowledgments. When a listener does not understand something, a clarification is requested. Careful planning is not the rule in conversational discourse. When speakers pause too long before talking, they will usually be interrupted. Despite this time pressure to speak, misunderstandings are infrequent; when they occur, they are easily resolved by repeating or rephrasing the message. Nonverbal communication acts, such as gestures, facial expressions, and body postures, can help to clarify messages. Speakers and listeners also share the same nonlinguistic setting. People and objects that are visible can be referred to by pronouns rather than by noun phrases (even without prior reference), and many adverbials and prepositions can be expressed by *here, there,* and *like this.*

In contrast, writing and reading are often individual endeavors. The writer receives no prompting about what to write and no immediate feedback on the clarity of the writing. But the writer is generally under less severe time constraints and can thus take more time to search for the best way to express a message. The writer can also correct and revise a text until a final copy is produced. Such care and precision is necessary in writing because there are no contextual and nonverbal cues to aid comprehension. The written text thus has to bear the whole burden of communication, which is one reason why writing is usually more precise than talking.

Functional Differences

One of the earliest needs to generate a writing system was to retain accurate records of property, commercial transactions, and legal judgments. A Chinese proverb holds that "The palest ink is better than the best memory." Writing has enabled the knowledge of centuries to accumulate, thus allowing each new generation to build on the ideas, discoveries, and inventions of the generation or generations before. Many academic subjects, such as history, geography, the physical sciences, and social sciences, owe their very existence to writing (Perera, 1984, p. l64). Another function not served by speech is labeling. Although speech is used to label objects in a referential sense, written labels serve more of an information function. Consider such labels as street names, signposts, nameplates on theaters and public buildings, brand labels, and danger warnings. Written language can also serve a variety of communicative functions, such as relating stories, events, and experiences or sharing information and making requests. Finally, a specialized function of writing is found in literature. Societies have oral literatures, but oral literatures are restricted to a few types, such as ballads, epic poetry, drama, folk stories, and myths. Essays, novels, diaries, and memoirs are some of the genres that are particular to writing.

Perera (1984) has suggested that the most basic uses of writing involve the recording of facts, ideas, and information. Although speech also has an informative function, an equally important function of speech is the role it plays in establishing and maintaining human relationships. A large part of everyday speech with friends, acquaintances, and other individuals serves social-interpersonal functions rather than intellectual ones. E-mail and instant messaging now serve this role as well.

One advantage writing has over speech, according to Perera (1984, p. l65), is that it allows ideas to be explored at leisure and in private. Writing can thus become a means of extending and clarifying one's thinking and ideas. Often in conversation when a controversial topic is raised, there is a tendency for opinions to polarize. Someone who tries to take both sides of a issue might be pressed to select one particular view. In writing, however, one can take time to develop a line of thought, weigh opposing arguments, notice errors in reasoning, and develop new lines of thinking.

Form Differences

The most obvious difference in form is that speech consists of sounds, whereas written language consists of letters. As indicated earlier, this would not be so much of a problem if speech sounds (i.e., phonemes) stood in one-to-one correspondence with written letters. Form differences between spoken and written language are not limited to the discrete segments (i.e., phonemes and letters) that make up speech and text. Spoken and written language also differ in how they represent suprasegmental, paralinguistic, and prosodic features. *Paralinguistic features* include pitch and timbre differences that distinguish male and female voices; general voice quality, such as breathiness, hoarseness, or nasality; and the general manner of how an utterance is produced, such as shouted, whispered, or spoken. Perera has pointed out that these features do not usually affect the actual meaning of an utterance; however, they may reflect the speaker's attitude about what is being said.

Prosodic features include intonation, stress, and rhythm. Perera (1984) presented four functions of prosodic features: (1) to enable the communicative intent of an utterance to differ from its grammatical form (e.g., *He's lost it* versus *He's lost it?*), (2) to group words into information units, (3) to place emphasis, and (4) to convey the speaker's attitude. These functions differ in the extent to which they can be reflected in writing. Whereas punctuation effectively changes the communicative intent of an utterance, it is not so effective in signaling which words belong together in information units. Italics, underlining, and the use of capital letters are some ways to distribute emphasis throughout a written utterance. But heavy use of these devices in formal writing is usually discouraged. Expressing attitudes in writing is clearly difficult. Perera (1984, p. 178) provided an example of how much attitudinal information is conveyed by prosodic features in the following quote of a journalist who listened to one of the Watergate tapes:

> Once you hear the tapes, and the tone in which he (Nixon) uttered the comments which previously have only been available in a neutral transcript, any last shred of doubt about his guilt must disappear.

Perera (1984) goes on to consider the extent to which the writing system represents the segmental and suprasegmental aspects of speech. Among other things, she pointed out that graphemes represent the "citation" (well-spoken) form of words rather than the degraded productions that often occur in fast speech (e.g., compare "did you know" to [dIdʒəno]). Punctuation can signal the grammatical function of a sentence and mark some prosodic boundaries. The writer, however, has no conventional way to express voice quality, volume, rate of speech, rhythm, and into national patterns.

Vocabulary Differences

One would expect that there would be differences in the vocabulary used in spoken and written language because writing provides more time and, therefore, more resources to select words. The additional time allows writers to choose words that communicate meanings clearly. Clear, unambiguous writing is necessary to ensure that the author's intended meaning is derived. Readers, unlike listeners, don't have the luxury of requesting clarification when the message is unclear. In contrast, conversational speech provides little opportunity to consider alternative word choices, and though one can revise a word choice once it is spoken, too much fumbling detracts from effective communication (Chafe & Danielewicz, 1987). With writing, time is often not a factor; one can spend seconds, minutes, hours, or days finding the appropriate word or expression, and even after a selection is made, the writer is free to revise without anyone noticing. Word processing programs do not keep track of earlier drafts.

The consequence of these differences is that the vocabulary of spoken language tends to be more limited in variety. A simple way to demonstrate this is by calculating type-token ratios (TTRs) for spoken and written language. TTR is calculated by dividing the number of different words by the total number of words in a sample. Chafe and Danielewicz (1987) show that TTRs for spoken language are consistently lower than for written language. Interestingly, the ratio for academic lectures is about the same as in conversations (.19/.18), indicating that rapid production of spoken language produces less varied vocabulary, regardless of the kind of speaking involved. The frequent use of nonspecific terms (e.g., *thing, whatever,* "doohickey," "whatchamacallit"), hedges (*sort of, kind of*), and maze behaviors (interjections, disfluencies, false starts, repetitions) are all indications of the processing demands of spoken language. Chafe and Danielewicz also show how spoken language has less referential explicitness than written language. Nonspecific third person pronouns (*it, this, that*) are used frequently in spoken language and are one of the factors that differentiate good from poor writing.

The lexicon that speakers and writers choose from is also not the same for writing and speaking. There is a literate lexicon (Nippold, 2007) that writers draw from in formal writing. For example, conjunctive adverbs like *thus, therefore, hence,* and *accordingly* are rarely used in spoken language. Chafe and Danielewicz (1987) suggest that spoken language compensates for its restricted lexical variety by assigning a premium to freshness. Speakers must stay current. *Cool* may have been cool 10 or 20 years ago, but not now. Freshness of vocabulary is less important in writing, where there is more of a premium on choosing the right word to convey a particular meaning. Not surprisingly, conversations and academic papers differ considerably in their use of literary and colloquial vocabulary (Chafe & Danielewicz, 1987). Academic papers had only 1 instance per 1,000 words of colloquial vocabulary (e.g., *kid bike, figure out*), whereas conversations had 27. Lectures and letters fall somewhere in the middle, indicating that there is nothing in the nature of speaking that prevents a speaker from using literary vocabulary and nothing in the nature of writing that prevents a writer from using colloquial vocabulary. Lectures are thus more literary than conversations, whereas letters are more conversational than academic papers.

Grammatical Differences

Samples of spoken language uncover relatively high frequencies of coordination, repetition, and rephrasing. Conversational discourse is typically low in lexical density and high in redundancy. Lexical items are spaced out and separated by grammatical words, and a high number of total words are used to convey a relatively small amount of information. Written language, in contrast, is high in lexical density and low in redundancy. This results from the use of grammatical structures that decrease redundancy and increase lexical density.

Studies (e.g., Chafe & Danielewicz, 1987) have shown that in conversation it is more common to provide smaller amounts of information at a time. Most written language, by contrast, is denser lexically as well as propositionally. Conversations, because of their interactive nature, are generally less coherent than writing. Speakers are free to change the subject at almost any point in a conversation. Topics need not be related in any logical way. In writing, however, an overall theme is necessary. Topic changes must be justified and explicitly made. Writing also has prescribed rules for organizing content. These rules cover the use of topic sentences, paragraph structure, and introductory and concluding statements.

Processing Differences

Earlier in this chapter, we talked about top-down processing models, discourse-level comprehension processes, and the higher-level knowledge schemas that contribute to comprehension of spoken and written language. The focus in these sections was on the commonalities between understanding speech and text. There are very important differences, however, in the contribution higher-level processes make to spoken and written language comprehension. The role of higher-level processes or context effects in reading has received considerable research attention and caused much confusion. One reason for this confusion is that researchers often fail to distinguish between the use of context to facilitate word recognition and the use of context to facilitate text comprehension. Context plays an important role in facilitating text comprehension; it plays a very limited role, however, in facilitating word recognition in good readers.

Support for the limited role of higher-level processes in word recognition comes from eye-movement experiments. Research using various eye-movement methodologies has been consistent in finding that the vast majority of content words in text receive a direct visual fixation (Just & Carpenter, 1987; Rayner & Pollatsek, 1989). Short function words may be skipped, but even many of these receive a direct visual fixation. The span of effective visual information during a fixation is thus quite small, meaning that text is sampled in a very dense manner, even when the words are highly predictable (Balota & Chumbley, 1985).

Based in part on evidence from these eye-movement studies, most models of reading have expectancy-based, top-down processes functioning after words have been recognized (Seidenberg, 1985; Till, Mross, & Kintsch, 1988). Higher-level contextual information plays more of a role in speech perception or language processing because of the well-documented ambiguity in decontextualized speech. For example, isolated words from normal conversation are often not recognized out of context. This is not the case, however, for written language. Fluent readers can identify written words out of context with near-perfect accuracy. As Stanovich (1986) has noted, the physical stimulus alone completely specifies the lexical representation in writing, whereas this is not always true in speech. It is more important in reading, therefore, for the input systems involved in word recognition to deliver a complete and accurate representation of words to higher level processes. Paradoxically, then, poor readers who have difficulty accurately decoding words must rely more on contextual information than good readers who have proficient word recognition skills. We will say more about the use of good and poor readers' use of contextual information in subsequent chapters.

BASIC FACTORS IN READING AND LANGUAGE DEVELOPMENT

It should be clear that although there is considerable overlap in the processes involved in spoken and written language, there are also many important differences between the two. These differences explain to a large extent why learning to read is not a simple derivative of learning to talk and understand. In the definition of language given earlier in this chapter, language learning and use were said to be determined by the interaction of biological, cognitive, psychosocial, and environmental factors. Learning to read is also determined by the interaction of these four factors. However, the relative importance or weight of these factors for learning to read is not the same as it is for learning spoken language.

Biological factors are crucial in learning spoken and written language. As indicated earlier, however, one important difference between learning to talk and learning to read is that the analysis of the speech stream is carried out below the level of consciousness by evolutionary old and highly adapted auditory processes. In contrast, the human visual system is not biologically adapted to process written text. By itself, this difference does not necessarily make learning to read more difficult than learning to talk; it does suggest, however, that learning to read requires more attentional resources than learning to talk.

Environmental factors play different but equally important roles in learning spoken and written language. As noted previously, almost all humans are reared in environments in which spoken language is the principal means of communication. The social–environmental forces to use language to communicate are just as crucial for language learning as the physical, perceptual, and cognitive mechanisms that make speech, hearing, and language possible. Children deprived of early exposure to language input will eventually develop some language abilities once normal input is provided, but they will never be normal language users, as the tragic cases of Genie and other severely deprived children have shown (Curtiss, 1977). Although it is rare to find examples of extreme deprivation of language input, there are still many societies in the world that place little importance or value on literacy. These societies account for the high rates of illiteracy (40 percent) in the world. Most of the individuals reared in these societies will have little exposure to print and no formal instruction in reading.

Because the biological and social bases of reading are not as strong as they are for spoken language, psychosocial factors, such as motivational and attentional states, often play a more important role in learning to read than in learning to talk. Unless a child has a severe emotional disorder, such as autism, language learning will be relatively unaffected by motivational and attentional states. This is not the case in learning to read because reading requires a considerable amount of motivational and attentional resources. Reading difficulties in individuals with motivational and attentional problems have been well documented (e.g., Guthrie et al., 2009; Willcutt & Pennington, 2000).

Cognitive factors play a fundamental role in learning spoken and written language because spoken and written language are essentially cognitive achievements. Both rely on basic cognitive processes to encode, store, and retrieve information. In addition, the same store of linguistic and conceptual knowledge is tapped by readers as by speakers and listeners. Metacognitive abilities, however, play a more important role in learning to read than in learning to talk and understand. This is because learning to read requires awareness of the phonological properties of speech, whereas learning to talk requires little if any explicit metalinguistic knowledge. By the time children are able to make explicit metalinguistic judgments—around age 4 or 5—they have progressed through the various developmental language stages.

Summary

It should be clear that there are similarities as well as differences in the knowledge and processes that underlie spoken and written language. The similarities between spoken and written language are most evident in the vocabulary both share. Readers and listeners also rely on common sources of structural, propositional, and world knowledge and have attentional and memory limitations that influence how readily spoken and written language is processed. The most fundamental differences between spoken and written language involve the perceptual and biological/social bases of spoken language and the explicit phonological awareness required to become a proficient reader. Because reading is not a biologically endowed human ability, attentional, instructional, and motivational factors play a central role in learning to read. These differences explain to a large extent why learning to read is not a simple derivative of spoken language as well as why some children have difficulty learning to read. In the next chapter, we consider what is involved in becoming a proficient reader.

References

American Speech-Language-Hearing Association (ASHA). Committee on Language. (1983, June). Definition of language. *ASHA, 25,* 44.

Balota, D., & Chumbley, J. (1985). The locus of word-frequency effects in the pronunciation task: Lexical access and/or production? *Journal of Memory and Language, 24,* 89–106.

Bever, T. (1970). The cognitive basis for linguistic structures. In J. R. Hayes (Ed.), *Cognition and the development of language* (pp. 279–352). New York: Wiley.

Brown, A. (1987). Metacognition, executive control, self-regulation and other more mysterious mechanisms. In F. Weinert & R. Kluwe (Eds.), *Metacognition, motivation, and understanding* (pp. 65–116). Hillsdale, NJ: Erlbaum.

Carroll, D. (1994). *Psychology of language.* Pacific Grove, CA: Brooks/Cole.

Catts, H. (2009). The narrow view of reading promotes a broad view of comprehension. *Language, Speech, and Hearing Services in Schools, 40,* 178–184.

Chafe, W. (1970). *Meaning and the structure of language.* Chicago: The University of Chicago Press.

Chafe, W., & Danielewicz, J. (1987). Properties of spoken and written language. In R. Horowitz & S. Samuels (Eds.), *Comprehending oral and written language* (pp. 83–113). New York: Academic Press.

Clark, H., & Clark, E. (1977). *Psychology and language.* New York: Harcourt Brace Jovanovich.

Collins, A., & Loftus, E. (1975). A spreading activation theory of semantic processing. *Psychological Review, 82,* 407–428.

Collins, A., & Quillian, M. (1969). Retrieval time from semantic memory. *Journal of Verbal Learning and Verbal Behavior, 8,* 240–248.

Coltheart, M., Curtis, B., Atkins, P., & Haller, M. (1993). Models of reading aloud: Dual-route and parallel-distributed-processing approaches. *Psychological Review, 100,* 589–608.

Crowder, R. (1982). *The psychology of reading.* New York: Oxford University Press.

Curtiss, S. (1977). *Genie: A psycholinguistic study of a modern-day "Wild Child."* New York: Academic Press.

Dollaghan, C., & Kaston, N. (1986). A comprehension monitoring program for language-impaired children. *Journal of Speech and Hearing Disorders, 51,* 264–271.

Fodor, J., & Garrett, M. (1967). Some syntactic determinants of sentential complexity. *Perception and Psychophysics, 2,* 289–296.

Frazier, L. (1987). Sentence processing: A tutorial review. In M. Coltheart (Ed.), *Attention and performance, Vol. XII. The psychology of reading* (pp. 559–586). Hillsdale, NJ: Erlbaum.

Gates, A. (1949). Character and purposes of the yearbook. In N. Henry (Ed.), *The forty-eighth yearbook of the National Society for the Study of Education: Part II. Reading in the elementary school* (pp. 1–9). Chicago: University of Chicago Press.

Gernsbacher, M. (1996). The structure-building framework: What it is, what it might also be, and why. In B. Britton & A. Graesser (Eds.), *Models of understanding text* (pp. 289–312). Mahwah, NJ: Erlbaum.

Gibbs, R. (1996). Metaphor as a constraint on text understanding. In B. Britton & A. Graesser, (Eds.), *Models of understanding text* (pp. 215–240). Mahwah, NJ: Erlbaum.

Gleitman, L., & Rozin, P. (1977). The structure and acquisition of reading, 1: Relations between orthographies and the structure of language. In A. Reber & D. Scarborough (Eds.), *Toward a psychology of reading* (pp. 1–53). The proceedings of the CUNY conferences. New York: Wiley.

Gough, P., & Tunmer, W. (1986). Decoding, reading, and reading disability. *Remedial and Special Education, 7,* 6–10.

Graesser, A., & Britton, B. (1996). Five metaphors for text understanding. In A. Graesser & B. Britton (Eds.), *Models of understanding text* (pp. 341–351). Mahwah, NJ: Erlbaum.

Guthrie, J. T., McRae, A., Coddington, C. S., Klauda, S. L., Wigfield, A., & Barbosa, P. (2009). Impacts of comprehensive reading instruction on diverse outcomes of low-achieving and high-achieving readers. *Journal of Learning Disabilities, 42,* 195–214.

Hirsch, E. D. (2006). *The knowledge deficit: Closing the shocking education gap for American children.* New York: Houghton Mifflin.

Hoover, W., & Gough, P. (1990). The simple view of reading. *Reading and Writing: An Interdisciplinary Journal, 2,* 127–160.

Just, M., & Carpenter, P. (1987). *The psychology of reading and language comprehension.* Boston: Allyn & Bacon.

Kamhi, A. (2009a). Prologue: The case for the narrow view of reading. *Language, Speech, and Hearing Services in Schools, 40,* 174–178.

Kamhi, A. (2009b). Epilogue: Solving the reading crisis—Take 2: The case for differentiated assessment. *Language, Speech, and Hearing Services in Schools, 40,* 212–215.

Kintsch, W. (1974). *The representation of meaning in memory.* Hillsdale, NJ: Erlbaum.

Kintsch, W. (1988). The role of knowledge in discourse comprehension: A construction-integration model. *Psychological Review, 95,* 163–182.

Kintsch, W. (1998). *Comprehension: A paradigm for cognition.* New York: Cambridge University Press.

Kintsch, W., & Keenan, J. (1973). Reading rate as a function of the number of propositions in the base structure of sentences. *Cognitive Psychology, 5,* 257–274.

Kintsch, W., & van Dijk, T. (1978). Toward a model of text comprehension and production. *Psychological Review, 85,* 363–394.

Kucan, L., & Beck, I. (1997). Thinking aloud and reading comprehension research: Inquiry, instruction, and social interaction. *Review of Educational Research, 67,* 271–279.

Laing, S., & Kamhi, A. (2002). The use of think-aloud protocols to compare inferencing abilities in average and below-average readers. *Journal of Learning Disabilities, 35,* 436–447.

Liberman, I. (1983). A language-oriented view of reading and its disabilities. In H. Myklebust (Ed.), *Progress in learning disabilities* (pp. 81–101). New York: Grune and Stratton.

Lieberman, P. (1973). On the evolution of language: A unified view. *Cognition, 2,* 59–94.

Long, D., Seely, M., Oppy, B., & Golding, J. (1996). The role of inferential processing in reading ability. In B. Britton & A. Graesser (Eds.), *Models of understanding text* (pp. 189–214). Mahwah, NJ: Erlbaum.

Lund, N., & Duchan, J. (1993). *Assessing children's language in naturalistic contexts* (3rd ed.). Englewood Cliffs, NJ: Prentice Hall.

Mandler, J., & Johnson, N. (1977). Remembrance of things parsed: Story structure and recall. *Cognitive Psychology, 9,* 111–151.

Mannes, S., & St. George, M. (1996). Effects of prior knowledge on text comprehension: A simple modeling approach. In B. Britton & A. Graesser (Eds.), *Models of understanding text* (pp. 115–140). Mahwah, NJ: Erlbaum.

National Reading Panel (NRP). (2000). *Teaching children to read: An evidence-based assessment of the scientific literature on reading and its implications for reading instruction.* Washington, DC: National Institute of Child Health and Human Development.

Nippold, M. (2007). *Later language development: School-age children, adolescents, and young adults* (3rd ed.). Austin, TX: Pro-Ed.

Nittrouer, S. (1996). The relation between speech perception and phonemic awareness: Evidence from low-SES children and children with chronic OM. *Journal of Speech and Hearing Research, 39,* 1059–1070.

Nittrouer, S., Manning, C., & Meyer, G. (1993). The perceptual weighting of acoustic cues changes with linguistic experience. *Journal of the Acoustical Society of America, 94,* S1865.

Patterson, K., & Coltheart, V. (1987). Phonological processes in reading: A tutorial review. In M. Coltheart (Ed.), *Attention and performance* (Vol. 12, pp. 421–447). London: Erlbaum.

Perera, K. (1984). *Children's writing and reading: Analysing classroom language.* Oxford: Blackwell.

Perfetti, C. (1985). *Reading ability.* New York: Oxford University Press.

Perfetti, C. (1986). Cognitive and linguistic components of reading ability. In B. Foorman & A. Siegel (Eds.), *Acquisition of reading skills* (pp. 1–41). Hillsdale, NJ: Erlbaum.

Rayner, K., & Pollatsek, A. (1989). *The psychology of reading.* Englewood Cliffs, NJ: Prentice Hall.

Reitsma, P. (1990). Development of orthographic knowledge. In P. Reitsma & L. Verhoeven (Eds.), *Acquisition of reading in Dutch* (pp. 43–64). Dordrecht: Foris.

Rumelhart, D. (1977). Toward an interactive model of reading. In S. Dornic & P. Rabbit (Eds.), *Attention and performance VI* (pp. l83–221). Hillsdale, NJ: Erlbaum.

Schiffrin, D. (1994). *Approaches to discourse.* Cambridge, MA: Blackwell.

Seidenberg, M. (1985). The time course of information activation and utilization in visual word recognition. In D. Besner, T. Waller, & G. MacKinnon (Eds.), *Reading research: Advances in theory and practice* (Vol. 5, pp. 199–252). New York: Academic Press.

Seidenberg, M. (1995). Visual word recognition: An overview. In J. Miller & P. Eimas (Eds.), *Speech, language, and communication* (pp. 137–179). San Diego: Academic Press.

Seidenberg, M., & McClelland, J. (1989). A distributed, developmental model of word recognition and naming. *Psychological Review, 96,* 523–568.

Share, D., & Stanovich, K. (1995). Cognitive processes in early reading development: Accommodating individual differences into a model of acquisition. *Issues in Education, 1,* 1–57.

Simmons, D., Kame'enui, E., Harn, B., Coyne, M., Stoolmiller, M., Santoro, L., et al. (2007). Attributes of effective and efficient kindergarten reading intervention: An examination of instructional time and design specificity. *Journal of Learning Disabilities, 40,* 331–348.

Stanovich, K. (1985). Explaining the variance in reading ability in terms of psychological processes: What have we learned? *Annals of Dyslexia, 35,* 67–96.

Stanovich, K. (1986). Matthew effects in reading: Some consequences of individual differences in the acquisition of literacy. *Reading Research Quarterly, 21,* 360–406.

Stanovich, K. (1991). Word recognition: Changing perspectives. In R. Barr, M. Kamil, P. Mosenthal, & P. D. Pearson (Eds.), *Handbook of reading research, Volume II* (pp. 418–452). White Plains, NY: Longman.

Stein, N., & Glenn, C. (1979). An analysis of story comprehension in elementary school children. In R. Freedle (Ed.), *New directions in discourse processing* (pp. 53–l20). Norwood, NJ: Ablex.

Stolz, W. (1967). A study of the ability to decode grammatically novel sentences. *Journal of Verbal Learning and Verbal Behavior, 6,* 867–873.

Thomson, M. (1984). *Developmental dyslexia: Its nature, assessment, and remediation.* Baltimore: Edward Arnold.

Till, R., Mross, E., & Kintsch, W. (1988). Time course of priming for associate and inference words in a discourse context. *Memory & Cognition, 16,* 283–298.

Trabasso, T., & Magliano, J. (1996). Conscious understanding during comprehension. *Discourse Processes, 21,* 255–287.

Turner, A., Britton, B., Andraessen, P., & McCutchen, D. (1996). A predication semantics model of text comprehension and recall. In B. Britton & A. Graesser (Eds.), *Models of understanding* (pp. 33–72). Mahwah, NJ: Erlbaum.

UNESCO Institute for Statistics. (September 2010). Adult and youthliteracy: Global trends in gender parity. Retrieved from http://www.uis.unesco.org/template/pdf/Literacy/Fact_Sheet_2010_Lit_EN.pdf

van den Broek, P., Risden, K., Fletcher, C., & Thurlow, R. (1996). A "landscape" view of reading: Fluctuating patterns of activation and the construction of a stable memory representation. In B. Britton & A. Graesser (Eds.), *Models of understanding text* (pp. 165–188). Mahwah, NJ: Erlbaum.

van Dijk, T., & Kintsch, W. (1983). *Strategies of discourse comprehension.* Cambridge, MA: MIT Press.

Whitney, P. (1998). *The psychology of language.* New York: Houghton Mifflin.

Willcutt, E., & Pennington, B. (2000). Co-morbidity of reading disability and attention-deficit/hyperactivity disorder: Differences by gender and subtype. *Journal of Learning Disabilities, 33,* 179–182.

Willingham, D. (2006). How knowledge helps: It speeds and strengths reading comprehension, learning—and thinking. *American Educator, Spring 2006,* 1–12.

Chapter 2

Reading Development

Alan G. Kamhi and Hugh W. Catts

For many years, the focus in learning to read was on what the teacher did or should have done, rather than on what happened or should happen in the child (Gibson & Levine, 1975). Beginning in the 1980s, considerable progress has been made in understanding the reading acquisition process. This progress has occurred because researchers began to focus on the processes, traits, and skills children need to become proficient readers (e.g., Ehri, 1991; Juel, 1991; Share, 1995). Progress was not made when the sole focus was on teachers and methods.

This is not to say that research on methods of teaching is unimportant. Teachers need information about which instructional methods work best for particular children and classes. But, as Juel (1991) has noted, "[T]he lens through which we view reading instruction should be opened more widely to include not just the method in isolation, but factors that accompany the method" (p. 761). Examples of these factors include time spent reading, the kinds of texts that are read, the social setting for instruction, and patterns of interaction. To understand how children learn to read, it is thus important to focus on what children are learning as well as on what teachers and parents are teaching.

Children's path on the road to proficient reading begins well before they have formal reading instruction in school and continues until they can recognize words accurately and with little effort. Most typically developing readers develop accurate, effortless word recognition skills in the first few years of elementary school. The knowledge and skills that underlie the development of proficient word recognition skills are the focus of the first part of this chapter. The second part of the chapter considers the development of reading comprehension abilities.

Like the other chapters in the first part of this book, this chapter was a collaborative effort. The chapter is written in the first person to avoid the cumbersome language that would be needed to relate personal anecdotes about family members.

EMERGENT LITERACY PERIOD (BIRTH–KINDERGARTEN)

From birth until the beginning of formal education, children growing up in literate cultures accumulate knowledge about letters, words, and books. In theories of reading development, the period of time before children go to school is usually referred to as the emergent literacy period. How much literacy knowledge children acquire during this period depends on how much exposure they have to literacy artifacts and events, as well as their interest and facility in learning. At one end of the continuum are children from low-print homes who have little exposure to literacy artifacts and events. These children begin school with little literacy knowledge. At the other end of the continuum are children from high-print homes who enjoy everything about language and literacy. Some of these children may have a sizable sight word vocabulary and be able to decode some novel words by the time they enter school. How much literacy knowledge children acquire during the emergent literacy period is thus highly variable. Most children will not acquire all the knowledge discussed in this section, but because some do, it seems important to know what children can learn about literacy, language, and reading before they have any formal instruction.

The term "literacy socialization" has been used to refer to the social and cultural aspects of learning to read. Van Kleeck and Schuele (1987) discuss three specific areas of literacy socialization: (1) literacy artifacts, (2) literacy events, and (3) the types of knowledge children gain from literacy experiences. Most children growing up in middle- and upper-class homes are surrounded by literacy artifacts from the time of birth. Characters from nursery rhymes decorate walls. Sheets and crib borders often have pictures and writing, alphabet blocks and books might be on the shelf, and T-shirts often have slogans or city names printed on them. In addition to the child's own possessions, homes are filled with items such as books, newspapers, magazines, mail, pens, crayons, and writing pads.

Joint Book Reading

More important than literacy artifacts are the literacy events children participate in and observe and the knowledge they acquire from these events. The most instructionally organized literacy event is joint book reading. In 1985, the Commission on Reading of the National Institute of Education called joint book reading "the single most important activity for developing the knowledge required for eventual success in reading" (p. 23). In some mainstream homes, parents begin reading to their children as soon as babies are born. In some families, mothers may even begin reading to their unborn fetuses. In most mainstream homes, parents are reading to their infants by 5 to 6 months, which, not coincidentally, is the time when infants are able to sit up and focus at least some attention on a book. From these interactions with books, babies learn that books are important to adults in their world, and lots of talk surrounds books. They may also realize that their parents work hard to get and keep their attention on these curious objects and delight in their slightest attempts to participate. Before babies can even talk, they may be turning pages of books and spending considerable time looking at pictures in books.

Because babies do not understand much of the language they hear, van Kleeck reasons that we might expect parents to read a lot of rhyming books that de-emphasize meaning. But this does not appear to be the case. Van Kleeck and her colleagues found that 14 middle-class mothers chose rhyming books less than 10 percent of the time with their 6- to 12-month-old infants (van Kleeck, Gillam, Hamilton, & McGrath, 1995, cited in van Kleeck, 1995). Mothers did, however, use a rhythmic, singsong cadence, presumably to get and maintain the infant's attention. Even with babies, parents labeled pictures, actions, and events and related the information in the book to the child's life. The focus for parents is primarily on meaning and comprehension.

As infants get older, parents gradually introduce input that is more cognitively demanding. For example, Snow and Goldfield (1981) showed that parents decreased their labeling and increased discussion of events as their children got older (2 years; 6 months to 3 years; 6 months). As children mature, they are also expected to play more of an active role in the book-reading activity. One way children become more active is their ability to respond to so-called test questions. Heath (1982), for example, found that there were three kinds of information children learn to talk about during book-reading routines: (1) *what* explanations, (2) *reason* explanations, and (3) *affective* explanations. Learning to respond to these kinds of questions prepares children for the types of questions they will encounter from teachers and on tests once they enter school.

Children have a lot of help in learning to respond to test questions and provide various kinds of explanations about what they read. Parents who are attuned to the child's developmental level will provide questions and answers that the child can understand. Adults will also modify or scaffold a text to ensure that the child is able to make sense of it. Proficient scaffolders are able to reduce vocabulary and syntactic complexity as well as provide explanations and interpretations that the child understands. As children get older, the process of "sense making" becomes more of a shared enterprise (Heath, 1982; van Kleeck, 1995). One important characteristic of this shared enterprise is that children learn how to ask questions about the texts they are reading. The answers they receive to their questions are a key source for the development of conceptual knowledge and reasoning skills during the preschool years. Another important source for conceptual and reasoning skills is the books themselves, which become more sophisticated and complex as children get older.

Joint book reading not only affects children's conceptual and reasoning skills, but it also exposes children to specific components of print and book conventions. This exposure inevitably contributes to and facilitates the learning of letter names, shapes, and sounds (e.g., Burns, Griffin, & Snow, 1999). In some cases, the literacy artifacts and joint book-reading activities may lead preschoolers to the discovery of the underlying alphabetic principle—that words consist of discrete sounds that are represented by letters in print.

One could easily get the impression in this section that joint book reading experiences are all children need to learn to read. Despite the commonsense appeal of the importance of joint book reading, there is some controversy in the literature about the impact joint book reading actually has on early reading ability. Scarborough and Dobrich (1994) reviewed three decades of research on the influence of joint book reading on language and literacy development. The observed effects in this research were quite variable within and between samples. Demographics, attitudes, and skill levels seemed to make stronger direct contributions to early reading success than joint book reading.

Scarborough and Dobrich's (1994) findings have been challenged in another study by Bus, van Ijzendoorn, and Pellegrini (1995). Using a more extensive body of studies and a quantitative analysis, Bus and colleagues found support for the hypothesis that book reading had a direct impact on learning to read. There were hardly any studies with negative effects. Although book reading only explained about 8 percent of the variance in the outcome measures, the effect size of .59 was fairly strong. Importantly, the effects were not dependent on the socioeconomic status of the families. Even in lower-class families with (on average) low levels of literacy, book reading had a beneficial effect on literacy skills. Because book reading seems to make the start at school easier, it may be particularly important for children from low socioeconomic families.

It is surprising that direct effects of shared book reading have been somewhat difficult to prove, although a recent study did find that joint book reading improved expressive vocabulary in toddlers (Richman & Columbo, 2007). It seems that there would have to be some kind of threshold for the beneficial effects of book reading. Scarborough and Dobrich (1994) come to the same conclusion: "It might matter a great deal whether a preschooler experiences little or no shared reading with a responsive partner, but beyond a certain threshold level, differences in the quantity or quality of this activity may have little bearing" (p. 285). There is some empirical support for threshold effects in a study by Stevenson and Fredman (1990). These authors found that reading, spelling, and IQ scores of a sample of 550 13-year-olds were strongly predicted by the frequency with which their parents reported reading to them as preschoolers. However, there was a cutoff point at which children who were read to fewer than four times a week performed more poorly than children who were read to more regularly.

Another possible confounding factor in joint book-reading studies is children's interest or facility in literacy activities. A child who would prefer playing video games may get little out of joint book-reading activities. For such children, it is conceivable that too much shared reading might have some negative consequences because they may develop a negative attitude toward reading and other literacy events. The possibility of the negative effects of book reading is an intriguing one. Scarborough and Dobrich (1994, p. 295) use the notion of broccoli effects to refer to this issue. Will serving broccoli to a child who dislikes it make the child into a broccoli lover, or will it serve to reinforce and solidify the child's negative attitude? There is some evidence that negative attitudes can impact on early reading ability. Wells (1985), for example, has found that 11 percent of preschoolers did not like being read to. He also found that preliteracy knowledge scores at age 5 were strong predictors of subsequent reading achievement at ages 7 and 10 (Wells, 1985, 1986). These preliteracy scores were significantly correlated with parental reports of the child's perceived interest in literacy ($r = .45$), the degree of concentration exhibited when engaged in literacy experiences ($r = .56$), and the amount of time spent on literacy activities ($r = .65$).

Importantly, negative attitudes may not have long-term effects on reading achievement. A former neighbor, who is a school librarian, has a child who did not like to be read to when he was young. She would often come down to my house and see my wife reading to my daughter and wonder what she was doing wrong. She kept trying different approaches to get her son interested in books, but he preferred any activity to reading. Now, as a young adult, he still does not like to read books, especially novels. Preference and ability, however, are not the same thing. Although this young adult does not read many books, he does reads articles and texts related to his profession, computer science. Although his parents and schooling have been unable to instill a favorable attitude toward reading books, they have helped him achieve a high level of literacy. This example suggests that negative attitudes toward joint book reading may not prevent children from becoming good readers, but such attitudes may affect how long it takes these children to achieve high literacy levels.

Studies of precocious readers provide additional evidence for the important role early attitudes and motivation have on learning to read. Scarborough and Dobrich (1994) cite several studies showing that precocious readers preferred literacy-related toys and that the greater amount of instruction provided by parents was prompted by the child's desires rather than the parents' preset goals. My older daughter, Alison, was one of these highly motivated children. She loved everything to do with literacy. In addition to the usual literacy events and artifacts, she actually enjoyed doing reading workbooks filled with "phonics" activities. She also loved playing the phonological awareness "games" that Hugh and I used in our studies. I got so tired of the games, especially on long car rides, that I sometimes wished Alison could be more like my neighbor's child, who never tired of playing video games. But Alison's interest in literacy activities paid off; she was reading by age 5.

A positive attitude and motivation to read play an important role in how much preschool children learn about the form of printed language. Most parents would probably not go out and buy phonics workbooks for their preschool children or play phonological awareness games unless their children enjoyed these activities. There must be a basic interest in language and literacy for children to seek out these activities. This interest is sustained, however, by the ability to achieve high levels of success in these activities. If, for example, Alison struggled with the workbook activities or phonological awareness games, I doubt she would have kept doing them. My younger daughter, Franne, learned to read by age $6^1/_2$, about a year and a half later than Alison. On the surface, Franne appeared to show less interest than Alison in phonics activities, especially before she turned 4. The difference, I think, was not so much in Franne's interest level, but in the difficulty she had doing the activities. As soon as Franne began to achieve some success with phonics activities, she pursued these activities with as much enthusiasm as Alison did. Interest and motivation are thus linked at least in part to ability level.

Learning About Print

As discussed in the previous section, joint book reading contributes to and facilitates the learning of letter names, shapes, and sounds. In homes where children are exposed to literacy artifacts and events (high-print homes), there are many other opportunities for young children to learn about print. For example, one of the first songs many children learn is the alphabet song. I have vivid memories of Alison, at age 2, entertaining several rows of passengers on a plane by reciting the alphabet song over and over again. After all the letter names are mastered, children begin to learn the letter shapes. In high-print homes children are continually exposed to print through the multitude of literacy artifacts and toys that parents buy. Alison, like many of her friends, had a little desk with magnetic alphabet letters that she could place on the board. She began by learning all the capital letters, and once she mastered these, we bought her the magnetic lowercase letters. She also had access to a keyboard with its slightly different orthography.

Adams (1990), in her seminal book on early reading, reviewed evidence showing that letter recognition accuracy and speed were critical determinants to reading proficiency. Letter recognition speed and accuracy are important for reading because a child who can recognize most letters will have an easier time learning about letter sounds and word spellings than a child who has to devote attentional resources to remember which letter is what. Learning sound–letter correspondences depends on solid knowledge of letters. Individuals who continue to have difficulty recognizing letters will inevitably have decoding problems, which in turn could lead to comprehension difficulties and frustration with the whole reading process.

The exposure to a variety of literacy artifacts, frequent joint book reading, and various experiences with letter names and sounds may lead preschoolers to the discovery of the alphabetic principle. The insight that letters stand for individual sounds in words requires knowing something about letters (e.g., their names, shapes, and sounds) and the awareness that words consist of discrete sounds. Much has been written about the importance of phonological awareness for early reading (see Adams, 1990; Gillon, 2004; Torgeson, Wagner, & Rashotte, 1994). The important role phonological awareness plays in reading has led to an interest in how children become aware that words consist of discrete sounds. Children as young as 2 years old begin to show some appreciation of the sound system. This awareness is seen in children's spontaneous speech repairs, rhyming behaviors, and nonsense sound play. One of my favorite examples of early phonological awareness is when Alison, at around age 2, put a plastic letter *T* in a cup and said, "Look, Daddy, I'm pouring tea." This example indicates that Alison was able to make a correspondence between the word "tea" and the letter *T*. Her interest in how words sound was also seen in her interest in nursery rhymes and word games. Rhyming activities typically reflect awareness of syllabic and subsyllabic units, such as onsets and rimes (e.g., c-at, h-at, b-at).

Interest in rhyming and developing knowledge of rimes and onsets may lead some children to become interested in and aware of all the sounds in words. Children like Alison soon go beyond simple rhyming games to more challenging "letter and sound" games. One of Alison's favorite car games was to think of words beginning with a certain letter. When this game got too easy, we changed it to thinking of words ending with certain letters. Children like Alison demonstrate that it is possible to acquire phoneme awareness without systematic formal instruction. Although her specific experiences with phonological awareness games may be unique, her early reading proficiency is not particularly noteworthy. Each year I ask my graduate students how many of them were able to read when they entered kindergarten. A surprisingly high percentage (20 to 25 percent) of the students raise their hands. Not surprising is that they have strong memories of their mothers (not fathers) reading to them. Graduate students are obviously not a random sample of the population, so it is fair to say that most children need some formal instruction to become aware of phonemes. Because this instruction typically does not occur until kindergarten, many children may not show adequate phoneme awareness until sometime in the first grade (Catts, Petscher, Schatshneider, & Bridges, 2009).

So much attention has been devoted to the importance of joint book-reading activities, letter recognition, and phonological awareness that the importance of general language and cognitive factors for reading sometimes get overlooked. Although language and cognitive abilities may not be highly correlated to early reading ability, they play an important role in reading comprehension (e.g., Adlof, Catts, & Lee, 2010). Consider, for example, that during the emergent literacy period, children acquire considerable knowledge about language. This knowledge enables them to be fairly competent communicators by the time they enter school. By 5 years of age, children can express abstract conceptual notions involving temporal, spatial, and causal relations. These notions are often expressed in complex sentence structures that include multiple embeddings of subordinate, relative, and infinitive clauses. By 5 years of age, children also have considerable knowledge of familiar scripts and story structure. Children are also developing cognitively during the preschool years, and their increasingly sophisticated reasoning and problem-solving abilities begin to be reflected in measures of reading comprehension during the middle elementary school years.

Summary

It should be apparent that young children learn a great deal about literacy during the emergent literacy period. It is not uncommon for children from high-print homes to enter kindergarten with the ability to recite the alphabet, recognize letters, use a computer, write their name and a few other words, and sight-read a dozen or more written words. It is also not uncommon for a precocious child who enjoys literacy activities to enter school with fairly sophisticated decoding skills. Children who begin school with such extensive knowledge about literacy obviously have a considerable advantage over children who enter school without this knowledge and experience. Teachers need to be aware that children with limited literacy knowledge and experiences are not slow learners or reading disabled. They will, however, be at risk for reading difficulties if they enter kindergarten or first grade with limited early literacy experiences. The last 15 years has seen an explosion in research and educational programs to reduce the number of children at risk for reading difficulties (e.g., Justice et al., 2010; Snow, 1999). The risk of reading difficulties is significantly reduced for children who are enrolled in preschools that have language- and literacy-rich curriculums (Justice et al., 2010). Unfortunately, many at-risk children are not in preschool environments that foster language and literacy development.

THE DEVELOPMENT OF WORD RECOGNITION SKILLS

In considering how emergent readers become proficient readers, it is necessary to understand what it means to be a proficient reader. It is generally agreed that a proficient reader can recognize words accurately and with little effort. Accurate, effortless word recognition requires knowledge of letter sequences or orthographic patterns. Although phonological decoding skills are necessary to develop proficient word recognition, these skills are rarely used by the mature fluent reader. With all the emphasis on phonological awareness and decoding/phonics approaches in recent years, we sometimes forget that proficient word recognition seldom involves sounding words out. Proficient word recognition relies primarily on visual, orthographic information rather than phonological information. If you don't believe this, think about how you read the last sentence. Did you sound out the particular words in the sentence? Imagine sounding out a word like *proficient,* p-r-o-f-i-c-i-e-n-t. Sounding out words, letter by letter or even syllable by syllable, would make reading an incredibly tedious endeavor. Accurate, effortless word recognition requires the ability to use a direct visual route without phonological mediation to access semantic memory and word meaning.

Mature readers, of course, are still capable of sounding out words, but they rarely need to break down a word into its individual sounds to decode it. Even novel words usually have familiar syllable structures or orthographic sequences that can facilitate decoding. For example, most people would probably have little difficulty decoding an unfamiliar name like "Stackenberg" because it contains familiar syllable structure and letter sequences. However, a name like "Kamhi" would be more likely to be sounded out and mispronounced because there is no English word with the orthographic or spelling sequence "a-m-h-i." One has to decide between the various pronunciations of the two vowels, whether the "h" is aspirated or silent, and stress (first or second syllable). Even family members disagree about the pronunciation. Most prefer "kām-eye" like me, but some prefer "kām-ie" because it is more similar to the original Hebrew and Arabic pronunciations, where the final vowel is /i/. The Hebrew is best transliterated as Kimchi (ch = velar fricative), the Arabic as kam hī (aspirated /h/ and second-syllable stress).

How children become automatic fluent readers has intrigued theorists for years. Stage models are a common way to capture the changes that occur in the acquisition of complex behaviors such as reading. Most reading specialists are probably familiar with Chall's (1983) stage theory of reading. Although stage theories have a number of shortcomings that will be discussed later, they provide a useful framework for understanding the basic developmental changes that occur as children learn to read.

Logographic Stage

Most stage theories of reading acknowledge an initial visual or logographic stage in learning to read (Ehri, 1991, 2005; Frith, 1985). Frith (1985), for example, has proposed a "logographic stage" to mark the end of the emergent literacy period and a transition to a phonetic or alphabetic stage of reading. In this stage, children construct associations between unanalyzed spoken words and one or more salient graphic features of the printed word or its surrounding context. During this stage, children do not use knowledge of letter names or sound–letter relationships to recognize words. Ehri (1991, p. 387) has suggested that if readers use letters as cues, they do so because their shapes are visually salient, not because the letters correspond to the sounds in the word. As a result, they cannot read new words and can be easily fooled by switching visual cues. For example, when the Coca-Cola logo was pasted on a Rice Krispies box, more than half the preschoolers tested thought that it said "Rice Krispies" (Masonheimer, Drum, & Ehri, 1984). When one letter was changed in the Pepsi logo to read Xepsi, 74 percent of preschoolers read the label as Pepsi.

The role of logographic reading for the development of word recognition skills is controversial. Share and Stanovich (1995) have suggested that it has no functional value because it ignores correspondences between print and sound at a sublexical level. If logographic reading had any functional value, one would expect to find positive correlations with reading ability. Share and Stanovich (1995) cited numerous studies that found no relationship between logographic reading and letter reading ability, suggesting that from the standpoint of acquiring proficient word recognition skills, the logographic stage may best be regarded as prereading. Because logographic reading has no apparent developmental role in reading, children do not have to read logographically to begin to read phonetically. Most children from high-print homes probably go through a clearly defined period when they read logographically, but there would be no reason to teach children to read logographically if they entered school with limited literacy knowledge. The first "true" stage of word recognition would have to involve the use of at least some phonetic cues to recognize words.

Alphabetic Stage

Stage theorists differ in the number of stages it takes to develop proficient word recognition skills (Chall, 1983; Ehri, 2005; Frith, 1985). There is general agreement that when children begin to read words by processing sound–letter correspondences, they move into the alphabetic stage. Theorists differ, however, in the number of phases that exist in the development of automatic sight word recognition. Ehri (2005), for example, has identified four phases of children's developing knowledge of the alphabetic system: pre-alphabetic, partial alphabetic, full alphabetic, and consolidated alphabetic. The pre-alphabetic phase corresponds to the logographic stage. Whether one identifies one phase of alphabetic knowledge or many, the fundamental aspect of this stage remains the ability to use sound–letter correspondences to decode novel words. Most theories of reading development acknowledge that constructing associations between sounds and letters is the fundamental task facing the beginning reader. Importantly, productive learning of sound–letter correspondences involves more than just recognizing letters and coupling them with appropriate sounds. It is not enough to memorize the sounds that go with each letter. To make use of those sounds, the child must realize that they are the sounds that make up spoken language. The child needs to link the letters to the particular set of phonemic sounds that comprise spoken language (see Adams, 1990). This is the alphabetic insight that underlies the ability to phonologically decode words.

The alphabetic insight, like other insights, is a one-time occurrence. Having the insight does not make the task of learning all the sound–letter correspondences any easier. The sounds or phonemes that children must associate with letters are abstract linguistic concepts rather than physically real entities and, as such, do not always correspond to discrete and invariant sounds. As a result of coarticulation, the sound segments of speech blend together in running, conversational speech. Sounds that are less affected by coarticulation are thus inherently easier to associate with letters than sounds that are affected by coarticulation. This is why continuant sounds and letters (e.g., /s/, /f/, /m/) are often taught before stop sounds (/b/, /d/, /g/). In the word *see*, for example, it is easy to have the child listen for the /s/ sound (s-s-s-s-s) and separate it from the vowel (eeeeee). For the word *bat,* however, it is not possible to separate the /b/ from its accompanying vowel. Without a vowel, the *b* in *bat* is nothing more than a burst of air that is more similar to a bird's chirp than the "buh" [b] sound many people think a *b* makes. But if *b* was really a [b] then the word *bat* would be pronounced "buh-at" not "bat."

There are many examples of the lack of correspondence between sounds and letters in English. This lack of correspondence makes learning to read a slow process and makes learning to spell even more difficult. Consider, for example, the words *writer* and *rider.* Most people think that the difference in these two words is in the medial consonant. *Writer* has a *t* whereas *rider* has a *d.* But if you say these two words to yourself and don't affect a British accent, the *t* and *d* in the two words are pronounced the same, as an alveolar flap /ɾ/. The two words sound different because the first vowel is longer in *rider* than it is in *writer.* Another frequently cited example is the *tr* in *truck.* It is difficult to say *tr* at a normal rate of speech without turning the /t/ into an affricate. Listen carefully, and you will hear something resembling the "ch" sound. A common early spelling of *truck* is thus "ch-u-k." Children's so-called invented spellings often reflect how words actually sound, which means they are not invented at all. Spelling words like they sound is a good thing because it indicates that children have phonological awareness. If a young child spelled words with random strings of letters (e.g., truck = *s-p-a-l-k),* parents and teachers should be concerned.

Learning sound–letter correspondences is further complicated by the allophonic variations of many English phonemes. In the *writer–rider* example given earlier, the alveolar flap /ɾ/ is an allophonic variation of /t/ and /d/. Many teachers incorrectly assume, however, that phonemes have only one phonetic form. But many English phonemes have several phonetic variations depending on where they occur in words and the sounds around them. The phoneme /t/, for example, is produced in its canonical form with aspiration only before stressed vowels (e.g., *top, attack*). But as we saw with the word *writer,* an intervocalic /t/ is always flapped. A syllable final /t/ as in *pot* or *Kaitlin* may be unreleased. In s-clusters (e.g., *stop*), the /t/ actually sounds more like a /d/ than a /t/, and in words like *bottle,* the /t/ may become a glottal stop. These examples illustrate how phonemes can have several different phonetic variations. These phonetic variations make the task of learning what are actually phoneme–grapheme (rather than sound–letter) correspondences a difficult one.

Once one gets beyond the word level, there is even less correspondence between sounds and letters because the effects of coarticulation are greater in sentences and conversational speech. For example, in normal conversation, the phrase *did you know* is pronounced [dɪdʒəno]. A child who was told that the letter *y* corresponds to the "ya" sound would have difficulty constructing an association between this sound and letter because there is no "ya" sound in this sentence.

Another considerable obstacle facing young children is the irregularities of English spelling. Children must learn that many letters do not always sound like they should. There are 251 different spellings for the 44 sounds of English (Horn, 1926). Consider, for example, all the different spellings of the vowel sound /i/—ie, e, ei, i, y, ea, ee—or the consonant /f/—f, ff, gh, ph. Children also have to learn that each grapheme (letter) may have a number of different forms. Most graphemes have different upper- and lowercase forms and a different script form. Some graphemes may also have a different typewritten form (e.g., lowercase *a*), meaning that a particular grapheme might have as many as four or five different letter forms.

Despite these obstacles, young children gradually begin to move beyond the inefficient strategy of sounding out every word. Whereas the alphabetic insight and learning of phoneme–grapheme correspondences mark the transition into the alphabetic stage and the true beginning of word recognition, orthographic knowledge is necessary to develop automatic, effortless sight word recognition skills. This stage is discussed in the next section.

Orthographic Stage and Automatic Sight Word Recognition

The orthographic stage is characterized by the use of letter sequences and spelling patterns to recognize words by sight without phonological decoding. The ability to use a direct visual route without phonological mediation to access semantic memory and word meaning is crucial for developing automatic sight word recognition skills. Although some theorists disagree about what to call this final stage of word recognition (e.g., orthographic or automatic), there is consensus that orthographic knowledge is necessary for automatic, effortless word recognition. Without orthographic knowledge, readers would continue to sound out long multisyllabic words and rely on the more inefficient and time-consuming indirect phonological route to access semantic memory.

According to Ehri (1991, 2005) and Frith (1985), the orthographic or consolidated phase begins when children accumulate sufficient knowledge of spelling patterns so that they are able to recognize the words visually without phonological conversion. Orthographic knowledge accumulates as readers phonologically decode different words that share similar letter sequences, recognize these similarities, and store this information in memory. If readers are not able to phonologically decode all the letters in a word, they will have difficulty learning to recognize letter patterns that occur in different words (Ehri, 1991).

What kinds of orthographic patterns do readers detect? It seems obvious that readers will most likely learn patterns that occur frequently. Morphemes *(-ing, -ed, -able, -ment, -ity),* with their consistent spelling and function, present an excellent starting point to focus on orthographic rather than phonological sequences. Ehri (1991, p. 405) cited a study by Becker, Dixon, and Anderson-Inman (1980) in which they analyzed 26,000 high-frequency English words into root words and morphemes. They found about 8,100 different root words and about 800 different morphemes that occurred in at least 10 different words.

The other place to look for orthographic regularities is in words that share letter sequences. These words may be thought of as belonging to a particular word family or orthographic neighborhood. For example, *teach, reach, each,* and *preach* all have the common stem *-each,* whereas *cake, bake, take, make,* and *lake* all have the common stem *-ake.* In Chapter 5 of this book, Al Otaiba and her colleagues list some common spelling patterns that are found at the end of single-syllable words: *-ack, -ight, -eat, -ay, -ash, -ip, -ore,* and *-ell.* As readers begin to focus on common spelling sequences, they begin to use an analogy strategy to read new words (Goswami, 1986). Rather than sounding out a new word sound by sound, mature readers compare the letter sequence of a new word to letter sequences of familiar words in semantic memory. Al Otaiba and her colleagues give several examples of reading by analogy in their chapter. For example, the word *cart* might be read by noticing the word *car* and adding a /t/ sound at the end. A long word like *fountain* might initially be read by noticing its similarity to *mountain.*

As noted earlier, orthographic knowledge is crucial for the development of automatic word recognition skills because knowledge of letter sequences enables readers to set up access routes in memory to read words by sight. Although many theorists have characterized fluent sight word recognition as an automatic process, the concept of automaticity is not a simple one. Stanovich (1990, 1991) has discussed the difficulty involved in "unpacking" what automatic word recognition actually involves. He argues that the question of whether word recognition is automatic is not a good one because it confounds aspects of word recognition that can be differentiated such as speed, capacity usage, conscious control, obligatory execution, and influence of higher-level knowledge. Development of each of these factors does not coincide.

The concept of modularity provides a better way to characterize developing word recognition proficiency. A modular process is one that operates quickly and is not controlled or influenced by higher-level processes. Fodor (1983), who first proposed the concept of modularity, described modular systems as having functional autonomy and being cognitively impenetrable. Proficient word recognition fits the definition of a modular process because it is fast, requires little capacity and conscious attention, and is not affected by higher-level knowledge sources. In support of a modular view of word recognition, context effects have been shown to decrease as word recognition skills become more proficient (see Gough, 1983). In other words, children rely less on higher-level knowledge sources as their word recognition skills become more modularized. Although most reading theorists and practitioners will probably continue to talk about automatization of word recognition, it may be useful to attempt to incorporate modular notions in characteristics of proficient sight word recognition skill.

Problems with Stage Theories of Word Recognition

Although the stages of word recognition described in the previous section accurately portray the kinds of knowledge and skills required to become a proficient reader, the actual stages do not seem to be supported by empirical evidence (Ehri, 2005; Share & Stanovich, 1995). One consistent problem with stage theories is that the focus is primarily on what knowledge children need to become proficient readers rather than the mechanisms that underlie changes in reading proficiency. Another problem with stage theories is that each stage is associated with only one type of reading (logographic, alphabetic, orthographic), which implies that all words are read with the same approach at a particular stage. Although stage theorists often mention beginning and end points of stages, little attention is typically devoted to the actual development of the knowledge that characterizes these stages. For example, a common description of the alphabetic stage is that a child has little alphabetic knowledge at the beginning of the stage and is able to phonologically decode most words by the end of the stage. How a little knowledge becomes a lot of knowledge is often not addressed by most stage theorists (e.g., Spear-Swerling & Sternberg, 1996). Ehri (1991, 2005) is a notable exception. Another limitation of stage theories is that they tend to oversimplify development and obscure individual differences. Although there are certain things that all children must learn to become proficient readers, children may take different paths to becoming good readers.

The Self-Teaching Hypothesis

Share (1995) and Share and Stanovich (1995) offered an alternative to stage-based theories. The key notion in what they refer to as the "self-teaching hypothesis" is that phonological decoding functions as a self-teaching mechanism that enables the learner to acquire the detailed orthographic representations necessary for fast and accurate visual word recognition and for proficient spelling. Although direct instruction and contextual guessing may play some role in developing orthographic knowledge, Share and Stanovich argue that only phonological decoding offers a viable means for the development of fast, efficient visual word recognition.

Direct instruction cannot account for orthographic learning because children encounter too many unfamiliar words. The average fifth grader, for example, encounters around 10,000 new words per year (Nagy & Herman, 1987); there is no way teachers, parents, or peers can help children with all these unfamiliar words. The problem with contextual guessing is that the primary purpose of text is to convey nonredundant information, not redundant information. Sentences like *We walked into the restaurant and sat down at a* ___ are rare because they violate a basic communicative convention of conveying new or nonredundant information. Gough (1983) has referred to context as a false friend because it helps you when you least need it. It works best for high-frequency function words, but not very well for content words.

To further support the inadequacy of contextual guessing, Share and Stanovich cited data from a study by Finn (1977/78) indicating that the average predictability of words when they were deleted was 29.5 percent. Guesses were thus twice as likely to be wrong than right. The inadequacy of contextual guessing is caused in part by the large number of synonyms or near-synonyms in English and the fact that most of the predictable words are function words (e.g., determiners) that contribute little to the meaning of the sentence or text. But even if children are successful in guessing the correct word, this strategy is not a viable one to develop proficient sight word recognition skills because children are not focusing on particular spelling patterns of the words.

Because of the inadequacy of direct instruction and contextual guessing for the development of efficient sight word reading, Share and Stanovich (1995) contended that the ability to phonologically decode words and associate printed words with their spoken equivalents must play a pivotal role in the development of fluent sight word recognition. In their own words,

> According to the self-teaching hypothesis, each successful decoding encounter with an unfamiliar word provides an opportunity to acquire the word-specific orthographic information that is the foundation of skilled word recognition and spelling. In this way, phonological recoding acts as a self-teaching mechanism or built-in teacher enabling the child to independently develop knowledge of specific word spellings and more general knowledge of orthographic conventions. (p. 18)

The self-teaching hypothesis attempts to explain one of the long-standing puzzles of how children learn to read. I remember years ago wondering how my older daughter Alison seemed to change overnight from a slow plodding reader, asking about every other word, to a fluent reader. I read somewhere a long time ago that the transition to fluent, proficient decoding is like magic. I knew that helping Alison with unfamiliar words could not turn her into a fluent reader, so I just waited and assumed some day it would all come together. When the day finally came, I had no idea what the underlying factors were that led Alison (and other young children) to finally automatize the word recognition process.

The answer according to Share and Stanovich (1995) is that children teach themselves to read fluently. What makes learning to read seem magical is that parents and most professionals never could satisfactorily explain how children seemed to become proficient sight word readers overnight. One reason that it has taken so long for a self-teaching theory of reading to be proposed and will take many more years to be accepted is that we have always assumed that teachers taught children to read. But as will become clear later, it is difficult to teach children all they need to know to become proficient sight word readers.

There are four features of the self-teaching role of phonological decoding: (1) item-based as opposed to stage-based role of decoding in development, (2) early onset, (3) progressive "lexicalization" of word recognition, and (4) the asymmetric relationship between primary phonological and secondary orthographic components in the self-teaching process. Each of these features is discussed in more detail.

The stage theories reviewed in the previous section propose that all words are initially phonologically decoded with a later developmental shift to visual access using orthographic information. In reviewing the research that addresses the phonological-to-orthographic shift, Share and Stanovich (1995, p. 14) noted that it is consistently inconsistent. Some studies find evidence of direct visual access in early grades with no indication of a transition from a phonological to a visual-orthographic stage (e.g., Barron & Baron, 1977). Other studies, in contrast, found evidence in support of the developmental phonological to visual-orthographic shift (e.g., Backman, Bruck, Hebert, & Seidenberg, 1984).

To resolve the conflicting findings, Share (1995) suggested that it is more appropriate to ask how children read individual words. Whether a child needs to phonologically decode a word or is able to recognize it by sight depends on how often a child has been exposed to a particular word and the nature and success of phonologically decoding the particular word. Familiar high-frequency words are recognized visually with minimal phonological decoding, whereas novel or low-frequency words for which the child has yet to develop orthographic representations will be more dependent on phonological decoding. The frequency of phonological decoding will thus vary according to children's familiarity with words in particular texts. If the text is at the child's reading level or a little above, "a majority of the words will be recognized visually, while the smaller number of low-frequency unfamiliar words will provide opportunities for self-teaching with minimal disruption of ongoing comprehension processes" (Share, 1995, p. 155). Importantly, the self-teaching opportunities with these unfamiliar words represent the "cutting edge" of reading development not merely for the beginner, but for readers throughout the ability range (p. 156).

Evidence of self-teaching can be found at the very earliest stage of word recognition. For self-teaching to occur, children need to have at least some sound–letter knowledge, some phonological awareness, some vocabulary knowledge, and the ability to use contextual information to determine exact word pronunciations based on partial decodings. The key point here is that children do not need to have accurate phonological decoding skills to develop orthographic-based representations. These orthographic representations may, however, be somewhat incomplete or primitive, but the primitive nature of these representations does not prevent them from being used for direct (visual) access to meaning.

The lexicalization of phonological decoding is a central aspect of the self-teaching hypothesis. Early decoding skill is based on simple one-to-one correspondences between sounds and letters. There is little sensitivity to orthographic and morphemic context. Share and Stanovich (1995, p. 23) suggested that with print exposure, these early sound–letter correspondences become *lexicalized*; that is, they come to be associated with particular words. As the child becomes more attuned to spelling regularities beyond the level of simple one-to-one phoneme–grapheme correspondences, this orthographic information is used to modify the initial lexicalizations children develop. The outcome of this process of lexicalization, according to Share and Stanovich, "is a skilled reader whose knowledge of the relationships between print and sound has evolved to a degree that makes it indistinguishable from a purely whole-word mechanism that maintains no spelling–sound correspondence rules at the level of individual letters and digraphs" (pp. 23–24).

The notion of lexicalization resolves one of the classic enigmas of word recognition—that the rules required for proficient sight word reading are very different from the simplistic and sometimes incorrect rules (e.g., /b/ = "buh") taught to beginning readers. Basic knowledge of simple sound–letter correspondences is a logical starting point for the beginning reader, but it is impossible to become a proficient sight word reader using these rules. These simple rules are used as a bootstrap or scaffold for developing the "complex lexically constrained knowledge of spelling–sound relationships that characterize the expert reader" (Share & Stanovich, 1995, p. 25).

The final claim that the self-teaching hypothesis makes is that phonological skills are the primary self-teaching mechanism for the acquisition of fluent word recognition. The contribution of visual/orthographic factors is secondary and "largely parasitic upon the self-teaching opportunities provided by decoding and print exposure" (Share & Stanovich, 1995, p. 26). Phonological decoding causes children to look at all the letters in a word, and this attention gradually leads to recognition of common letter sequences and other orthographic patterns. The evidence in support of this claim is found in studies documenting the strong relationship between pseudoword reading and word recognition (e.g., Stanovich & Siegel, 1994). Correlation coefficients typically exceed .70, indicating that a large part of the variance in word recognition is accounted for by the ability to phonologically decode. One possible point of confusion is that phonological decoding can occur on different size units of speech, such as phonemes, syllables, rimes/onsets, and morphemes. The most straightforward type of decoding involves identifying and blending together the individual sounds in words. Because simple one-to-one sound blending is a very inefficient way to decode long words and words with irregular spellings, children will try to find larger units to phonologically decode. For example, they may divide words into onsets and rimes. It is much easier to phonologically decode *fight* as f-ight and *bought* as b-ought than it is to sound out individual letters. As children begin to notice common morphemes in different words, they will use these language-based units to decode unfamiliar words. Once they get to this point, they should also be able to decode novel words by making analogies to other words that they already know (cf. the *mountain/fountain* example discussed earlier). As novel words become familiar, children will be able to visually recognize the whole word without having to phonologically decode any part of the word.

Share and Stanovich (1995) make it very clear that phonological decoding skill is no guarantee of self-teaching: "It only provides the opportunities for self-teaching. Other factors such as the quantity and quality of exposure to print together with the ability and/or inclination to attend to and remember orthographic detail will determine the extent to which these opportunities are exploited" (p. 25). In other words, there is a lot of room for individual differences in reading ability. At one end of the continuum, there will be cases of children with severe deficits in visual/orthographic memory. Even with good phonological decoding skill, these children would have to tackle every word as if they were seeing it for the first time. At the other extreme are children who may recall word-specific letter patterns after only a single exposure. These children should become proficient readers at a relatively early age given adequate exposure to print.

Evaluating the Self-Teaching Hypothesis

In the 15 years since Share first proposed the self-teaching hypothesis, considerable research has investigated whether phonological decoding is in fact the primary mechanism of learning to read. Not surprisingly, the research conducted by Share and his colleagues strongly supported this hypothesis (e.g., de Jong & Share, 2007; Share, 1999, 2004; Shatil & Share, 2003). Share (1999), for example, found that pure visual exposure to a novel word did not facilitate orthographic learning. As the self-teaching hypothesis predicts, phonological decoding was critical to the acquisition of word-specific orthographic representations.

In other studies, self-teaching was tested by asking children to read novel words embedded in stories. For example, the word *yait* was introduced in a story as the name of the coldest city in the world. After a number of repetitions and decoding attempts, children were asked to choose the correct spelling of the word from four alternatives, including a homophone foil (e.g., *yate*). If children used phonological recoding skills, they would be as likely to choose *yate* as *yait*, but studies (Nation, Angell, & Castles, 2007; Share, 2004) have shown that young children show evidence of rapid orthographic learning. These studies also find that for some children, a single exposure was sufficient for long-term orthographic learning, and this newly acquired knowledge was maintained for at least one month (Share, 2004). Orthographic learning also occurs in silent reading (Bowey & Muller, 2005; de Jong & Share, 2007).

Recent studies have found that spelling is a powerful self-teaching tool in the formation of word-specific orthographic representations (Shahar-Yames & Share, 2008). This should come as no surprise. Writing forces children to think about sound–letter correspondences, the relation of print to spoken language, and orthographic/spelling patterns. Adams, Treiman, and Pressley (1996) provide an excellent discussion of the impact of writing on learning to read.

Despite the attractiveness of the self-teaching hypothesis, some prominent reading theorists feel that it does not provide a complete account of orthographic learning. The hypothesis predicts that there should be a strong relationship between children's ability to decode a novel word correctly and their ability to recognize the word in a test of orthographic learning. Although a significant relationship has been found between decoding skill and orthographic learning ($r = .53$ in Cunningham, Perry, Stanovich, & Share, 2002, and $r = .3$ in Nation et al., 2007), many instances were found of decoding success and orthographic learning failure and vice versa. The absence of a strong relationship at an item (word) level suggests that factors other than phonological decoding influence learning word-specific orthographic representations (Nation, 2008; Nation et al., 2007). Factors that have been examined to date include semantic knowledge (Castles & Nation, 2008; Nation & Cocksey, 2009), morphological knowledge (e.g., Carlisle, 2003; Jarmulowicz, Hay, Taran, & Ethington, 2008), general language competence (Nation, 2008), and experience-based episodic knowledge (Nation, 2008). The research of Nation and her colleagues, which is summarized in Nation (2008), suggests that children's general language competence and experience-based episodic knowledge may have more of an impact on children's development of proficient sight word reading than deep semantic knowledge.

THE DEVELOPMENT OF READING COMPREHENSION

In Chapter 1, the processes involved in reading comprehension were reviewed. To assign meaning to texts, readers rely on previously stored knowledge about language and the world as well as specific knowledge about different text structures and genres. As reflected in the Simple View of reading, the ability to understand spoken language is the foundation for reading comprehension. Children cannot construct meanings of sentences and texts without understanding key vocabulary, and implicit knowledge of syntactic forms seems necessary to comprehend particular grammatical constructions. Background knowledge and basic reasoning abilities, such as making analogies and inferences, as well as metacognitive abilities, knowledge of text structure, interest, and attention, also play important roles in reading comprehension. A detailed discussion of how children acquire the knowledge and reasoning abilities to construct elaborate meanings and interpretations of texts is beyond the scope of this chapter. It is important to consider, however, what such a discussion would need to entail.

When children are first learning to read and their word recognition skills are inefficient, their ability to understand spoken discourse is necessarily much better than their ability to understand written texts. The development of proficient word recognition skills frees up attentional resources to focus on text comprehension and learning. Chall's (1983) stage theory of reading reflects this change in focus. In Chall's second stage of reading, children became unglued from print. In her third stage, which begins in about third grade and continues through middle school, children begin the long course of reading to learn. Chall noted that in traditional schools, children in the third/fourth grade begin to study the so-called subject areas, such as history, geography, and science. Content subjects such as these are not introduced until children have presumably become relatively proficient sight word readers.

Chall's "reading to learn" stage describes children's increasing ability to understand more sophisticated texts. Although the distinction between learning to read and reading to learn is appealing, it cannot be accurate. Even before children are actually reading, they are learning from the books that are read to them. As they are developing their word-reading abilities, they can still learn. As Hirsch (2006) has argued, knowledge of science, history, and other subjects can and should be taught to young children. Current reports show, however, that in most schools, teachers spend too much time teaching basic reading and math skills and not enough time on content areas like science and social studies (Pianta, Belsky, Houts, & Morrison, 2007).

As discussed in the previous section, stage theories typically do not address how processes become more proficient. To read more sophisticated texts, children need more than accurate, efficient word recognition. In addition to rapid lexical access, other aspects of linguistic processing, such as assigning syntactic/semantic roles, need to take place in a timely manner (Carlisle, 1991; Nation, 2008; Oakhill & Cain, 2007). Efficient linguistic processing plays an important role in one's ability to integrate ideas within and across sentences, paragraphs, and larger discourse units.

Children's facility for understanding texts also increases as they become more familiar with the particular structure and function of different text genres (Kintsch, 1998; Richgels, McGee, Lomax, & Sheard, 1987). When children start school, their experience with different kinds of discourse genres is often fairly limited. As Carlisle (1991) has noted, they are most familiar with running commentaries of their playmates, explanations of events or simple phenomena, and narratives encountered in shared story reading with adults. In school, they gradually become exposed to different genres, such as biography, drama, poetry, and the various kinds of expository texts used in science and social studies, but comprehension of expository texts has been found to consistently lag behind comprehension of narrative texts using formal assessments (Duke, 2000; National Center for Educational Statistics, 2001; Rasool & Royer, 1986).

Any attempt to explain the development of reading comprehension must also consider what it means to understand a text. Does it mean understanding particular words, sentences, paragraphs, or chapters? Does it mean understanding plot, purpose, theme, character motives, or author's intent? Or does it mean the ability to construct analytic and creative interpretations of texts? Standardized tests of reading comprehension typically assess information reflected in the first two questions through multiple-choice or fill-in-the blank (cloze-type) questions. Consider, though, if one's view of comprehension development was based on the way in which students responded to the following questions:

1. What made the book interesting?
2. Did you like the book? Why or why not?
3. Are there characters in the book who you would like to have as friends?
4. What other things would you like to see happen in the book?
5. If you were the main character, what would you have done different in the story?
6. If you could meet the author of the book, what would you say?
7. What things would you change in the story?
8. Have you ever experienced some of the events or feelings that the characters in the book experienced?

Questions such as these require informational knowledge as well as interpretation and reasoning skills. In addition, answering aesthetic questions requires the ability to explain and justify why one likes or doesn't like a particular text. A theory of how reading comprehension develops thus must address not only how students develop language, background knowledge, metacognitive skills, and reasoning abilities, but also how they learn to explain and justify their aesthetic responses to texts.

Misconceptions about Comprehension Development

It should be apparent that reading comprehension is too complex and influenced by too many factors (reader, text, and task) to be viewed as a unitary, invariant skill that develops in a nice, linear developmental trajectory. Although it may be possible to find aspects of language (e.g., vocabulary) and cognitive abilities that appear to develop incrementally throughout the school years, the ability to construct meanings of different texts cannot develop incrementally because the thinking and reasoning processes used to construct meaning are content or subject specific (Hirsch, 2006; Kintsch, 1998). This is why one of the best predictors of comprehension is often familiarity with content knowledge domains (Hirsch, 2006; Willingham, 2006). The domain specificity of comprehension means that the ability to extract meaning from text often does not generalize across content or subject areas (Hirsch & Pondiscio, 2010).

Unfortunately, the way comprehension is measured by standardized tests and characterized by grade-level benchmarks promotes the misconception that comprehension is a unitary, easily measurable skill that develops in discrete measurable increments over the school years. Standardized tests of reading comprehension do so by rank-ordering comprehension abilities into discrete age divisions, whereas grade-level benchmarks do so by fostering the misconception that comprehension is a unitary, generalizable skill that can be applied equally well to all texts.

To rank-order students, standardized measures of comprehension must use easy-to-score test items that normally distribute students at each age level. Easy-to-score test items require that there is only one correct answer for each question, but many texts, especially complex ones, have more than one plausible interpretation. If texts did not have more than one plausible interpretation, literary scholars would not still be writing academic articles and books about Shakespeare's plays and other works of literature. When tests and teachers assume that each text has only one correct or best interpretation, students learn that to perform well in class and on tests, they simply need to reconstruct or restate the meaning of the text as presented by the teacher or guidebook. It should come as no surprise, then, that studies (e.g., Purves, 1992) have shown that high school students view English classes as part of a game that involves reading to take comprehension tests. The students did not read for enjoyment or to enlarge their understanding; instead they focused on ways to get the information to pass tests. Performance turned out to be influenced by which period in the day students had English class: Those that had class in later periods did better than students who had class in first or second period because the later-period students got the test questions from their friends who had already taken the test.

Although grade-level comprehension benchmarks also promote a unitary, linear view of comprehension development, benchmarks may be useful in helping educators think about the qualities of good comprehension and the skills and strategies that may facilitate understanding. There has been considerable research on strategies that promote good comprehension (e.g., Barr, Blachowicz, Katz, & Daufman, 2002; National Institute of Child Health and Human Development [NICHD], 2000; Pressley, Graham, & Harris, 2006). Barr et al. (2002), for example, identified five strategies that good comprehenders use to help them understand different texts.

1. Good comprehenders use what they know. They realize that reading is more than remembering exact words from the text; it also involves reasoning and adding to their knowledge.

2. Good comprehenders self-question to establish what they don't know and what they want and need to know. Asking good questions helps them make hypotheses, draw analogies from experience, and set some purposes and guidelines for reading.
3. Good comprehenders integrate information across texts, add information by making inferences to build cohesion, and use structure to organize their comprehension.
4. Good comprehenders monitor their reading.
5. Good comprehenders respond thoughtfully to what they read. They respond personally to what they read and exhibit high degrees of critical and analytic thinking.

There is little doubt that readers who are able to do these things will be better comprehenders than readers who do not, but as discussed previously, the ability to extract meaning from text often will not generalize across content or subject areas (Hirsch & Pondiscio, 2010; Kintsch, 1998). So, although it is possible to describe what good comprehenders do to construct meanings of texts, this does not mean that a particular individual will always be a good (or poor) comprehender. Comprehension performance will vary based on the reader's background knowledge, interest level, the type of comprehension response required, and other reader and text factors.

The multifaceted nature of comprehension and its variability means that any attempt to provide a unifying theory of comprehension development is not just a futile endeavor; it is a misguided one. The complexity and variability of comprehension must be appreciated and understood to decide which assessments and interventions should be used to improve student performance. Chapters 6 and 7 should help educators and practitioners deal with the challenge of deciding what to assess and what to teach. In Chapter 6, I present a model of comprehension followed by a discussion of strategy instruction, content goals, and disciplinary literacy. In Chapter 7, Carol Westby provides an in-depth discussion of the language and inferencing aspects of comprehension.

Summary

In this chapter, I have attempted to provide a road map for the development of proficient reading. The primary focus in the chapter has been on the development of proficient word recognition skills because one can restrict the discussion to how children acquire specific phonological and orthographic knowledge. The importance of the emergent literacy period was emphasized followed by a discussion of the three basic stages in the development of word recognition skills. Share and Stanovich's (1995) self-teaching hypothesis was offered as an alternative to the stage theory of development. Although the self-teaching hypothesis does not provide a complete account of orthographic learning (Nation, 2008), it remains a viable explanation for how children learn to read.

The story of comprehension development is much more difficult to tell than the story of how children become proficient word-level readers. Rather than provide a model of comprehension development, which is not possible given its complexity and variability, I focused instead on the factors, skills, and knowledge that affect understanding. I also spent some time addressing the common misconception that comprehension is a unitary, invariant skill that develops in a nice, linear developmental trajectory. This misconception is fostered by the way comprehension is measured by standardized tests and grade-level comprehension benchmarks. Helping students construct literal, analytic, and creative interpretations of texts, a goal we all have, depends in large part on understanding the complexity and variability of comprehension.

References

Adams, M. (1990). *Beginning to read: Thinking and learning about print*. Cambridge, MA: MIT Press.

Adams, M., Treiman, R., & Pressley, M. (1996). Reading, writing, and literacy. In I. Sigel & A. Renninger (Eds.), *Mussen's handbook of child psychology: Volume 4. Child psychology in practice* (pp. 1–124). New York: Wiley.

Adlof, S. A., Catts, H., & Lee, J. (2010). Kindergarten predictors of second vs. eighth grade reading comprehension impairments. *Journal of Learning Disabilities, 43*, 332–345.

Backman, J., Bruck, M., Hebert, J., & Seidenberg, M. (1984). Acquisition and use of spelling-sound correspondences in reading. *Journal of Experimental Child Psychology, 38*, 114–133.

Barr, R., Blachowicz, C., Katz, C., & Daufman, B. (2002). *Reading diagnosis for teachers: An instructional approach* (4th ed). Boston: Allyn & Bacon.

Barron, R., & Baron, J. (1977). How children get meaning from printed words. *Child Development, 48*, 587–594.

Becker, W., Dixon, R., & Anderson-Inman, L. (1980). *Morphographic and root word analysis of 26,000 high-frequency words*. Eugene, OR: University of Oregon College of Education.

Bowey, J., & Muller, D. (2005). Phonological recoding and rapid orthographic learning in third-graders' silent reading: A critical test of the self-teaching hypothesis. *Journal of Experimental Child Psychology, 92*, 203–219.

Burns, M., Griffin, P., & Snow, C. (1999). *Starting out right: A guide to promoting children's reading success*. Washington, DC: National Academy Press.

Bus, A., van Ijzendoorn, M., & Pellegrini, A. (1995). Joint book reading makes for success in learning to read: A meta-analysis on intergenerational transmission of literacy. *Review of Educational Research, 65*, 1–21.

Carlisle, J. (1991). Planning an assessment of listening and reading comprehension. *Topics in Language Disorders, 12*, 17–31.

Carlisle, J. (2003). Morphology matters in learning to read: A commentary. *Reading Psychology, 24*, 291–322.

Castles, A., & Nation, K. (2008). Learning to be a good orthographic reader. *Journal of Research in Reading, 31*, 1–7.

Catts, H., Petscher, Y., Schatschneider, C., & Bridges, M. (2009). Floor effects in universal screening and their impact on the early identification of reading disabilities. *Journal of Learning Disabilities, 42*, 163–176.

Chall, J. (1983). *Stages of reading development*. New York: McGraw-Hill.

Commission on Reading. (1985). *Becoming a nation of readers: The report of the Commission on Reading*. Washington, DC: The National Institute of Education.

Cunningham, A., Perry, K., Stanovich, K., & Share, D. (2002). Orthographic learning during reading: Examining the role of self-teaching. *Journal of Experimental Child Psychology, 82*, 185–199.

de Jong, P., & Share, D. (2007). Orthographic learning during oral and silent reading. *Scientific Studies of Reading, 11*, 55–71.

Duke, N. K. (2000). 3.6 minutes per day: The scarcity of informational texts in first grade. *Reading Research Quarterly, 35*, 202–224.

Ehri, L. (1991). Development of the ability to read words. In R. Barr, M. Kamil, P. Mosenthal, & P. Pearson (Eds.), *Handbook of reading research, Volume II* (pp. 1–417). White Plains, NY: Longman.

Ehri, L. (2005). Learning to read words: Theory, findings, and issues. *Scientific Studies of Reading, 9*, 167–188.

Finn, P. (1977/78). Word frequency, information theory, and cloze performance: A transfer feature theory of processing in reading. *Reading Research Quarterly, 23*, 510–537.

Fodor, J. (1983). *The modularity of mind*. Cambridge, MA: MIT Press.

Frith, U. (1985). Beneath the surface of developmental dyslexia. In K. Patterson, J. Marshall, & M. Coltheart (Eds.), *Surface dyslexia* (pp. 1–330). London: Erlbaum.

Gibson, E., & Levine, H. (1975). *The psychology of reading*. Cambridge, MA: MIT Press.

Gillon, G. (2004). *Phonological awareness: From research to practice*. New York: Guilford Press.

Goswami, U. (1986). Children's use of analogy in learning to read: A developmental study. *Journal of Experimental Child Psychology, 42*, 73–83.

Gough, P. (1983). Context, form, and interaction. In K. Rayner (Ed.), *Eye movements in reading* (pp. 1–211). New York: Academic Press.

Heath, S. (1982). What no bedtime story means: Narrative skills at home and at school. *Language in Society, 11*, 49–76.

Hirsch, E. D., Jr. (2006). *The knowledge deficit: Closing the shocking education gap for American children*. Boston: Houghton Mifflin.

Hirsch, E. D., Jr., & Pondiscio, R. (2010, July/August). There's no such thing as a reading test. *The American Prospect, 21*, A13–A15. Retrieved September 7, 2010, from http://www.prospect.org/cs/digital_edition_jul_aug2010.

Horn, E. (1926). *A basic writing vocabulary.* University of Iowa Monographs in Education, No. 4. Iowa City: University of Iowa Press.

Jarmulowicz, L., Hay, S., Taran, V., & Ethington, C. (2008). Fitting derivational morphophonology into a developmental model of reading. *Reading and Writing, 21,* 275–297.

Juel, C. (1991). Beginning reading. In R. Barr, M. Kamil, P. Mosenthal, & P. Pearson (Eds.), *Handbook of reading research* (Vol. 2, pp. 1–788). White Plains, NY: Longman.

Justice, L., McGinty, A., Cabell, S., Kilday, C., Knigton, K., & Huffman, G. (2010). Language and literacy curriculum supplement for preschoolers who are academically at risk: A feasibility study. *Language, Speech, and Hearing Services in Schools, 41,* 161–178.

Kintsch, W. (1998). *Comprehension: A paradigm for cognition.* Cambridge, MA: Cambridge University Press.

Masonheimer, P., Drum, P., & Ehri, L. (1984). Does environmental print identification lead children into word reading? *Journal of Reading Behavior, 16,* 257–271.

Nagy, W., & Herman, P. (1987). Breadth and depth of vocabulary knowledge: Implications for acquisition and instruction. In M. McKeown & M. Curtis (Eds.), *The nature of vocabulary acquisition* (pp. 1–35). Hillsdale, NJ: Erlbaum.

Nation, K., (2008). Learning to read words. *The Quarterly Journal of Experimental Psychology, 61,* 1121–1133.

Nation, K., Angell, P., & Castles, A. (2007). Orthographic learning via self-teaching in children learning to read English: Effects of exposure, durability, and context. *Journal of Experimental Child Psychology, 96,* 71–84.

Nation, K., & Cocksey, J. (2009). The relationship between knowing a word and reading it aloud in children's word reading development. *Journal of Experimental Child Psychology, 103,* 296–308.

National Center for Education Statistics. (2001). *International comparisons in fourth-grade reading literacy: Findings from the progress in international reading literacy study (PIRLS) of 2001.* Retrieved May 27, 2003, from http://nces.ed.gov.

National Institute of Child Health and Human Development (NICHD). (2000). *Report of the National Reading Panel. Teaching children to read: An evidence-based assessment of the scientific research literature on reading and its implications for reading instruction: Reports of the subgroups* (NIH Publication No. 00-4754). Washington, DC: U.S. Government Printing Office.

Oakhill, J., & Cain, K. (2007). Introduction to comprehension development. In K. Cain & J. Oakhill (Eds.), *Children's comprehension problems in oral and written language: A cognitive perspective* (pp. 1–40). New York: Guilford Press.

Pianta, R., Belsky, J., Houts, R., & Morrison, F. (2007). Teaching: Opportunities to learn in American classrooms. *Science, 315,* 1795–1796.

Pressley, M., Graham, S., & Harris, K. (2006). The state of educational intervention research as viewed through the lens of literacy intervention. *British Journal of Educational Psychology, 76,* 1–19.

Purves, A. (1992). Testing literature. In J. Langer (Ed.), *Literature instruction: A focus on student response* (pp. 1–34). Urbana, IL: National Council of Teachers of English.

Rasool, J., & Royer, J. (1986). Assessment of reading comprehension using the sentence verification technique: Evidence from narrative and descriptive texts. *Journal of Educational Research, 79,* 180–184.

Richgels, D., McGee, L., Lomax, R., & Sheard, C. (1987). Awareness of four text structures: Effects on recall of expository texts. *Reading Research Quarterly, 22,* 177–196.

Richman, W. A., & Columbo, J. (2007). Joint book reading in the second year and vocabulary outcomes. *Journal of Research in Childhood Education, 21,* 242–253.

Scarborough, H., & Dobrich, W. (1994). On the efficacy of reading to preschoolers. *Developmental Review, 14,* 245–302.

Shahar-Yames, D., & Share, D. (2008). Spelling as a self-teaching mechanism in orthographic learning. *Journal of Research in Reading, 31,* 22–39.

Share, D. (1995). Phonological recoding and self-teaching: *Sine qua non* of reading acquisition. *Cognition, 55,* 151–218.

Share, D. (1999). Phonological recoding and orthographic learning: A direct test of the self-teaching hypothesis. *Journal of Experimental Child Psychology, 72,* 95–129.

Share, D. (2004). Orthographic learning at a glance: On the time course and developmental onset of self-teaching. *Journal of Experimental Child Psychology, 87,* 267–298.

Share, D., & Stanovich, K. (1995). Cognitive processes in early reading development: Accommodating individual differences into a model of acquisition. *Issues in Education, 1,* 1–57.

Shatil, E., & Share, D. (2003). Cognitive antecedents of early reading ability: A test of the modularity hypothesis. *Journal of Experimental Child Psychology, 86,* 1–31.

Snow, C. (1999). Facilitating language development promotes literacy learning. In L. Eldering & P. Leseman (Eds.), *Early education and culture* (pp. 1–162). New York: Falmer Press.

Snow, C., & Goldfield, B. (1981). Building stories: The emergence of information structures from conversation.

In D. Tannen (Ed.), *Analyzing discourse: Text and talk.* Washington, DC: Georgetown University Press.

Spear-Swerling, L., & Sternberg, R. (1996). *Off track: When poor readers become "learning disabled."* Boulder, CO: Westview Press.

Stanovich, K. (1990). Concepts in developmental theories of reading skill: Cognitive resources, automaticity, and modularity. *Developmental Review, 10,* 1–29.

Stanovich, K. (1991). Word recognition: Changing perspectives. In R. Barr, M. Kamil, P. Mosenthal, & P. Pearson (Eds.), *Handbook of reading research, Volume II* (pp. 1–452). White Plains, NY: Longman.

Stanovich, K., & Siegel, L. (1994). The phenotypic performance profile of reading-disabled children: A regression-based test of the phonological-core variable-difference model. *Journal of Educational Psychology, 86,* 24–53.

Stevenson, J., & Fredman, G. (1990). The social environmental correlates of reading ability. *Journal of Child Psychology and Psychiatry, 31,* 681–698.

Torgesen, J., Wagner, R., & Rashotte, C. (1994). Longitudinal studies of phonological processing and reading. *Journal of Learning Disabilities, 27,* 276–286.

van Kleeck, A. (1995). Emphasizing form and meaning separately in prereading and early reading instruction. *Topics in Language Disorders, 16,* 27–49.

van Kleeck, A., & Schuele, C. (1987). Precursors to literacy: Normal development. *Topics in Language Disorders, 7,* 13–31.

Wells, G. (1985). Preschool literacy-related activities and success in school. In D. Olson, N. Torrance, & A. Hildyard (Eds.), *Literacy, language, and learning: The nature and consequences of reading and writing* (pp. 1–255). New York: Cambridge University Press.

Wells, G. (1986). *The meaning makers.* Portsmouth, NH: Heinemann.

Willingham, D. T. (2006, Spring). How knowledge helps: It speeds and strengthens reading comprehension, learning—and thinking. *American Educator, 30,* 1–12.

Chapter 3

Defining and Classifying Reading Disabilities

Hugh W. Catts, Alan G. Kamhi, and Suzanne M. Adlof

The development of reading is one of the major achievements of the early school years. For most children, learning to read is an enjoyable experience and one that comes without hardship. As noted in Chapter 2, some children enter school with a rich preschool history of literacy and in a few short months are well on their way to becoming skilled readers. Other children begin school with more limited literacy experiences, but with appropriate instruction, they go on to become competent readers as well. Some children, on the other hand, experience significant difficulty learning to read and struggle for years with written language. These children are the primary concern of this book. In this chapter, we begin by providing a historical perspective of reading disabilities that reflects our interest in the language basis of reading. After a brief summary of terminology, prevalence, and gender differences, we provide an in-depth discussion of the definitional and classification issues associated with reading disabilities.

HISTORICAL BASIS OF READING DISABILITIES

There is no such thing as an unbiased historical perspective. Historical reviews usually reflect the theoretical biases of the reviewer. One's biases influence not only the interpretation of the literature reviewed, but also what body of literature is reviewed. Some time ago, the second author (Kamhi, 1992) was asked to respond to Sylvia Richardson's historical perspective of dyslexia (Richardson, 1992). Richardson's medical orientation and background were clearly reflected in her review. She traced the roots of dyslexia to the medical literature of 100 years ago, wherein dyslexia was first viewed as a type of aphasia. She presented a brief history of aphasia, highlighting the work of Broca, Wernicke, and Jackson, and then discussed the early accounts of dyslexia by other medical professionals such as Hinshelwood and Orton. Whereas Richardson's medical background influenced her historical perspective of dyslexia, our language background influences our historical perspective. The story we will tell about reading disabilities traces how reading problems have come to be viewed as a language-based disorder. There are, of course, other stories one could tell about reading disabilities. One could, for example, tell the story of the emergence of the field of learning disabilities and its relationship to reading disabilities (Lerner, 1985; Torgesen, 1991) or focus on perceptual-motor and visual correlates of reading disabilities (Benton, 1991).

In some respects, the different stories one can tell about reading disabilities should begin and end at the same place. It is hard to begin a story of reading disabilities without mention of Morgan and Hinshelwood, and it is hard to end the story without acknowledging the critical role of language factors in the disability. With these points in mind, here is our story of reading disabilities.

Early Reports

Reports of children with reading disabilities first began to appear in the late 1890s (Morgan, 1896). The identification of reading disabilities at that time was due, in part, to more widespread mandatory school attendance. As more and more children attended school on a regular basis, children who were experiencing difficulties learning to read despite adequate instruction became more apparent to educators. Some of these children were subsequently referred to physicians and other related professionals. However, most physicians did not recognize the significance of these learning difficulties until the late 1800s. Children with reading problems were generally thought to be poorly motivated or of low intelligence. Toward the end of the nineteenth century, reports began to be published that described patients who had lost spoken and/or written language abilities as the result of brain injury or illness (e.g., Berlin, 1887; Brodbent, 1872; Kussmaul, 1887). These accounts demonstrated that individuals could lose language abilities but retain other aspects of intelligence. Physicians and other professionals soon began to recognize the similarities between acquired reading disabilities and the reading problems experienced by some children. This recognition led to the publication of scholarly reports of reading disabilities in children.

W. Pringle Morgan, an English physician, is generally given credit for the first published paper on developmental reading disabilities (Morgan, 1896). In this paper, he described the case of a bright 14-year-old boy who was "quick at games," but had great difficulty learning to read. Morgan reported that despite 7 years of laborious and persistent instruction in reading, the boy could only read or spell the simplest of words. He described the boy's condition as *congenital word blindness*, a term coined by Hinshelwood (1895), a Scottish ophthalmologist, who had used *word blindness* to refer to the problems experienced by a schoolteacher with an acquired reading problem. Morgan found many similarities between the boy and the schoolteacher, but the boy's problems were not the result of an injury or illness. Because there was no obvious cause for the boy's reading problem, Morgan concluded that this problem must be congenital in nature.

Soon after Morgan's report, Hinshelwood (1900, 1917) published several accounts of congenital word blindness. He argued that the condition was the result of neurological deficits that impaired children's ability to remember visually presented letters and words. He also noted that the disorder ran in families and was probably hereditary. Hinshelwood also had some specific views on treatment and prognosis of the disorder. He believed strongly that all children with the disorder could learn to read and advocated for daily one-on-one instruction using the "old-fashioned" phonics method of teaching reading, rather than the look-and-say method that was commonly used at the time. He also recommended the use of multisensory input.

Hinshelwood's views about treatment are remarkably consistent with current views on this subject (see Chapter 5).

Orton

One of the earliest accounts of developmental reading disabilities in the United States was by Samuel T. Orton. As the director of a mental health clinic in Iowa, Orton encountered a number of children whose primary problem was difficulty in learning to read. In 1925, he discussed these children's difficulties in a paper entitled "Word Blindness in School Children" (Orton, 1925). Following the publication of this paper, Orton began a comprehensive research program that included an investigation of speech and reading problems in children. In 2 years, he and his research team, employing a mobile clinic, examined more than 1,000 children across the state (J. Orton et al., 1975). This research and his subsequent work in private practice in New York laid the foundation for his seminal book, *Reading, Writing, and Speech Problems in Children* (Orton, 1937).

As a result of his extensive research, Orton recognized that reading disabilities were more common than generally thought. He believed that the prevalence rate was much higher than the 1/1000 estimate that had been reported by Hinshelwood and others. Orton's higher prevalence figure was due primarily to the way he defined the disability. Whereas others only recognized the most severe cases as instances of reading disabilities, he believed that reading disabilities were distributed along a graded continuum with no clear demarcation between the most and least severe cases. He maintained, as many do today, that the problems experienced by children with the most severe cases of reading disabilities are not qualitatively different from those found in the less severe cases.

Orton also attempted to explain the cause of reading disabilities. Rather than propose deficits in a specific area of the brain as Hinshelwood did, Orton argued that reading problems resulted from a failure to develop cerebral dominance for language in the left hemisphere. His theory is perhaps best known for its explanation of the reversal (e.g., *b/d*) and sequencing errors (e.g., *was/saw*) that had been observed in dyslexic individuals. Orton thought that insufficient cerebral dominance caused occasional confusion between the mirror images of words that he mistakenly believed were represented in each hemisphere. This confusion led to reversal or sequencing errors. Although this account of reading errors is clearly inaccurate, many of Orton's other insights into the nature of reading disabilities are quite consistent with what we know today. In his 1937 book, he offered a classification system that included different types of spoken and written language disorders. He viewed reading disabilities as part of a larger set of developmental language disorders. He noted that many children who had problems in reading also had difficulties in spoken language or had a history of spoken language difficulties. Orton's language-based view of reading disabilities was clearly way ahead of its time. In fact, it was so ahead of its time that it was ignored for decades.

Orton also developed a program of intervention for reading disabilities. Like Hinshelwood, he recommended a multisensory approach that involved explicit instruction in phoneme–grapheme associations. Children were first taught to link letters with their sounds and names. Once phoneme–grapheme correspondence was firmly established, children were taught to blend letter sounds together to form words. Orton believed all children with reading disabilities could learn to read using this approach. He later collaborated with Anna Gillingham to develop the Orton–Gillingham Approach. Currently, this program and ones like it are among the most popular methods of instruction for children with severe reading disabilities.

The important insights Orton and Hinshelwood made about the nature of reading disabilities had little impact on the prevailing views of reading disabilities held by most educators and other professionals of their time. In Orton's case, this was probably because he was more known for his theory of cerebral dominance than for his language-based view of reading development. In any event, it would take about 50 years for researchers to begin to accumulate convincing evidence in support of a language-based view of reading. During these years, reading disabilities were attributed to an assortment of intellectual, perceptual, environmental, attitudinal, and/or educational problems (Critchley, 1970; Torgesen, 1991).

Johnson and Myklebust

Doris Johnson and Helmer Myklebust's contributions are of particular relevance to a language-based perspective of reading disabilities. Johnson and Myklebust were affiliated with the Institute for Language Disorders at Northwestern University. This institute was one of the first in which language specialists worked in conjunction with other professionals in the treatment of children with reading disabilities. Johnson and Myklebust's work at the Institute led to a seminal book on learning disabilities (Johnson & Myklebust, 1967). In this book, they offered a description and classification system for children with spoken and written language disorders. Among the problems described was auditory dyslexia, the term they used for a prominent form of reading disabilities. They reported that in addition to reading problems, children with auditory dyslexia had problems perceiving the similarities in the initial and final sounds in words. These children also had problems breaking words into syllables and phonemes, retrieving the names of letters and words, remembering verbal information, and pronouncing phonologically complex words in speech (e.g., pronouncing *enemy* as *emeny*). In providing this description of children with reading disabilities, Johnson and Myklebust were the first to clearly delineate the extent of the phonological processing deficits experienced by these children. As will be discussed throughout this book, phonological processing deficits are now known to be strongly associated with developmental reading disabilities.

The Modern Era

The work of Orton and Johnson and Myklebust laid the foundation for the now widely accepted view that reading problems generally reflect limitations in language, rather than limitations in general cognitive abilities or visual perception. This view began to be espoused in the early 1970s by Mattingly (1972), Lerner (1972), and Shankweiler and Liberman (1972). Evidence in support of language-based theories of reading accumulated rapidly during the 1970s and 1980s. Lower-level phonological correlates of reading, as well as higher-level syntactic and semantic correlates, were studied in this work (Bradley & Bryant, 1983; Perfetti, 1985; Vellutino, 1979; Wagner & Torgesen, 1987). This research is discussed in several chapters of this book.

The change from visually based theories of reading disabilities to language-based theories opened the door for language specialists to become involved in reading problems. Speech-language pathologists with their knowledge and training in language and language disorders have become increasingly involved in the identification, assessment, and treatment of individuals with reading disabilities. The contribution a language specialist can make in serving individuals with reading disabilities is becoming recognized by teachers, reading specialists, special educators, and psychologists. This recognition has led to an increase in the collaborative efforts between these professionals and language specialists.

Collaborative efforts have been encouraged and supported by writings and presentations from well-known language specialists. It is now more than 35 years since Norma Rees (1974) and Joel Stark (1975) began writing about the role of the speech-language pathologist in reading disabilities. It was another 10 years before Wallach and Butler (1984) published their seminal book on language and learning disabilities. This book represented the first comprehensive attempt to integrate research on language development and disorders with research on learning and reading disabilities. Like the present book, contributors were language specialists. This book provided an important link for professionals involved in serving children and adolescents with language-based learning disorders. One of our goals in writing our first book on reading disabilities (Kamhi & Catts, 1989) was to make this link even stronger by focusing more closely on the language basis of reading disabilities. This role was highlighted as well in Catts and Kamhi (1999, 2005) and in this revision.

TERMINOLOGY

Many different terms have been used to refer to individuals with reading disabilities (RD). As noted earlier, *congenital word blindness* was the first term to be employed. Other terms include *dyslexia, developmental dyslexia, specific reading disability*, and *reading disability*. The term *disability* is often used interchangeably with *disorder, impairment,* and, in some cases, *retardation.* More general terms such as *learning disability* and *poor reader* are also used to characterize individuals with reading problems. The term *language-learning disability* has also been used by some to describe school-age children who have spoken and written language deficits (Gerber, 1993; Wallach & Butler, 1994). Occasionally, the word *developmental* is added to clarify that the disability is not an acquired problem, but rather one of initial learning.

Of all the terms used to refer to individuals with RD, the term *dyslexia* has been the most confusing and the most misunderstood. Etymologically, dyslexia means difficulty with words. Dyslexia was first used in the late nineteenth century to label reading problems associated with brain injury or illness (Berlin, 1887). The term was later applied to developmental reading disabilities where there was no evidence of brain damage. Dyslexia, however, eventually became a popular label for children who made reversal *(b/d)* or sequencing errors *(was/saw)*. Most people outside the field of reading disabilities continue to think of dyslexia as reading or writing backwards. Although children with dyslexia do make reversal and sequencing errors, these errors represent only a small proportion of the total errors they make. More important, normally developing readers as well as nondyslexic poor readers also make these kinds of errors, so the occurrence of these errors has little diagnostic value (see Chapter 4 for more discussion of this issue). Despite the confusion surrounding the term *dyslexia*, it remains a popular label among researchers and clinicians who deal specifically with reading disabilities.

The standard educational term used to categorize children with RD in the United States is *learning disabled.* Although the majority of children labeled learning disabled have received this designation on the basis of their poor reading skills, the term is also used for other learning problems (e.g., math difficulties). Because of the heterogeneity of children with learning disabilities, most investigators and clinicians agree that the term learning disability is too broad to be used to refer to reading disabilities. The term *language-learning disability* suffers from some of the same problems as the term *learning disability.* Use of this term is primarily restricted to speech-language pathologists, though some reading theorists have also embraced the term (Ceci & Baker, 1978). In the past, the term has not been well defined and has included a variety of problems beyond reading disabilities. Despite these problems, by focusing attention on the language basis of many learning problems, the term *language-learning disability* has played an important role in getting language specialists involved in serving children with reading and other learning disabilities.

Throughout this book, we primarily use the term *reading disabilities*. This term is a common term used by researchers and practitioners to refer to a heterogeneous group of children who have difficulty learning to read. We also use the terms *dyslexia* and *specific comprehension deficit* to refer to more specific types of reading problems. These latter terms are defined later in this chapter.

PREVALENCE

What is the prevalence of reading disabilities? For many years, it was thought that this question could be answered in a rather straightforward manner. Reading abilities were assumed to be distributed bimodally, with normal readers constituting one group and children with RD the other. The reading achievement scores of the normal readers were thought to be distributed along a normal bell-shaped curve, whereas children with RD were thought to have reading scores that clustered together and formed a "hump" at the low end of the normal distribution. Children with RD could, therefore, be clearly distinguished from typically developing children, and the prevalence of reading disabilities could be easily determined.

Early support for the existence of a hump in the reading achievement distribution was provided by Rutter and Yule (1975) and Yule, Rutter, Berger, and Thompson (1974). In the 1960s, Rutter, Yule, and their colleagues conducted a large epidemiological study on the Isle of Wight in England. The study included the entire population of about 3,500 9- to 11-year-old children living on the island. One of the many goals of this investigation was to determine the prevalence of reading disabilities. A reading disability was operationally defined as performance on a reading achievement test (word recognition or reading comprehension) that was at least two standard deviations below normal. If scores were normally distributed without a hump in the low end, it would be predicted that 2.3 percent of the population of children should perform two standard deviations below the mean. Depending on how reading was measured (i.e., word recognition or reading comprehension) and the age of the children, the results indicated that between 3.1 and 4.4 percent of the subjects obtained reading scores more than two standard deviations below the mean. Yule and colleagues (1974) also reported that in a comparative group of children from London, the prevalence rate was 6.3 to 9.3 percent. The researchers concluded that there was evidence of a hump at the low end of the reading achievement distribution and that this indicated the distinct nature of reading disabilities.

A number of investigators questioned the validity of the prevalence data from the Isle of Wight study (Rodgers, 1983; Shaywitz, Escobar, Shaywitz, Fletcher, & Makuch, 1992; van der Wissel & Zegers, 1985). The primary criticism concerned the possible ceiling effects of the Neale Analysis of Reading Ability, the instrument used to measure reading achievement in this study. This reading test had an upper age limit of 12 years, which was exceeded by many of the subjects in the study. Van der Wissel and Zegers (1995) argued that such a ceiling effect could result in an apparent hump in the low end of the reading distribution. To test this, they ran a computer simulation in which a ceiling effect was artificially imposed. This resulted in a hump at the low end of the distribution much like that reported by Rutter and Yule (1975) and Yule and colleagues (1974).

Shaywitz and coworkers (1992) attempted to replicate the results from the Isle of Wight study in their data from the Connecticut Longitudinal Study, an investigation involving approximately 400 Connecticut children who entered kindergarten in 1983. Their results indicated that regardless of the way in which reading disabilities were defined or the grade at which they were examined (first to sixth grade), there was no evidence of an excess of poor readers at the low end of the distribution. In other words, children with RD did not represent a distinct group. They were simply at the low end of the reading ability continuum (also see Rodgers, 1983; Share, McGee, McKenzie, Williams, & Silva, 1987).

These results have important implications for the notion of the prevalence of reading disabilities. These results indicate that the distinction between normal children and those with RD is arbitrary. It depends on the specific cutoff score selected by the researcher or clinician. For example, if one standard deviation below the mean is selected as the sole criterion for defining a reading disability, then the prevalence of reading disabilities would be about 16 percent. If two standard deviations is selected as the dividing line, then the prevalence of reading disabilities would decrease to 2.3 percent.

Just because the notion of prevalence is a relative one, it does not mean that reading disabilities are not real phenomenon. This point has been made very clearly by Ellis (1985), who noted that a reading disability is like obesity. He stated that for any given age and height there is an uninterrupted continuum from painfully thin to inordinately fat. Where on the continuum obesity falls is entirely arbitrary, but the arbitrariness of the distinction between overweight and obese does not mean that obesity is not a real and worrysome condition, nor does it prevent research into the causes and cures of obesity from being both valuable and necessary (Ellis, 1985). Although the prevalence of reading disabilities, like obesity, depends on where one draws the line, reading disabilities are as real as obesity.

Gender Differences

It has been commonly assumed that the prevalence of reading disabilities is higher in boys than in girls (Critchley, 1970; Golderberg & Schiffman, 1972; Thomson, 1984). Most early studies of reading disabilities supported this assumption. For example, the boy-to-girl ratio of reading disabilities reported by Naidoo (1972) was 5:1 and by Rutter and colleagues (Rutter, Tizard, & Whitmore, 1970) was 3.3:1. Subsequent studies, however, failed to find such large gender differences in the prevalence of reading disabilities (e.g., Prior, Sanson, Smart, & Oberklaid, 1995; Shaywitz, Shaywitz, Fletcher, & Escobar, 1990). Shaywitz and colleagues (1990) attributed the conflicting results in prevalence figures to whether the sample selected for study was identified by schools/clinics or by research. School and clinic samples typically showed a higher prevalence of boys with reading disabilities. Research-identified samples, they argued, were more likely to show no gender bias because objective criteria based on reading performance were used to identify the children with RD. They hypothesized that the reason for the large gender bias in schools or clinics was that factors other than reading performance were often used for diagnostic or classification purposes. For example, children's attention, level of activity, or classroom behavior could influence identification. Shaywitz and colleagues noted that boys are more active, more inattentive, and more disruptive than girls. Research has also shown that boys have a higher rate of clinically significant hyperactivity than girls (Willcutt & Pennington, 2000). Poor readers with behavior and attention problems are more likely to be referred for an evaluation and subsequently identified as reading or learning disabled than poor readers without behavior and attention problems.

Shaywitz and colleagues (1990) tested this explanation in two samples of poor readers from the Connecticut Longitudinal Study. One sample included all children in the study whose reading achievement score was 1.5 standard deviations or more below their IQ (research-identified sample). The other sample consisted of all children who were classified by the school district as reading/learning disabled and who were receiving special services for their reading problems (school-identified sample). Consistent with their predictions, the researchers found a 4:1 ratio in favor of boys in the school-identified sample compared with a 1.3:1 ratio in a re-search-identified sample. These results suggested that a selection bias might have accounted for the earlier findings of more boys than girls with reading disabilities.

Until recently, most studies had employed samples of children with RD who have been identified by schools or clinics. More recent studies relying on large, population-based samples have usually found gender differences in prevalence of dyslexia in boys versus girls, with boys slightly more likely to be identified than girls (Katusic, Colligan, Barbaresi, Shaid, & Jacobsen, 2001; Rutter et al., 2004; but see Siegel & Smythe, 2005). However, these differences are typi-cally small and can sometimes be explained by statistical properties of the tests used to identify reading difficulties (Share & Silva, 2003; Siegel & Smythe, 2005). Thus, converging evidence suggests that if a low score on a reading achievement test is used as the primary criterion to iden-tify a reading disability, then one should expect to find nearly as many girls with reading disabil-ities as boys.

DEFINING READING DISABILITY

It should be clear after the discussions of prevalence and gender that the way children with RD are defined has significant theoretical implications. Indeed, the validity of research on reading disabilities depends in large part on the operational definitions used to select participants for study. At least some of the inconsistencies in the literature can be attributed to the lack of uniformity in the criteria used to identify students with RD. As noted in the previous section, the reliance on school or clinic designations of reading/learning disabilities has led to the inclusion of children with behavior and attention problems in studies of children with RD. Research that has used such heterogeneous samples of poor readers has produced a host of questionable associations between reading disabilities and behavioral, cognitive, and environmental variables.

Definitions also affect the identification, assessment, and treatment of children with RD. Definitions are used to determine who is eligible for remedial services. Definitions of reading/learning disabilities vary from state to state and from school district to school district. This variability significantly influences whether a given child will receive remedial services. A particular child may qualify for special services in one state or school district, but not another. Definitions can also give direction for intervention. Specifying the nature of the problems associated with reading disabilities in a definition can lead professionals to areas of difficulty that should be considered in planning intervention. Clearly, definitions are not simply trivial matters for scholars to debate.

Defining reading disabilities has not proven to be an easy task, in part because several different disciplines are interested in reading disabilities. Reading problems have been the concern of special educators, reading specialists, physicians, optometrists, psychologists, and speech-language pathologists. These individuals have different orientations and theoretical biases that influence the way they define reading disabilities. As a result, different professionals may focus on different aspects of the problem. Despite these different orientations and theoretical biases, most professionals agree that the term *reading disability* should not be used to refer to all children who have problems in learning to read. For example, children who have had inadequate instruction are not considered reading disabled. In addition, children with severe visual impairment or mental retardation are seldom classified as reading disabled. Most professionals also agree that a group of children exists who have reading problems despite normal or above-average levels of intelligence. The terms *specific reading disability* and *dyslexia* have typically been used to characterize this group of children. In the sections that follow, we begin by considering the exclusionary criteria that have traditionally been used to define reading disabilities. The remaining sections consider the advantages of using inclusionary criteria to define reading disabilities and our attempt to differentiate between children with specific reading disabilities and those with more general language-learning problems. In these sections, we will use the term *dyslexia* to refer to children with a specific reading disability because much of the literature uses this label. This term also seems to be more appropriate for labeling a condition whose symptoms are seldom limited to reading problems. In the sections that follow, we will first address the definition of dyslexia. This will be followed by a consideration of other language-based reading problems.

Exclusionary Factors

Traditionally, definitions of dyslexia have focused heavily on exclusionary factors. For the most part, definitions have provided as much, if not more, information about what dyslexia is not than what it is. Consider, for example, an influential definition of dyslexia proposed by the World Federation of Neurology (Critchley, 1970):

> Dyslexia is a disorder manifested by difficulty learning to read despite conventional instruction, adequate intelligence, and socio-culture opportunity. It is dependent upon cognitive disabilities which are frequently of constitutional origin. (p. 11)

The World Federation definition excludes a number of causal factors from dyslexia. Although stated in a positive manner, inadequate instruction, lack of opportunity, and low intelligence are ruled out as potential causes of the reading problems found in dyslexia. Other definitions exclude sensory deficits such as impairments in hearing or visual acuity (Lyon, 1995; Miles, 1983). Emotional disturbances and brain damage are also sometimes ruled out in definitions of dyslexia (Heaton & Winterson, 1996).

SENSORY/EMOTIONAL/NEUROLOGICAL FACTORS.   Generally, hearing and visual acuity are assessed. For children to be labeled dyslexic, they must have sensory abilities within normal limits (this includes corrected vision). In some cases, children with sensory deficits can be diagnosed as dyslexic, provided their reading problems go beyond those predicted on the basis of the hearing or visual handicap. Identification of dyslexia also typically requires that emotional and behavioral problems be ruled out as the cause of the reading difficulties. Poor readers, for example, with autism, childhood schizophrenia, or significant behavioral problems, are not considered dyslexic. Finally, neurological impairments caused by injury or illness are excluded from the diagnosis of dyslexia.

INSTRUCTIONAL FACTORS.   To be identified as dyslexic, poor readers also must have had adequate literacy experience. Unlike the acquisition of spoken language, the development of reading requires explicit instruction. Therefore, an individual who has not had adequate opportunity and instruction should clearly not be labeled reading disabled. Operationalizing this exclusionary criterion, however, can be difficult. Practitioners and researchers have most often relied on enrollment in an age-appropriate grade as evidence of adequate literacy experience and instruction. However, such a criterion is often not sufficient. In many inner-city schools, a large percentage of children in age-appropriate classrooms are reading well below national norms. Although these children clearly have reading problems, we do not consider them to be reading disabled.

Research suggests that the use of enrollment in an age-appropriate grade as an exclusionary criterion for reading disability may not even be sufficient for children attending middle-class schools. In a longitudinal study, Vellutino and colleagues (Vellutino, Scanlon, Sipay et al., 1996) sampled children from middle- and upper-middle-class school districts in Albany, New York. From this sample, a group of poor readers was identified on the basis of first-grade reading achievement. The poor readers were subsequently provided with 15 weeks of daily one-on-one tutoring (30 minutes per session). Following this intervention phase, the poor readers were divided into those who were hard to remediate and those who were easy to remediate. Vellutino and coworkers suggested that the former had a true reading disability whereas the latter simply lacked adequate literacy experience. The researchers further found that the the children with true RD (and not the readily remediated children) differed significantly from normal readers in cognitive abilities closely linked with reading development (namely, phonological processing). Vellutino and colleagues suggested that the diagnosis of dyslexia might be reserved for those children with phonological processing deficits who do not respond to short-term intervention efforts.

The role of instruction in defining reading disabilities has become especially prominent as the result of provisions within the reauthorization of the Individuals with Disabilities Education Improvement Act (IDEA 2004; PL 108-446). This act allows for the identification of children with RD based on their failure to respond to scientifically based instruction. As a result, a response to intervention (RTI) framework is now being employed in many schools to identify children with RD. This framework relies on high-quality reading instruction in general education and universal screening to identify children at risk for reading failure. At-risk children are then provided with supplemental small-group or individual instruction. Only after these adaptations have failed do children become eligible for learning disability classification and special education placement. Further monitoring is also recommended to evaluate the appropriateness of this placement.

The RTI approach appears on the surface to better address lack of appropriate instruction as a cause of a reading disability. This approach, however, is not without its challenges (Mastropieri & Scruggs, 2005; Scruggs & Mastropieri, 2002). It is unclear at the present time whether the RTI approach can be applied across the age spectrum and can effectively address the multifaceted nature of reading disabilities. For example, because each phase of the approach requires multiple, short, and reliable assessments of a target ability, it may work well for less severe reading disabilities or those that involve difficulties with word recognition but not other areas such as reading comprehension or spelling. Multiple baseline assessments are available to evaluate such behaviors as accuracy and fluency of word recognition (e.g., Good, Simmons, & Smith, 1998). However, the measurement of reading comprehension does not readily lend itself to this type of assessment, particularly in older poor readers. There is also the issue of availability of instructional adaptations. Although some reading-instruction adaptations for the general education classroom have been developed, much work is still needed to identify and validate interventions that target decoding, fluency, and comprehension difficulties. These and other issues will need to be resolved before problems in instruction can be ruled out in defining and identifying reading disabilities.

INTELLIGENCE.   Among exclusionary factors, intelligence has been given the most attention by practitioners. To be diagnosed as dyslexic, an individual traditionally had to demonstrate a significant difference between measured intelligence (IQ) and reading achievement. This was referred to as an IQ-achievement discrepancy. Generally, this meant that to be diagnosed as dyslexic, the individual must show poor reading achievement but normal or above normal intelligence. Poor readers with low IQs and children who did not meet IQ-achievement discrepancy criteria were variously labeled backward readers (Jorm, Share, Maclean, & Matthews, 1986; Rutter & Yule, 1975), low achievers (Fletcher et al., 1994), or garden-variety poor readers

(Gough & Tunmer, 1986; Stanovich, 1991). A common justification for the use of IQ-achievement discrepancy was that it differentiated children who had specific reading problems (i.e., dyslexics) from those who had more general learning difficulties.

Serious concerns have been raised about the use of IQ in definitions of dyslexia (Fletcher, Francis, Rourke, Shaywitz, & Shaywitz, 1992; Siegel, 1989; Stanovich, 1991, 1997; Stuebing et al., 2002). There are, for example, numerous methodological problems associated with selecting intelligence and achievement tests and comparing test performances. The tests used to measure IQ and achievement have been shown to significantly influence the magnitude of the discrepancy obtained. For example, Rudel (1985) found that a sample of 50 children referred for reading disabilities had a mean discrepancy of 23.9 months between mental age and reading age using the Gray Oral Reading Test, a timed test. In contrast, these same children had a mean discrepancy of only 8.6 months using the Wide Range Achievement Test, which tests the reading of single words and is untimed. Another measurement issue concerns potential problems involving statistical regression. Because of regression toward the mean, the calculation of IQ-achievement discrepancy can result in the overidentification of dyslexia in students with high IQs and underidentification of those with low IQs (cf. Fletcher, 1992; Francis, Espy, Rourke, & Fletcher, 1987; Francis et al., 2005).

Researchers have also shown that for some children, it can take several years of reading difficulty before the gap between a child's IQ and reading achievement scores grows large enough to meet discrepancy-based criteria. This problem has led some to refer to IQ-discrepancy approaches reading disabilities as "wait to fail" methods (Fletcher, Coulter, Reschly, & Vaughn, 2004; Fletcher et al., 1998; Lyon et al., 2001).

Another problem with the use of IQ in defining dyslexia is that IQ tests do not directly measure potential for reading achievement. Rather, they assess current cognitive abilities, some of which overlap with abilities important in reading. This is particularly true for verbal IQ tests that assess vocabulary and comprehension. Because of the overlap in the abilities measured by these tests and reading tests, many poor readers will have lower IQ levels than good readers. In addition, poor readers generally read less than good readers, and thus, they may acquire less of the knowledge measured by verbal IQ tests. As a result, verbal IQ tests may underestimate the intelligence of poor readers and make it harder for them to show an IQ-achievement discrepancy (Siegel, 1989).

The problem with verbal IQ tests has led some investigators to argue for the use of nonverbal IQ measures to identify children with dyslexia. However, performance on nonverbal IQ tests has little direct relationship to reading achievement (Stanovich, 1991). Knowing how well a child matches block designs or perceives the missing parts of pictures tells us little about how he or she should read words. Such an argument calls into question the practice of some language specialists who insist on using nonverbal IQ measures to estimate potential (or IQ-achievement discrepancy) of children with language-based reading disabilities.

Research has also challenged some of the basic assumptions associated with the use of IQ in defining dyslexia. Inherent to this approach is the belief that dyslexics have different profiles in reading and reading-related abilities than do poor readers with low IQs (Siegel, 1989; Stanovich, 1991, 1997). Contrary to this assumption, research has shown that dyslexics and low achievers typically have similar problems in learning to read (Fletcher et al., 1994; Flowers, Meyer, Lovato, Wood, & Felton, 2001; Francis, Fletcher, Shaywitz, Shaywitz, & Rourke, 1996; Share, 1996; Siegel, 1992). Both groups of children have difficulty learning to use the phonological route to decode words. Dyslexics and low achievers have also been shown to exhibit similar cognitive deficits, particularly in phonological processing (Das,

Mensink, & Mishra, 1990; Das, Mishra, & Kirby, 1994; Hoskins & Swanson, 2000; Hurford, Schauf, Bunce, Blaich, & Moore, 1994; Naglieri & Reardon, 1993; O'Malley, Francis, Foorman, Fletcher, & Swank, 2002; Stuebing et al., 2002; but see Eden, Stein, Wood, & Wood, 1995; Wolf & Obregon, 1989). There is also limited evidence of any distinct qualitative differences between dyslexics and low achievers in terms of heritability of reading problems and the neurological basis of these problems (Olson, Rack, Conners, DeFries, & Fulker, 1991; Pennington, Gilger, Olson, & DeFries, 1992; Steveson, Graham, Fredman, & McLoughlin, 1987; but see Knopik et al., 2002; Olson, Datta, Gayan, & DeFries, 1999; Wadsworth, Olson, Pennington, & DeFries, 2000).

A primary justification for the use of IQ in defining dyslexia has been its presumed prognostic value. It has been assumed that dyslexics, with their higher IQs, respond better to intervention than low achievers. Because of this assumption, dyslexics have often received special education, whereas low achievers typically have not. This practice, unfortunately, has gone unchecked for years. Recently, however, researchers have begun to investigate intervention outcome in relation to IQ. In general, studies have failed to find an association between improvement in reading (primarily word recognition) and IQ (Hatcher & Hulme, 1999; Share et al., 1987; Stage, Abbott, Jenkins, & Berninger, 2003; Torgesen, Wagner, & Rashotte, 1997; Vellutino, Scanlon, & Lyon, 2000). Torgesen et al. (1997), for example, found that IQ was not a good predictor of outcome in children at risk for reading disabilities who were participating in a two-and-one-half-year intervention study.

It should be clear that there are a number of serious problems associated with the use of IQ in defining dyslexia. These problems have led some leading scholars to argue that IQ should not be used in defining or diagnosing dyslexia (Aaron, 1991; Lyon et al., 2001; Siegel, 1989; Stanovich, 1991, 1997, 2005). The reauthorization of IDEA in 2004 also declared that states are no longer required to use IQ assessments in identifying children with learning disabilities. The abandonment of IQ as an exclusionary factor, however, has been slow to gain acceptance, which is really not surprising, given that normal or above-normal intelligence has always been a defining characteristic of dyslexia. In addition, IQ tests often have played a fundamental role in determining eligibility and placement for special education services. Because IQ is so entrenched in our definitions and practice involving reading disabilities, it is probably unrealistic to expect that researchers and practitioners would readily abandon its use. One way, however, to move beyond definitions based heavily on IQ-achievement discrepancy is to turn to definitions that specify inclusionary factors. By focusing on what dyslexia *is* and the inclusionary characteristics that define the disorder, we should be able to reduce the reliance on exclusionary factors such as IQ when identifying children with RD.

IDA Definition

Recent definitions of dyslexia have provided more information concerning inclusionary factors. These definitions specify the nature of the reading problems and the cognitive deficits associated with these problems. Prominent among more inclusionary definitions of dyslexia is the most recent definition proposed by the International Dyslexia Association (IDA; formerly the Orton Dyslexia Society), a professional organization devoted to the study of dyslexia. IDA defines dyslexia in the following manner:

> Dyslexia is a specific learning disability that is neurobiological in origin. It is characterized by difficulties with accurate and/or fluent word recognition and by poor spelling and decoding abilities. These difficulties typically result from a deficit in the phonological component of

language that is often unexpected in relation to other cognitive abilities and the provision of effective classroom instruction. Secondary consequences may include problems in reading comprehension and reduced reading experience that can impede growth of vocabulary and background knowledge. (Lyon, Shaywitz, & Shaywitz, 2003)

This definition is a significant improvement over traditional definitions and has the potential to provide needed guidance for research and practice. In the sections that follow, we discuss the various components of the IDA definition and point out some of its strengths and weaknesses.

Dyslexia as a Specific Learning Disability

The IDA classifies dyslexia as a specific type of learning disability and distinguishes it from other types of learning disabilities (e.g., math, reading comprehension) on the basis of particular symptoms and causal factors. By referring to dyslexia as a specific learning disability, the IDA definition places dyslexia within the diagnostic category used most often in educational settings. Traditionally, the term *dyslexia* has been employed most often by medical-related professionals. It has seldom been used in the schools to label children with RD, especially, in the United States. IDA is clearly hoping that educators will consider using *dyslexia* to refer to children with learning disabilities who meet this definition. This could not only broaden the use of the term, but could also bring much-needed specificity to the LD classification system.

The statement concerning the neurobiological origin of dyslexia replaces reference to "constitutional origin" in many previous definitions and reflects the considerable research in recent years concerning differences in brain structure and function between typical readers and individuals with dyslexia. The recognition of the neurological basis of dyslexia is also in keeping with the belief that learning disabilities are also neurobiological in origin (see Chapter 4).

Problems in Word Recognition and Spelling

The IDA definition specifies that a prominent symptom of dyslexia is difficulties in word recognition. Historically, the term *dyslexia* has been most closely linked with difficulties learning to recognize printed words (Critchley, 1970; Miles, 1983). A very large body of research indicates that children with dyslexia have significant problems decoding printed words, which results in difficulties recognizing novel words and building a sight vocabulary (see Chapter 5). The IDA definition further acknowledges that problems in word recognition may involve difficulties in accuracy and/or fluency. The latter specification is important for several reasons. Research has shown that individuals with dyslexia can improve their word-reading accuracy, but generally continue to lack fluency (Shaywitz, 2003). Also, cross-linguistic research indicates that, in languages with more consistent sound–symbol correspondence than English, beginning readers with dyslexia are more likely to experience problems in fluency than accuracy (e.g., Wimmer, 1993).

The IDA definition also states that dyslexia is typically characterized by spelling problems. Spelling involves the encoding of phonological information and is a particular area of weakness for most individuals with dyslexia (Miles, 1983). Spelling problems are generally quite persistent, and even with intervention, may be present in adulthood (Clark & Uhry, 1995). Along with poor spelling, the definition includes poor decoding abilities. Reference to decoding deficits at this point seems unnecessary because decoding problems are generally subsumed under word recognition difficulties. The intent here, however, is to clearly highlight that individuals with dyslexia have significant problems in both phonological encoding (i.e., spelling) and decoding (i.e., reading).

eficits in Phonological Processing

ie IDA definition states that difficulties in word recognition and spelling typically are the result
a deficit in the phonological component of language. Research over the last 20 years clearly
demonstrates a strong causal connection between a phonological processing deficit and the reading problems found in dyslexia (Catts, 1989a; Stanovich, 1988; Wolf & Bowers, 1999). As such,
a phonological processing deficit is considered to lie at the core of dyslexia. It is this deficit that
is heritable (Olson & Byrne, 2005; Pennington & Lefly, 2001; Snowling, Gallagher, & Frith,
2003), not word recognition or spelling difficulties that are the most noticeable and educationally
relevant aspects of the disorder. Unlike reading and spelling difficulties that do not appear until
school age and may subside with intervention, problems in phonological processing appear early
and persist throughout the life span (Blalock, 1982; Felton, Naylor, & Wood, 1990; Pennington
& Lefly, 2001; Scarborough, 1990; Wilson & Lesaux, 2001).

As will be discussed in detail in Chapter 4, the phonological processing problems associated with dyslexia most often occur in four areas. These include phonological awareness, phonological memory, phonological retrieval, and phonological production. Although the exact
manifestations of the problems in each of these areas will vary somewhat across individuals, and
within an individual throughout the life span, the phonological processing deficit is remarkably
consistent. This consistency is further evidence for viewing a deficit in the phonological component of language as the core of dyslexia.

The recognition that a phonological processing deficit is the core of dyslexia has both theoretical and educational implications. Theoretically, it means that individuals who have reading
problems that are caused by other cognitive or perceptual factors cannot be considered to be
dyslexic. For example, children with more general language impairments will not meet this definition of dyslexia. By general language problems, we mean severe and persistent problems in aspects of language that go beyond phonological processing (e.g., grammar and text processing).
Although children with dyslexia may often show early delays in language development, these delays subside before school entry (Scarborough, 1990, 1991) or remain mild in nature (Snowling et
al., 2003). If these deficits were persistent and severe, they would represent an alternative or additional causal factor and thus violate the primary inclusionary characteristics of dyslexia.

A phonologically based definition of dyslexia will also exclude visual problems as the
cause of dyslexia. As discussed in Chapter 4, some researchers have suggested that visual
deficits also can cause word-reading difficulties, although the confirmatory evidence is still in-
conclusive at this point. However, if visual problems do turn out to be the primary cause of word-
reading/spelling difficulties in some poor readers, these children would be considered to have a
"visual-based reading disability," rather than dyslexia. Conversely, research may show that visual
deficits co-occur with a phonological processing deficit and reading problems, but are not
causally related to them. As such, visual deficits could be considered correlated problems and
possibly symptoms of dyslexia. Others have suggested a similar status for factors such as
left–right confusion (Miles, 1983) or motor and balance problems (Nicolson & Fawcett, 1995).
As more converging evidence becomes available on these and other factors, they may also become part of the definition of dyslexia.

The recognition that a phonological processing deficit is the core of dyslexia has an important educational implication. This view allows for much earlier identification of children with
dyslexia. When a word-reading problem is the primary criteria for identifying dyslexia, children
may not be identified until they are in the second or third grade and are experiencing significant
difficulties learning to read. Such a "wait to fail" approach can have many negative consequences

(Spear-Swerling & Sternberg, 1996). By focusing on phonological processing abilities, it is possible to identify children who are dyslexic and at high risk for reading failure before they begin reading instruction (Catts, Fey, Zhang, & Tomblin, 2001; Pennington & Lefly, 2001).

Unexpected Underachievement

Like many previous definitions, the definition proposed by IDA also includes exclusionary factors. Specifically, it rules out ineffective classroom instruction as a cause of dyslexia. As discussed earlier in the chapter, operationalizing this exclusionary factor has been difficult. However, more recent approaches such as RTI may better ensure that instructional factors have been controlled in the identification of dyslexia. The IDA definition also states that the core deficit in phonological processing is often unexpected in relation to other cognitive abilities. The intent of such a statement is to rule out more general cognitive deficits as a cause of dyslexia. Although we are generally in agreement with this intent, we believe this portion of the definition is problematic. The primary problem is that "other cognitive abilities" are not specified. No guidance is given about the specific cognitive abilities that should serve as the benchmark and how these abilities might be measured. Our concern is that some may interpret "other cognitive abilities" as intelligence and continue to use IQ-based discrepancy approaches. We have already discussed the problems with using these approaches to define dyslexia. Clearly, the IDA definition should not be interpreted in that way. However, without more specificity, the interpretation of this part of the definition is unclear.

Our preference is to specify listening comprehension as the benchmark for comparison. Individuals would be identified as having dyslexia if they have word-reading problems and a phonological processing deficit that is unexpected in relation to listening comprehension abilities. Listening comprehension is an appropriate benchmark because of the critical role it plays in reading (Catts, Hogan, & Adlof, 2005; Gough & Tunmer, 1986). Also, because problems in listening comprehension typically stem from more general language deficits, this approach would be in keeping with the intent to rule out broader-based deficits as the cause of dyslexia. In the second half of this chapter, we introduce a classification system that relies on listening comprehension and word recognition abilities to subgroup poor readers.

Secondary Consequences

The final statement in the IDA definition addresses possible secondary or "downstream" consequences of dyslexia, the most important of which is a deficit in reading comprehension. It is well recognized that difficulties in word recognition can negatively impact reading comprehension by limiting access to lexical information about word and text meaning. Word recognition problems can also have an indirect influence on reading comprehension. Individuals who are poor readers generally read less than good readers. This lack of reading experience can impede growth in vocabulary and background knowledge, which in turn can negatively impact reading comprehension.

CLASSIFYING DYSLEXIA AND OTHER LANGUAGE-BASED READING DISABILITIES

So far in this chapter we have focused primarily on dyslexia. However, dyslexia is not the only type of language-based reading disability. Many poor readers have language impairments that go well beyond phonological processing and include difficulties in vocabulary, grammar, and text-level processing (Catts, Adlof, & Ellis Weismer, 2006; Catts, Fey, & Tomblin, 1997; Nation, Clarke, Marshall, & Durand, 2004). As noted previously, children exhibiting these deficits will not meet the criteria for dyslexia. Nevertheless, language problems play a causal role in their reading disabilities.

For most of these children, language problems are apparent early in life. Many will meet the criteria of a specific language impairment (Tomblin, Records, & Zhang, 1996). If these deficits persist into the school years, difficulties in written language are inevitable (Catts, Fey, Tomblin, & Zhang, 2002). Some of these children will have a phonological processing deficit in addition to their other language impairments and, like those with dyslexia, will experience significant deficits in word recognition (Catts, Adlof, Hogan, & Ellis Weismer, 2005; Catts, Hogan, & Adlof, 2005; Kamhi & Catts, 1986). Others, however, may not exhibit problems in phonological processing or word recognition in the early grades, but will have significant difficulties in reading comprehension later on. The latter children may not be identified as poor readers until later in elementary school when the curriculum places more emphasis on comprehension (Catts, Adlof, & Ellis Weismer, 2006; Catts, Hogan, & Fey, 2003; Leach, Scarborough, & Rescorla, 2003; Lipka, Lesaux, & Siegel, 2006).

In traditional reading diagnostic models, many poor readers with more general language-based reading problems would be diagnosed as low achievers or garden-variety poor readers. Because of their poor verbal skills, they would not typically demonstrate the IQ-achievement discrepancy necessary for diagnosis of dyslexia. As suggested earlier, a measure of listening comprehension is the better way to differentiate children with dyslexia from those with other language-based reading disabilities. However, this measure should not be viewed as a substitute for IQ in a discrepancy formula to determine eligibility for services. The determination of eligibility should be based on reading achievement independent of cognitive or language reference points. There is no clinical or theoretical basis for using discrepancy formulas at all. These formulas have resulted in the provision of special services for children with dyslexia who meet the discrepancy criteria while denying services to children with equally severe language-based reading disabilities who do not meet the discrepancy criteria. Such practice is unfortunate because research has shown that the latter children benefit well from intervention. These children have been shown to respond as well to intervention directed at word recognition as children who meet discrepancy criteria (Hatcher & Hulme, 1999; Vellutino et al., 2000). Other studies have shown that more general language problems in school-age children are also amenable to intervention (Dollaghan & Kaston, 1986; Ellis Weismer & Hesketh, 1993). Therefore, we recommend that although children with dyslexia should be distinguished from those with other language-based reading disabilities, both groups of children should be identified early and provided with appropriate intervention.

Subtypes Based on the Simple View of Reading

Our preferred system for subgrouping children with RD involves distinguishing between poor readers who have deficits in word recognition, those with deficits in listening comprehension, and those who have deficits in both word recognition and listening comprehension. This distinction is based on the Simple View of Reading, a view of reading proposed by Gough and his colleagues (Gough & Tunmer, 1986; Hoover & Gough, 1990). According to this view, reading comprehension can be thought of as the product of word recognition and listening comprehension. It is argued that if one wants to know how well individuals understand what they read, one needs simply to measure how well they decode words and how well they understand those words (and sentences) when read to them. Hoover and Gough (1990) tested the Simple View of Reading in a longitudinal study of English–Spanish bilingual children in first through fourth grades. As predicted, they found that word recognition and listening comprehension accounted for independent variance in reading comprehension. Their results showed that a combination of these variables explained between 72 and 85 percent of the variance in reading comprehension across grades.

Others have also provided data in support of the Simple View of Reading (e.g., Aaron, Joshi, & Williams, 1999; Carver, 1993; Catts, Hogan, & Fey, 2003; de Jong & van der Liej, 2002). The first author and his colleagues tested the Simple View in a longitudinal study of approximately 600 monolingual children (Catts, Hogan, & Adlof, 2005; Adlof, Catts, & Little, 2006). In the 2006 study, which utilized latent regression models, we found that performance on measures of word recognition and listening comprehension explained nearly 100 percent of the reliable variance in reading comprehension in each of second, fourth, and eighth grades. In each grade, most of the explained variance in reading comprehension was shared between word recognition and listening comprehension. However, the unique contributions of each of these components changed across grades. In second grade, 59 percent of the variance in reading comprehension was shared between word recognition and listening comprehension. Word recognition uniquely explained 35 percent, and listening comprehension uniquely explained 5 percent. Thus, word recognition by itself could explain 94 percent of the variance in second-grade reading comprehension, whereas listening comprehension by itself could explain 64 percent. In fourth grade, the contributions of word recognition and listening comprehension were more similar: 62 percent of the explained variance was shared between the two constructs, 19 percent was uniquely explained by word recognition, and 17 percent was uniquely explained by listening comprehension. By eighth grade, all of the reliable variance (100 percent) in reading comprehension could be explained by listening comprehension, with approximately 62 percent shared with word recognition.

According to the Simple View, four subgroups of poor readers can be identified on the basis of their strengths and weaknesses in word recognition and listening comprehension. These include subgroups with problems in word recognition alone, problems in listening comprehension alone, problems in both areas, and problems in neither area. As shown in Figure 3.1, we refer to the subgroup of poor readers with problems in word recognition alone as having *dyslexia*. This is consistent with current definitions of dyslexia, in which word recognition deficits are the primary characteristic. Children who have problems in listening comprehension,

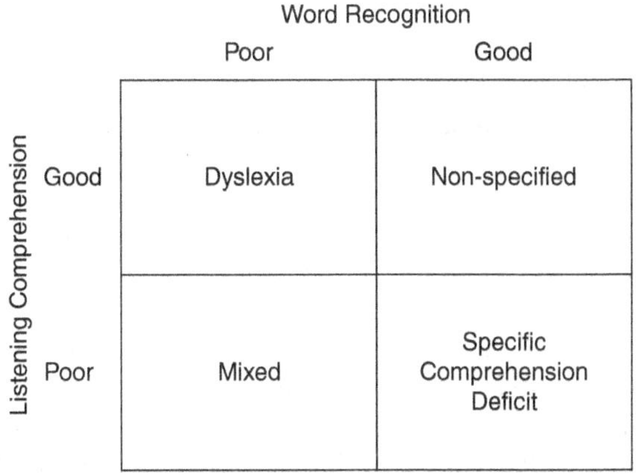

FIGURE 3.1 Subtypes Based on Word Recognition and Listening Comprehension

but not word recognition, are referred to as having a *specific comprehension deficit.* Children who have deficits in both word recognition and listening comprehension are referred to as having a *mixed* reading disability. Finally, the model allows for the possibility of a fourth subgroup of poor readers who have good word recognition and listening comprehension skills. This subgroup, referred to as *nonspecified,* includes children who have reading comprehension problems for reasons not predicted by the Simple View.

Previous research provides support for subgroups identified by the Simple View. Considerable attention has been devoted to the study of children with dyslexia. The problems individuals with dyslexia have in word recognition are well documented (Bruck, 1988; Rack, Snowling, & Olson, 1992; Snowling, 1981; Stanovich & Siegel, 1994). From the beginning, children with dyslexia have difficulties learning to phonologically decode words and to develop a sight-word vocabulary. As we discussed earlier, current definitions of dyslexia specify word recognition deficits as the primary symptom of the disorder. Most definitions also state that children with dyslexia have at least normal intelligence. Because intelligence is generally measured by verbally loaded tests, most children meeting the latter criterion would be expected to have normal listening comprehension abilities. Indeed, research confirms that, as a group, children defined as dyslexic have listening comprehension abilities that are within the normal range (Aaron, 1989; Ellis, McDougall, & Monk, 1996; Fletcher et al., 1994; Shankweiler et al., 1995). Bruck (1990) has further reported that in some cases, individuals with dyslexia may have exceptional listening comprehension abilities that allow them to compensate for their poor decoding skills. Consequently, these individuals' reading difficulties could be missed when using untimed tests of reading comprehension. Also, as was discussed earlier in the chapter, it is generally agreed that problems in phonological processing underlie the difficulties in word recognition. Therefore, although the Simple View does not explicitly include phonological processing abilities, these abilities play a role in this system by way of their influence on word recognition.

Children who have problems in both word recognition and listening comprehension (i.e., mixed RD) have also been the focus of research investigations. These children generally comprise groups of poor readers who fail to meet IQ-achievement discrepancy criterion for dyslexia. As noted earlier, they have been referred to as backward readers (Jorm et al., 1986; Rutter & Yule, 1975), low achievers (Fletcher et al., 1994), or garden-variety poor readers (Gough & Tunmer, 1986; Stanovich, Nathan, & Zolman, 1988). We prefer to call them children with mixed RD. Again, this is done to highlight the fact that they have problems in both word recognition and listening comprehension.

Studies have compared the reading and reading-related problems of children with dyslexia to those with mixed RD. These studies indicate that they have similar difficulties in word recognition (Ellis et al., 1996; Felton & Wood, 1992; Jorm et al., 1986; Stanovich & Siegel, 1994). Research also indicates that phonological processing deficits underlie many of the problems children with mixed RD have in recognizing printed words (Fletcher et al., 1994; Hurford et al., 1994; Shaywitz, Fletcher, Holahan, & Shaywitz, 1992). Unlike children with dyslexia, children with mixed RD have been shown to have significant deficits in language comprehension (Aaron et al., 1995; Ellis et al., 1996; Fletcher et al., 1994; Stanovich & Siegel, 1994). These problems are sometimes associated with more global cognitive deficits. In such cases, children have problems in both verbal and nonverbal processing. In other cases, however, difficulties are specific to language processing. These children may show deficits in vocabulary, morphosyntax, and text-level processing, but have normal nonverbal abilities (Catts, 1993; Catts, Adlof, Hogan, & Ellis Weismer, 2005; Catts, Fey, & Tomblin, 1997).

A third subgroup in this system is comprised of children with problems in listening comprehension, but with normal or above-normal word recognition abilities. This profile has sometimes been referred to as *hyperlexia* (Aaron, Frantz, & Manges, 1990; Aram & Healy, 1988; Elliott & Needleman, 1976; Silberberg & Silberberg, 1967). Hyperlexia, as it was originally conceived, was used to refer to children with exceptional word-decoding skills. Children with hyperlexia were observed to be quite precocious and learn "to read" before they entered school. Despite their exceptional word recognition abilities, hyperlexic children have been found to demonstrate significant problems in comprehension. Huttenlocher and Huttenlocher (1973) described the case of M. K., who by the age of 4 years, 6 months, had learned to read with minimal parental help. At 4 years, 10 months, he could read a third-grade passage fluently. M. K. enjoyed reading and, in fact, was quite compulsive about it. He would read any written material in sight. His comprehension of what he read, however, was severely impaired.

Aram (1997) reviewed research concerning hyperlexia. She reported that children with hyperlexia generally have exceptional phonological decoding skills. These children also have good sight-word-reading abilities. These abilities, however, may not be at the same level as those in phonological decoding. Aram further noted that children with hyperlexia typically have impairments in spoken language. Of particular significance are their deficits in listening comprehension. Children with hyperlexia have been shown to perform poorly on tests of semantic and syntactic processing (Aram, Ekelman, & Healy, 1984; Siegel, 1984). Hyperlexia, in its extreme case, has also been found to be associated with one or more developmental disabilities such as mental retardation, autism, and schizophrenia (see Aram & Healy, 1988). In some cases, it co-occurs with other "splinter skills" such as exceptional music talent or memory for names and dates.

Most poor readers who demonstrate good decoding skills but poor listening comprehension do not fit this description of hyperlexia. We prefer the term *specific comprehension deficit* to describe children with reading comprehension difficulties whose primary problem is in listening comprehension. This term is more inclusive and does not have the clinical connotations of hyperlexia. It has the added advantage of explicitly directing attention to children who have problems understanding language in the face of good word recognition skills. Much of the focus in the field of reading disabilities has been on children with word recognition problems. Although many poor readers have deficits in word recognition, emerging research indicates that a sizable number of poor readers, especially those in later grades, fall into the specific comprehension deficit subgroup (Catts, Hogan, & Adlof, 2005).

One area of possible confusion with the term *specific comprehension deficit* is that a similar term, *poor comprehenders,* is used in a somewhat different way by some researchers. For example, Nation and her colleagues (Nation, Adams, Bower-Crane, & Snowing, 1999; Nation et al., 2004; Nation & Snowling, 1998; see also Cain, Oakhill, Barnes, & Bryant, 2001) refer to children with good word recognition but poor *reading* comprehension as poor comprehenders. Although listening comprehension is not a defining characteristic of poor comprehenders, most of these children have difficulties in semantic and syntactic processing, inference making, and working memory, all of which are part of listening comprehension. The few poor comprehenders who do not have problems in listening comprehension would meet our criterion for the nonspecified group.

Classification Studies

Currently, only a few studies have attempted to classify groups of children with RD on the basis of word recognition and listening comprehension abilities. In one study, Aaron, Joshi, and

Williams (1999) examined the reading comprehension abilities of 139 children in third, fourth, and sixth grades and identified 16 children who were performing at least one standard deviation (SD) below the mean. They found that 13 of the 16 children with RD could be classified into subtypes on the basis of word recognition and/or listening comprehension deficits. Six of the 13 children had problems in word recognition but not listening comprehension (i.e., dyslexic). Four children were observed to have deficits in listening comprehension, but had normal word recognition abilities (i.e., specific comprehension deficit). In addition, three children performed poorly in both word recognition and listening comprehension (i.e., mixed RD). Aaron and colleagues also noted that two of the unclassified children had deficits primarily in reading rate. Consequently, they suggested that reading rate problems, particularly in older children, might qualify as another subgroup of poor readers. We will review this subgroup in the section on word recognition subtypes later in the chapter.

The first author and his colleagues have also used the Simple View to classify poor readers. In our first study (Catts, Hogan, & Fey, 2003), we identified from a sample of over 600 second-grade children 183 subjects who performed at least 1 SD below the mean in reading comprehension. These poor readers were subsequently divided into subgroups based on whether they had word recognition and/or listening comprehension deficits (defined as performance that was at least 1 SD below the mean of a normative group). We found that approximately 35 percent of the poor readers could be classified as having dyslexia and a similar percentage as having a mixed RD. The remaining 30 percent were about evenly divided in the specific comprehension deficit and nonspecified subgroups. Because these percentages were adjusted on the basis of epidemiologic data, they should be representative of the expected prevalences of subgroups among second-grade poor readers in the general population.

In a follow-up study, we further examined the poor reader subgroups (again selected from our large longitudinal sample) in fourth and eighth grades (Catts, Hogan, & Adlof, 2005). Our results showed that the prevalence of several subgroups changed significantly over grades. Specifically, the percentage of poor readers with dyslexia decreased to 22 percent in fourth grade and 13 percent in eighth grade, whereas the prevalence of poor readers with a specific comprehension deficit nearly doubled to about 30 percent in fourth and eighth grades. The prevalence of poor readers classified as having mixed RD showed little change across grades, whereas rates of those classified as nonspecific were similar in second and fourth grades, but somewhat higher in eighth grade (24 percent).

For the most part, the change in the prevalence of dyslexia and specific comprehension deficit subgroups from one grade to the next was not the result of participants shifting in subgroup placement. In fact, children in these subgroups were quite stable in their decoding/ listening comprehension profiles. The reduction in the percentage of children with dyslexia was more a reflection of the fact that children with this profile were less likely to have reading comprehension deficits in the later grades. For example, whereas the majority of second-grade children with dyslexia continued to show a similar profile in eighth grade, fewer than a third of these children were classified as poor readers at that time (i.e., did not have poor reading comprehension). A similar explanation can account for the large increase in children with a specific comprehension deficit from second to fourth/eighth grades. Our results showed that 77 percent of poor readers who were in the specific comprehension deficit subgroup in fourth/eighth grades had a similar profile in second grade. However, fewer than half of these children met the criterion for a poor reader at that time. In subsequent analyses of these children's tenth-grade performance, we found similar prevalence rates for each of the Simple View profiles as was observed in eighth grade.

Other Subtyping Methods Based on Word Recognition Skills

PHONOLOGICAL VS. SURFACE DYSLEXIA SUBGROUPS.   In the past, a great deal of attention was focused on classifying subgroups of children with dyslexia according to their relative strengths and weaknesses with different types of word recognition. Recall that there are two routes to word recognition: the phonological route, where words are decoded or "sounded out," and the visual route, where words are recognized automatically from their print forms. Typically, nonword reading measures have been used to assess children's phonological decoding skills, and exception-word-reading measures have been used to measure their visual word recognition skills. These two routes to word recognition present two possible sources of word recognition difficulty and three potential subgroups of children with word-reading difficulties.

Researchers from different fields have used different terms to refer to these different word-reading subgroups. For example individuals who show difficulties with nonword decoding but not with exception-word reading have been referred to as "audio-phonetic" (Ingram, 1964), "dysphonetic" (Boder, 1971, 1973), or "phonological" dyslexics (Coltheart, Patterson, & Marshall, 1980; Marshall & Newcombe, 1973). Individuals who show the opposite profile—difficulties with exception-word reading but not nonword decoding—have been referred to as "visuospatial" (Ingram, 1964), "dyseidetic" (Boder, 1971, 1973) or "surface" dyslexics (Coltheart et al., 1980; Marshall & Newcombe, 1973). Individuals with difficulties in both areas have been referred to as "alexic" (Boder, 1971, 1973) or "deep" dyslexics (Coltheart et al., 1980; Marshall & Newcombe, 1973).

Converging research indicates that intra-individual differences in nonword reading versus exception-word reading are relative, not absolute. Thus, children with dyslexia do not form distinct subgroups. Operationally, these abilities can be displayed on a scatter plot with performance on exception-word-reading measures plotted on one axis and scores on nonword reading measures plotted on the other. Ellis (1985) argued that if surface dyslexics were distinct from phonological dyslexics, there should be distinct "galaxies" of dyslexics within the scatter plot. Instead poor readers tend to be distributed continuously throughout this two-dimensional space (Ellis, 1985, p. 192; Ellis et al., 1996; Murphy & Pollatsek, 1994). Most individuals with dyslexia show at least some problems with both nonword and exception-word reading, whereas extreme or "pure" cases of phonological and surface dyslexia are rare (Castles & Coltheart, 1993; Stanovich, Siegel, & Gottardo, 1997).

Although few individuals display pure phonological or surface dyslexia, Castles and Coltheart (1993) argued that the identification of relative dissociations in nonword versus exception-word reading for individuals with dyslexia could have important implications for understanding and treating their word-reading disabilities, especially if different types of problems underlie these word-reading profiles. Murphy and Pollatsek (1994) speculated that instructional differences might contribute to some of these observed individual differences. They observed that several of the children showing the surface dyslexic profile in their study had been enrolled in intensive phonics programs that taught them to read nonwords and real words but few exception words. Such instruction could have led to the error pattern of a surface dyslexic.

A similar perspective was provided by Stanovich and colleagues (1997), who compared children with dyslexia to two different control groups: chronological-age-matched controls (CA), and reading-level-matched controls (RL), who were younger, typically developing children with the same level of reading ability as the children with dyslexia. Compared to CA controls, about one quarter of the children with dyslexia showed a phonological dyslexia profile, one quarter showed a surface dyslexia profile, and half showed problems in both areas. When compared to RL controls, one quarter could still be classified as phonological dyslexics, but only one child was identified as a surface dyslexic. That is, when children with dyslexia were compared to RL controls, the surface dyslexia group essentially disappeared. Similar findings have also been reported by Manis and others (Gustafson, 2001; Manis, Seidenberg, Doi, McBride-Chang, & Petersen, 1996; Manis et al., 1999). Based on these findings, Stanovich and colleagues (1997) concluded that the surface dyslexia profile is best characterized as a developmental lag. In other words, children with surface dyslexia develop along a normal trajectory, but at a slower pace than their peers. Stanovich hypothesized that surface dyslexia might result from mild phonological processing deficits combined with inadequate reading experience, whereas phonological dyslexia represented a true developmental disorder. Children with phonological dyslexia have severe phonological processing deficits, and their reading skills develop along a different trajectory.

Other evidence to support the notion that surface dyslexia is related to instruction and/or reading experience comes from RTI and genetics studies. In an early RTI study, Vellutino and colleagues found that some children with RD could be "readily remediated" with short-term intervention (Vellutino et al., 1996). These children, who Vellutino and colleagues believed to have instructional or experiential deficits (and who may have also had mild phonological processing deficits), may at least partially overlap with the surface dyslexics identified by Stanovich and his colleagues. Vellutino and colleagues also identified a contrasting group of "hard to remediate" poor readers who seemed to fit the profile of phonological dyslexics because they had deficits in phonological decoding and phonological processing. Similarly, Castles, Datta, Gayan, and Olson (1999) examined the genetic and environmental influences on word recognition subgroups. Both subgroups were significantly influenced by genetic and environmental factors. However, the influence of genetic factors was larger in phonological dyslexia, whereas the influence of environmental factors was larger in surface dyslexia (also see Gustafson, 2001).

Although many cases of surface dyslexia could be explained by mild phonological deficits combined with poor instruction or lack of experience, it does not seem to be the case that all can. Other types of cognitive processing deficits might be involved in such cases. Recent studies of written word learning in children and adults who show the surface dyslexia profile have found that these individuals are slower (and less accurate) than age and/or reading-level matched peers to learn novel written word forms, even when the amount and type of exposure is the same (Bailey, Manis, Pederson, & Seidenberg, 2004; Romani, Di Betta, Tsouknida, & Olson, 2008). More evidence is needed, but these results suggest that deficiencies in orthographic or visual processing skills could be implicated in the purest cases of surface dyslexia.

RATE VS. ACCURACY DISABLED SUBGROUPS.   Researchers have also examined subgroups of poor readers defined by discrepancies in accuracy versus speed of word recognition (e.g., Aaron et al., 1999; Adlof et al., 2006; Lovett, 1987). For example, Lovett (1987) distinguished children who were "accuracy-disabled," meaning they had difficulty accurately decoding words, from children who were "rate-disabled," meaning that they were accurate at decoding, but markedly slower than their typical peers. Lovett (1987) administered a large battery of tests of language, reading, and academic skills to 32 rate-disabled, 32 accuracy-disabled, and 32 control children who were matched to the other groups on chronological age, sex, and IQ. Children in the accuracy-disabled group showed the lowest levels of performance across all measures. They made more word-reading errors, read more slowly, and showed poorer comprehension than the other groups. They also showed deficits in morphological and syntactic knowledge, and they were slow at rapid automatic naming tasks. In contrast, children in the rate-disabled group were more selectively impaired. They performed like the readers in the control group in decoding and sight-word-reading accuracy, and they did not show large differences in comprehension skills. With respect to oral language abilities, the rate-disabled and normal readers were similar with one exception: The rate-disabled children were significantly slower on tasks measuring rapid automatic naming.

What actually underlies reading rate deficits is unclear at present. Some children with rate deficits may not have had an adequate amount of reading experience. This may be especially true for children whose accuracy deficits have recently been remediated. Because automaticity of word recognition increases with practice, they may lag behind their normal peers in speed of word recognition. Reading rate problems may also be related to phonological retrieval deficits. Lovett's (1987) results seem to confirm the problems these children have in the rapid retrieval of verbal labels. Wolf, Bowers, and Biddle (2000) have also reported a link between reading rate and naming speed. Based on results we describe next, we hypothesize that language and/or comprehension difficulties themselves can cause rate deficits.

Although it is possible to find children who are accurate but slow word readers, there is currently very little evidence that rate deficits, by themselves, actually lead to comprehension failure. We recently examined subgroups of children with accuracy, rate, and/or listening comprehension difficulties in second, fourth, and eighth grades using the large longitudinal database described earlier in the chapter (Adlof et al., 2006). In this study, children were identified as having a "rate deficit" if they performed above the 40th percentile on a standardized test of single-word reading accuracy and below the 25th percentile on a standardized test of connected text fluency. Over 500 children were tested in each grade, and of these, between 19 and 37 showed a rate deficit at any grade. The term "specific rate deficit" was used to refer to those children who met the rate deficit criteria and scored above the 40th percentile on a composite measure of listening comprehension. The prevalence of specific rate deficits was even smaller, with between 10 and 17 children fitting that profile at any given grade. The rate of reading comprehension difficulties in the rate deficit group was relatively low. More importantly, *all* children in the specific rate deficit group showed adequate reading comprehension skill, with no child scoring below the 25th percentile in reading comprehension at any grade. Thus, in over 500 children tested at several different time points, we could find no evidence that slow but accurate reading was associated with reading comprehension difficulties, unless oral language difficulties were also present.

Converging evidence is provided by a recent study of 9- to 14-year-old children with specific reading comprehension deficits (Cutting, Materek, Cole, Levine, & Mahone, 2009). Cutting and colleagues found that children with specific reading comprehension deficits did not differ from typical readers on a standardized test of single-word and nonword reading accuracy and rate. However, children with specific comprehension deficits were slower than typical readers when reading connected texts. These results suggest that comprehension difficulties themselves might lead to a slower rate while reading connected texts. Thus, the results of these investigations have brought us full circle, to the first subgrouping method we proposed in this chapter, based on distinctions between word-reading and listening comprehension skills. In the remaining sections of this chapter, we offer suggestions for applying these subgroups to research and clinical or educational practice.

Combining Subtypes in Research and Practice

In the previous sections, we have described several classification systems for subtyping children with RD. Although presented separately, these systems overlap quite a bit. We prefer to begin with the Simple View model, which divides poor readers into three primary subtypes: dyslexia, mixed RD, and specific comprehension deficit. Children with mixed RD and dyslexia both have deficits in word recognition; thus, they may further be characterized as primarily phonological or surface dyslexics, depending on their relative strengths and weaknesses in nonword decoding and exception-word reading. Because they display difficulty with word recognition accuracy, their reading rates are expected to be slower than typical children. Children with mixed RD and those with a specific comprehension deficit share deficits in listening comprehension. Children with specific comprehension deficits may also show slower rates of reading connected texts, as a result of their comprehension difficulties.

Whereas this combined classification system has some research support, further empirical validation is necessary. More comprehensive studies are needed to classify and compare sub-groups of poor readers. We need to know, for example, if children with mixed RD show the same profiles in word recognition abilities and phonological processing as children with dyslexia. Although some studies suggest they are similar (Ellis et al., 1996; Felton & Wood, 1992; Share, 1996; Stanovich & Siegel, 1994), further investigation is needed. We could find, for example, that because of their language deficits, children with mixed RD might show particular difficulties using context to develop a sight-word vocabulary. As a result, these children may be more likely to demonstrate a surface dyslexia profile. More research is also needed to investigate the relationship between reading rate and comprehension. That is, should rate be viewed as a predictor of comprehension, or rather, as the outcome of comprehension? Do specific rate deficits—those that occur in the absence of listening comprehension problems—require treatment, if reading comprehension is not affected? We also need to compare children with a specific comprehension deficit and mixed RD. Do these children show similar deficits in listening comprehension? Are there other subgroups within these groups? Listening comprehension is a complex process that consists of linguistic, conceptual, and metacognitive processes. At present, there do not appear to be homogeneous subtypes of listening comprehension difficulties (Catts et al., 2006; Nation et al., 2004), but further research is needed to investigate this issue.

Whereas comparative investigations can further our understanding of reading disabilities, theoretical advancements may better be made by treating variables of interest in a continuous rather than categorical fashion. Poor readers do not cluster together in terms of their word recognition abilities, but rather fall continuously along several dimensions. The same is true for listening comprehension and the factors that underlie it. Research designs and statistical analyses that examine the continuous relationships between reading ability, word recognition, listening comprehension, and related factors (cognitive and environmental variables) could provide us with a better understanding of reading disabilities.

Clinical Implications

The classification system presented here has some important clinical and educational implications. By considering children's strengths and weaknesses in listening comprehension and accuracy/rate of word recognition, practitioners may be better able to describe reading problems, plan intervention, monitor progress, and determine prognosis (Aaron, 1991). Our classification system suggests that all children with RD need an assessment that includes measures of word recognition, listening comprehension, and related cognitive processes. Word-recognition abilities can be evaluated by standardized tests such as the Woodcock Reading Mastery Tests—Revised Normative Update (Woodcock, 1998). This battery of tests provides an assessment of children's abilities to read real and nonsense words. These tests can be supplemented by lists of exception words to more directly evaluate reading by the visual route (see Manis et al., 1996). These measures should allow practitioners to uncover discrepancies between nonword and exception-word reading, however, local normative data must be gathered to fully appreciate the meaning of these discrepancies (Stanovich et al., 1997). Rate and fluency of word recognition may also need to be considered. In Chapter 5, Al Otaiba and colleagues discuss various ways to measure this aspect of word recognition. They also provide other suggestions for the assessment of word recognition and related language processes (e.g., phonological awareness).

Our classification system further suggests that assessment for reading disabilities should include an evaluation of children's listening comprehension abilities. This may involve the use of measures traditionally employed to assess receptive vocabulary and grammatical knowledge (Bishop, 2003; Carrow-Woolfolk, 1999; Dunn & Dunn, 2007; McGee, Ehrier, & DiSimoni, 2007). Norm-referenced tests are available to measure the comprehension of extended spoken texts (Newcomer, 2001; Semel, Wiig, & Secord, 2003; Wechsler, 2009; Woodcock, 1991), or criterion-referenced measures, such as the Qualitative Reading Inventory-5 presented in a listening format (Leslie & Caldwell, 2010), can also be used. Our research on reading subtypes suggests that it may be necessary to measure listening comprehension and related abilities in at-risk children prior to the emergence of reading problems. Recall that over half of the fourth- and eighth-grade poor readers with a specific comprehension deficit were not identified as poor readers in second grade. Thus, to identify children with a specific comprehension deficit in second grade or earlier, practitioners will need to examine these children's language abilities.

The proposed classification system should also help clinicians plan intervention programs. This system suggests that children with dyslexia or mixed RD share the need for intervention directed at word recognition abilities. However, this intervention could vary, depending on the specific problems a poor reader has in word recognition (e.g., nonword decoding, exception-word reading, and/or reading rate). Unfortunately, current research provides only limited direction for differential treatment of these subgroups. As more intervention studies consider the interaction between word recognition subtypes and treatment outcomes, we will be better able to design appropriate intervention programs. While awaiting these results, some insights may be taken from current research. This work suggests that children with phonological dyslexia can benefit from direct and explicit instruction in the use of the phonological route. In Chapter 5, Al Otaiba and colleagues describe intervention programs that have been effective in improving the nonword reading abilities of poor readers. If children with surface dyslexia have a developmental lag (Stanovich et al., 1997), they may be able to catch up with their peers with more instruction and practice in reading. They may also benefit from intervention directed at mild phonological processing problems (e.g., Vellutino et al., 1996). It is important not to assume that because surface dyslexics are like younger normal children, they will catch up on their own. They have significant reading problems, and without intervention, they may fall farther behind their peers. Poor readers with rate deficits may improve their automaticity of word recognition through repeated reading, continuous reading, and paired or imitative reading interventions (Clark & Uhry, 1995; O'Connor, White, & Swanson, 2007; Rashotte & Torgesen, 1985; Samuels, 1977). These activities may also give the poor reader a sense of success and appreciation for fluent reading.

Interventions for children with specific comprehension deficits as well as those with mixed RD will need to focus on comprehension skills. Again, research is needed to determine which types of comprehension interventions are most effective for different groups of students. Interventions to improve comprehension skills could include general oral language activities such as those focusing on increasing vocabulary knowledge or grammatical knowledge, or higher-level discourse activities that improve schema knowledge or teach the use of text structure and metacognitive strategies to aid comprehension. Chapters 6 and 7 offer suggestions for improving the reading comprehension skills of children with mixed RD or a specific comprehension deficit.

References

Aaron, P. G. (1989). Qualitative and quantitative differences among dyslexic, normal, and nondyslexic poor readers. *Reading and Writing: An Interdisciplinary Journal, 1,* 291–308.

Aaron, P. G. (1991). Can reading disabilities be diagnosed without using intelligence tests? *Journal of Learning Disabilities, 24,* 178–186.

Aaron, P. G., Frantz, S. S., & Manges, A. R. (1990). Dissociation between comprehension and pronunciation in dyslexic and hyperlexic children. *Reading and Writing: An Interdisciplinary Journal, 2,* 243–264.

Aaron, P. G., Joshi, M., & Williams, K. A. (1999). Not all reading disabilities are alike. *Journal of Learning Disabilities, 32,* 120–137.

Adlof, S. M., Catts, H. W., & Little, T. D. (2006). Should the Simple View of Reading include a fluency component? *Reading and Writing, 19,* 933–958.

Aram, D. (1997). Hyperlexia: Reading without meaning in young children. *Topics in Language Disorders, 17,* 1–13.

Aram, D. M., Ekelman, B. L., & Healy, J. M. (1984). *Reading profiles of hyperlexic children.* Paper presented at the International Neuropsychology Society, Aachen, Germany.

Aram, D. M., & Healy, J. M. (Eds.). (1988). *Hyperlexia: A review of extraordinary word recognition.* New York: Guilford Press.

Bailey, C. E., Manis, F. R., Pederson, W. C., & Seidenberg, M. S. (2005). Variation among developmental dyslexics: Evidence from a printed-word-learning task. *Journal of Experimental Child Psychology, 87,* 125–154.

Benton, A. (1991). Dyslexia and visual dyslexia. In J. Stein (Ed.), *Vision and visual dysfunction: Vol. 13. Visual dyslexia* (pp. 141–146). London: Macmillan Press.

Berlin, R. (1887). *Eine besondere art der wortblindheit: Dyslexia [A special type of wordblindness: Dyslexia].* Wiesbaden: J.F. Bergmann.

Bishop, D. (2003). *Test for Reception of Grammar-2.* San Antonio, TX: PsychCorp.

Blalock, J. W. (1982). Persistent auditory language deficits in adults with learning disabilities. *Journal of Learning Disabilities, 15,* 604–609.

Boder, E. (1971). Developmental dyslexia: Prevailing diagnostic concepts and a new diagnostic approach. In H. R. Myklebust (Ed.), *Progress in learning disabilities* (Vol. 2, pp. 293–321). New York: Grune & Stratton.

Boder, E. (1973). Developmental dyslexia: A diagnostic approach based on three atypical reading-spelling patterns. *Developmental Medicine and Child Neurology, 15,* 663–687.

Bradley, L., & Bryant, P. (1983). Categorizing sounds and learning to read: A causal connection. *Nature, 301,* 419–421.

Brodbent, W. H. (1872). On the cerebral mechanism of speech and thought. *Transactions of the Royal Medical and Chirurgical Society, 15,* 330–357.

Bruck, M. (1988). The word recognition and spelling of dyslexic children. *Reading Research Quarterly, 23,* 51–69.

Bruck, M. (1990). Word recognition skills of adults with a childhood diagnosis of dyslexia. *Developmental Psychology, 26,* 439–454.

Cain, K., Oakhill, J. V., Barnes, M. A., & Bryant, P. E. (2001). Comprehension skill, inference-making ability, and the relation to knowledge. *Memory and Cognition, 29,* 850–859.

Carrow-Woolfolk, E. (1999). *Test for Auditory Comprehension of Language-3.* Austin, TX: Pro-ED.

Carver, R. (1993). Merging the Simple View of Reading with reading theory. *Journal of Reading Behavior, 25,* 439–455.

Castles, A., & Coltheart, M. (1993). Varieties of developmental dyslexia. *Cognition, 47,* 149–180.

Castles, A., Datta, H., Gayan, J., & Olson, R. K. (1999). Varieties of developmental reading disorder: Genetic and environmental influences. *Journal of Experimental Child Psychology, 72,* 73–94.

Catts, H. W. (1989a). Defining dyslexia as a developmental language disorder. *Annals of Dyslexia, 39,* 50–64.

Catts, H. W. (1989b). Speech production deficits in developmental dyslexia. *Journal of Speech and Hearing Disorders, 54,* 422–428.

Catts, H. W. (1993). The relationship between speech-language impairments and reading disabilities. *Journal of Speech and Hearing Research, 36,* 948–958.

Catts, H. W., Adlof, S. M., & Ellis Weismer, S. (2006). Language deficits in poor comprehenders: The case for the Simple View of Reading. *Journal of Speech, Language, and Hearing Research, 49,* 278–293.

Catts, H. W., Adlof, S. M., Hogan, T. P., & Ellis Weismer, S. (2005). Are SLI and dyslexia distinct disorders? *Journal of Speech, Language, and Hearing Research, 48,* 1378–1396.

Catts, H. W., Fey, M., & Tomblin, B. (1997). *Language basis of reading disabilities.* Paper presented at the Society for the Scientific Study of Reading, Chicago.

Catts. H. W., Fey, M. E., Tomblin, J. B., & Zhang, Z. (2002). A longitudinal investigation of reading outcomes in children with language impairments. *Journal of Speech, Language, and Hearing Research, 45,* 1142–1157.

Catts, H. W., Fey, M. E., Zhang, X., & Tomblin, J. B. (2001). Estimating risk for future reading difficulties in kindergarten children: A research-based model and its clinical implications. *Language, Speech, and Hearing Services in Schools, 32,* 38–50.

Catts, H. W., Hogan, T. P., & Adlof, S. M. (2005). Developmental changes in reading and reading disabilities. In H. W. Catts & A. G. Kamhi (Eds.), *Connections between language and reading disabilities* (pp. 25–40). Mahwah, NJ: Erlbaum.

Catts, H. W., Hogan, T. P., & Fey, M. (2003). Subgrouping poor readers on the basis of reading-related abilities. *Journal of Learning Disabilities, 36,* 151–164.

Catts, H. W., & Kamhi, A. G. (Eds.). (2005). *Connections between language and reading disabilities.* Mahwah, NJ: Erlbaum.

Catts, H., & Kamhi, A. (Eds.). (1999). *Language and reading disabilities.* Boston: Allyn & Bacon.

Ceci, S., & Baker, S. (1978). Commentary: How should we conceptualize the language problems of learning disabled children? In S. Ceci (Ed.), *Handbook of cognitive, social, and neuropsychological aspects of learning disabilities* (pp. 102–115). Hillsdale, NJ: Erlbaum.

Clark, D. B., & Uhry, J. K. (1995). *Dyslexia: Theory and practice of remedial instruction.* Baltimore: York Press.

Coltheart, M., Patterson, K., & Marshall, J. (Eds.). (1980). *Deep dyslexia.* London: Routledge and Kegan Paul.

Critchley, M. (1970). *The dyslexic child.* Springfield, IL: Charles C Thomas.

Cutting, L. E., Materek, A., Cole, C. A. S., Levine, T. M., & Mahone, E. M. (2009). Effects of fluency, oral language, and executive function on reading comprehension performance. *Annals of Dyslexia, 59,* 34–54.

Das, J., Mensink, D., & Mishra, R. (1990). Cognitive processes separating good and poor readers when IQ is covaried. *Learning and Individual Differences, 2,* 423–436.

Das, J. P., Mishra, R. K., & Kirby, J. R. (1994). Cognitive patterns of children with dyslexia: A comparison between groups with high and average nonverbal intelligence. *Journal of Learning Disabilities, 27,* 235–242, 253.

de Jong, P. F., & van der Liej, A. (2002). Effects of phonological abilities and linguistic comprehension on the development of reading. *Scientific Studies of Reading, 6,* 51–77.

Dollaghan, C., & Kaston, N. (1986). A comprehension monitoring program for language-impaired children. *Journal of Speech and Hearing Disorders, 51,* 264–271.

Dunn, L., & Dunn, L. (2007). *Peabody Picture Vocabulary Test-4.* Circle Pines, MN: American Guidance.

Eden, G. F., Stein, J. F., Wood, M. H., & Wood, F. B. (1995). Verbal and visual problems in reading disability. *Journal of Learning Disabilities, 28,* 272–290.

Elliott, D. E., & Needleman, R. M. (1976). The syndrome of hyperlexia. *Brain and Language, 3,* 339–349.

Ellis, A. W. (1985). The cognitive neuropsychology of developmental (and acquired) dyslexia: A critical survey. *Cognitive Neuropsychology, 2,* 196–205.

Ellis, A. W., McDougall, S., & Monk, A. F. (1996). Are dyslexics different? II. A comparison between dyslexics, reading age controls, poor readers, and precocious readers. *Dyslexia: An International Journal of Practice and Research, 2,* 59–68.

Ellis Weismer, S., & Hesketh, L. (1993). The influence of prosodic and gestural cues on novel word acquisition by children with specific language impairment. *Journal of Speech and Hearing Research, 36,* 1013–1025.

Felton, R. H., Naylor, C. E., & Wood, F. B. (1990). Neuropsychological profile of adult dyslexics. *Brain and Language, 39,* 485–497.

Felton, R. H., & Wood, F. B. (1992). A reading level match study of nonword reading skills in poor readers with varying IQ. *Journal of Learning Disabilities, 25,* 318–326.

Fletcher, J. M. (1992). The validity of distinguishing children with language and learning disabilities according to discrepancies with IQ: Introduction to the special series. *Journal of Learning Disabilities, 25,* 546–548.

Fletcher, J. M., Coulter, W. A., Reschly, D. J., & Vaughn, S. (2004). Alternative approaches to the definition and identification of learning disabilities: Some questions and answers. *Annals of Dyslexia, 54,* 304–331.

Fletcher, J. M., Francis, D. J., Rourke, B. P., Shaywitz, S. E., & Shaywitz, B. A. (1992). The validity of discrepancy-based definitions of reading disabilities. *Journal of Learning Disabilities, 25,* 555–561, 573.

Fletcher, J. M., Francis, D. J., Shaywitz, S. E., Lyon, G. R., Foorman, B. R., Stuebing, K. K., et al. (1998). Intelligence testing and the discrepancy model for children with learning disabilities. *Learning Disabilities Research and Practice, 13,* 186–203.

Fletcher, J. M., Shaywitz, S. E., Shankweiler, D. P., Katz, L., Liberman, I. Y., Stuebing, K. K., Francis, D. J., Fowler, A. E., & Shaywitz, B. A. (1994). Cognitive profiles of reading disability: Comparisons of discrepancy and low achievement definitions. *Journal of Educational Psychology, 86,* 6–23.

Flowers, L., Meyer, M., Lovato, J., Wood, F., & Felton, R. (2001). Does third grade discrepancy status predict the course of reading development? *Annals of Dyslexia, 51,* 49–71.

Francis, D. J., Espy, K. A., Rourke, B. P., & Fletcher, J. M. (1987). Validity of intelligence test scores in the definition of learning disability: A critical analysis. In B. P. Rourke (Ed.), *Neuropsychological validation of learning disability subtypes* (pp. 15–44). New York: Guilford Press.

Francis, D. J., Fletcher, J. M., Shaywitz, B. A., Shaywitz, S. E., & Rourke, B. (1996). Defining learning and language abilities: Conceptual and psychometric issues with the use of IQ tests. *Language, Speech, and Hearing Services in Schools, 27,* 132–143.

Francis, D. J., Fletcher, J. M., Stuebing, K. K., Lyon, G. R., Shaywitz, B. A., & Shaywitz, S. E. (2005). Psychometric approaches to the identification of LD: IQ and achievement scores are not sufficient. *Journal of Learning Disabilities, 38,* 98–108.

Gerber, A. (1993). *Language-related learning disabilities: Their nature and treatment.* Baltimore: Brookes.

Golderberg, H., & Schiffman, G. (1972). *Dyslexia: problems of reading disabilities.* New York: Grune & Stratton.

Good, R. H., Simmons, D. C., & Smith, S. B. (1998). Effective academic interventions in the United States: Evaluating and enhancing the acquisition of early reading skills. *School Psychology Review, 27,* 45–56.

Gough, P. B., & Tunmer, W. E. (1986). Decoding, reading, and reading disability. *Remedial and Special Education, 7,* 6–10.

Gustafson, S. (2001). Cognitive abilities and print exposure in surface and phonological types of reading disability. *Scientific Studies of Reading, 5,* 351–375.

Hatcher, P. J., & Hulme, C. (1999). Phonemes, rhymes, and intelligence as predictors of children's responsiveness to remedial reading instruction: Evidence from a longitudinal intervention study. *Journal of Experimental Child Psychology, 72,* 130–154.

Heaton, P., & Winterson, P. (1996). *Dealing with dyslexia.* San Diego, CA: Singular.

Hinshelwood, J. (1895, December 21). Letter-word- and mind-blindness. *Lancet, 146*(3773), 1564–1569.

Hinshelwood, J. (1900). Congenital word-blindness. *Lancet, 1,* 1506–1508.

Hinshelwood, J. (1917). *Congenital word blindness.* London: H. K. Lewis.

Hoover, W. A., & Gough, P. B. (1990). The Simple View of Reading. *Reading and Writing: An Interdisciplinary Journal, 2,* 127–160.

Hoskins, M., & Swanson, L. (2000). Cognitive processing of low achievers and children with reading disabilities: A selective meta-analytic review of the published literature. *The School Psychology Review, 29,* 102–119.

Hurford, D. P., Schauf, J. D., Bunce, L., Blaich, T., & Moore, K. (1994). Early identification of children at risk for reading disabilities. *Journal of Learning Disabilities, 27,* 371–382.

Huttenlocher, P. R., & Huttenlocher, J. (1973). A study of children with hyperlexia. *Neurology, 23,* 1107–1116.

Ingram, T. T. S. (1964). The nature of dyslexia. In F. A. Young & D. B. Lindsley (Eds.), *Early experience and visual information processing in perceptual and reading disorders.* Washington, DC: National Academy of Sciences.

Johnson, D., & Myklebust, H. (1967). *Learning disabilities: Educational principles and practice.* New York: Grune & Stratton.

Jorm, A. F., Share, D. L., Maclean, R., & Matthews, R. (1986). Cognitive factors at school entry predictive of specific reading retardation and general reading backwardness: A research note. *Journal of Child Psychology and Psychiatry, 27,* 45–54.

Kamhi, A. G. (1992). Response to historical perspective: A developmental language perspective. *Journal of Learning Disabilities, 25,* 48–52.

Kamhi, A. G., & Catts, H. W. (1986). Toward an understanding of developmental language and reading disorders. *Journal of Speech and Hearing Disorders, 51,* 337–347.

Kamhi, A. G., & Catts, H. W. (1989). *Reading disabilities: A developmental language perspective.* Boston: Allyn & Bacon.

Katusic, S. K., Colligan, R. C., Barbaresi, W. J., Schaid, D. J., & Jacobsen, S. J. (2001). Incidence of reading disability in a population-based birth cohort, 1976–1982, Rochester, Minn. *Mayo Clinic Proceedings, 76,* 1081–1092.

Knopik, V. S., Smith, S. D., Cardon, L., Pennington, B., Gayán, J., Olson, R. K., & DeFries, J. C. (2002). Differential genetic etiology of reading component processes as a function of IQ. *Behavior Genetics, 32,* 181–198.

Kussmaul, A. (1887). Disturbances of speech. In H. von Ziemssen (Ed.), *Cyclopedia of the practice of medicine.* New York: William Wood.

Leach, J. M., Scarborough, H. S., & Rescorla, L. (2003). Late-emerging reading disabilities. *Journal of Educational Psychology, 95,* 211–225.

Lerner, J. W. (1972). Reading disability as a language disorder. *Acta Symbolica, 3,* 39–45.

Lerner, J. W. (1985). *Learning disabilities: Theories, diagnosis, and teaching strategies*. Boston: Houghton Mifflin.

Leslie, L., & Caldwell, J. (2001). *Qualitative Reading Inventory-III*. New York: Addison Wesley Longman.

Lipka, O., Lesaux, N. K., & Siegel, L. S. (2006). Retrospective analyses of the reading development of a group of grade 4 disabled readers: Risk status and profiles over 5 years. *Journal of Learning Disabilities, 39*, 364–378.

Lovett, M. W. (1987). A developmental approach to reading disability: Accuracy and speed criteria of normal and deficient reading skill. *Child Development, 58*, 234–260.

Lyon, G. R. (1995). Toward a definition of dyslexia. *Annals of Dyslexia, 4*, 3–30.

Lyon, G. R., Fletcher, J. M. Shaywitz, S. E., Shaywitz, B. A., Wood, F. B., Schulte, A., Olson, R. K., & Torgesen, J. K. (2001). Learning disabilities: An evidence-based conceptualization. In C. E. Finn, A. J. Rotherham, & C. J. Hokanson, Jr. (Eds.), *Rethinking special education for a new century* (pp. 259–287). Washington, DC: Fordham Foundation and Progressive Policy Institute.

Lyon, G. R., Shaywitz, S. E., & Shaywitz, B. A. (2003). A definition of dyslexia. *Annals of Dyslexia, 53*, 1–14.

Manis, F. R., Seidenberg, M. S., Doi, L. M., McBride-Chang, C., & Petersen, A. (1996). On the basis of two subtypes of developmental dyslexia. *Cognition, 58*, 157–195.

Manis, F. R., Seidenberg, M. S., Stallings, L., Joanisse, M., Bailey, C., Freedman, L., Curtin, S., & Keating, P. (1999). Developmental dyslexic subgroups: A one-year follow up. *Annals of Dyslexia, 49*, 105–137.

Marshall, J., & Newcombe, F. (1973). Patterns of paralexia: A psycholinguistic approach. *Journal of Psycholinguistic Research, 2*, 175–200.

Mastriopieri, M. A., & Scruggs, T. E. (2005). Feasibility and consequences of response to intervention: Examination of the issues and scientific evidence as a model for the identification of individuals with learning disabilities. *Journal of Learning Disabilities, 38*, 525–531.

Mattingly, I. (1972). Reading the linguistic process, and linguistic awareness. In J. Kavanaugh & I. Mattingly (Eds.), *Language by ear and by eye* (pp. 133–147). Cambridge, MA: MIT Press.

McGee, R. L., Ehrier, D. J., & DiSimoni, F. (2007). *The Token Test for Children-2*. Austin, TX: Pro-Ed.

Miles, T. (1983). *Dyslexia: The pattern of difficulties*. Springfield, IL: Charles C Thomas.

Morgan, W. (1896). A case of congenital word-blindness. *British Medical Journal, 2*(1), 378.

Murphy, L., & Pollatsek, A. (1994). Developmental dyslexia: Heterogeneity without discrete subgroups. *Annals of Dyslexia, 44*, 120–146.

Naglieri, J. A., & Reardon, S. M. (1993). Traditional IQ is irrelevant to learning disabilities—intelligence is not. *Journal of Learning Disabilities, 26*, 127–133.

Naidoo, S. (1972). *Specific dyslexia*. London: Pitman.

Nation, K., Adams, J. W., Bower-Crane, C. A., & Snowing, M. J. (1999). Working memory deficits in poor comprehenders reflect underlying language impairments. *Journal of Experimental Child Psychology, 73*, 139–158.

Nation, K., Clark, P., Marshall, C. M., & Durand, M. (2004). Hidden language impairments in children: Parallels between poor reading comprehension and specific language impairments. *Journal of Speech, Language, and Hearing Research, 47*, 199–211.

Nation, K., & Snowling, M. J. (1998). Individual differences in contextual facilitation: Evidence from dyslexia and poor reading comprehension. *Child Development, 69*, 996–1011.

Newcomer, P. (2001). *Diagnostic Achievement Battery-Third Edition*. Austin, TX: Pro-Ed.

Nicolson, R. I., & Fawcett, A. (1995). Dyslexia is more than phonological disability. *Dyslexia: An International Journal of Research and Practice, 1*, 19–36.

O'Connor, R. E., White, A., & Swanson, H. L. (2007). Repeated reading versus continuous reading: Influences on reading fluency and comprehension. *Exceptional Children, 74*, 31–46.

Olson, D., & Byrne, B. (2005). Genetic and environmental influences on reading and language ability and disability. In H. W. Catts & A. G. Kamhi (Eds.), *Connections between language and reading disabilities* (pp. 173–200). Mahwah, NJ: Erlbaum.

Olson, R. K., Datta, H., Gayan, J., & DeFries, J. C. (1999). A behavioral-genetic analysis of reading disabilities and component processes. In R. M. Klein & P. A. MacMullen (Eds.), *Converging methods for understanding reading and dyslexia*. (pp. 133–153). Cambridge, MA: MIT Press.

Olson, R. K., Rack, J., Conners, F., DeFries, J., & Fulker, D. (1991). Genetic etiology of individual differences in reading disability. In L. Feagans, E. Short, & L. Meltzer (Eds.), *Subtypes of learning disabilities* (pp. 113–135). Hillsdale, NJ: Erlbaum.

O'Malley, K. J., Francis, D. J., Foorman, B. R., Fletcher, J. M., & Swank, P. R. (2002). Growth in precursor and reading-related skills: Do low-achieving and IQ-discrepant readers develop differently? *Learning Disabilities Research & Practice, 17*, 19–34.

Orton, J. L., Thompson, L. J., Buncy, P. C., Bender, L., Robinson, M. H., & Rome, P. D. (1975). Samuel T. Orton, who was he: Part 1. Biographical sketch and personal memories. *Bulletin of Orton Society, 25,* 145–155.

Orton, S. (1925). Word-blindness in school children. *Archives of Neurology and Psychiatry, 14,* 581–615.

Orton, S. (1937). *Reading, writing and speech problems in children.* London, UK: Chapman Hall.

Pennington, B. F., Gilger, J. W., Olson, R. K., & DeFries, J. C. (1992). The external validity of age- versus IQ-discrepancy definitions of reading disability: Lessons from a twin study. *Journal of Learning Disabilities, 25,* 562–573.

Pennington, B. F., & Lefly, D. L. (2001). Early reading development in children at family risk for dyslexia. *Child Development, 72,* 816–833.

Perfetti, C. (1985). *Reading ability.* New York: Oxford University Press.

Prior, M., Sanson, A., Smart, D., & Oberklaid, F. (1995). Reading disability in an Australian community sample. *Australian Journal of Psychology, 47,* 32–37.

Rack, J. P., Snowling, M. J., & Olson, R. K. (1992). The nonword reading deficit in developmental dyslexia: A review. *Reading Research Quarterly, 27,* 28–53.

Rashotte, C. A., & Torgesen, J. K. (1985). Repeated reading and reading fluency in reading disabled children. *Reading Research Quarterly, 20,* 180–188.

Rees, N. S. (1974). The speech pathologist and the reading process. *ASHA, 16,* 255–258.

Richardson, S. O. (1992). Historical perspectives on dyslexia. *Journal of Learning Disabilities, 25,* 40–47.

Rodgers, B. (1983). The identification and prevalence of specific reading retardation. *British Journal of Educational Psychology, 3,* 369–373.

Romani, C., DiBetta, A. M., Tsouknida, E., & Olson, A. (2008). Lexical and nonlexical processing in developmental dyslexia: A case for different resources and different impairments. *Cognitive Neuropsychology, 25,* 798–830.

Rudel, R. (1985). The definition of dyslexia: Language and motor deficits. In F. H. Duffy & N. Geschwind (Eds.), *Dyslexia: A neuroscientific approach to clinical evaluation* (pp. 33–53). Boston: Little, Brown and Company.

Rutter, M., Caspi, A., Fergusson, D., Horwood, J., Goodman, R., Maughan, B., et al. (2004). Sex differences in developmental reading disability: New findings from 4 epidemiological studies. *Journal of the American Medical Association, 291,* 2007–2012.

Rutter, M., Tizard, J., & Whitmore, K. (1970). *Education, health and behaviour.* London: Longman.

Rutter, M., & Yule, W. (1975). The concept of specific reading retardation. *Journal of Child Psychology and Psychiatry, 16,* 181–197.

Samuels, S. J. (1977). The method of reacted reading. *The Reading Teacher, 32,* 403–408.

Scarborough, H. S. (1990). Very early language deficits in dyslexic children. *Child Development, 61,* 1728–1743.

Scarborough, H. S. (1991). Early syntactic development of dyslexic children. *Annals of Dyslexia, 41,* 207–220.

Scruggs, T. E., & Mastropieri, M. A. (2002). On babies and bathwater: Addressing the problems of identification of learning disabilities. *Learning Disability Quarterly, 25,* 155–159.

Semel, E., Wiig, E., & Secord, W. (2003). *Clinical Evaluation of Language Fundamentals–IV.* San Antonio, TX: The Psychological Corporation.

Shankweiler, D., Crain, S., Katz, L., Fowler, A. E., Liberman, A. M., Brady, S. A., Thornton, R., Lundquist, E., Dreyer, L., Fletcher, J. M., Stuebing, K. K., Shaywitz, S. E., & Shaywitz, B. A. (1995). Cognitive profiles of reading-disabled children: Comparison of language skills in phonology, morphology, and syntax. *Psychological Science, 6,* 149–156.

Shankweiler, D., & Liberman, I. (1972). Misreading: A search for causes. In J. Kavanaugh & I. Mattingly (Eds.), *Language by ear and by eye* (pp. 293–317). Cambridge, MA: MIT Press.

Share, D. (1996). Word recognition and spelling processes in specific reading disabled and garden-variety poor readers. *Dyslexia: An International Journal of Research and Practice, 2,* 167–174.

Share, D. L., McGee, R., McKenzie, D., Williams, S., & Silva, P. (1987). Further evidence relating to the distinction between specific reading retardation and general reading backwardness. *British Journal of Developmental Psychology, 5,* 35–44.

Share, D. L., & Silva, P. A. (2003). Gender bias in IQ-discrepancy and post-discrepancy definitions of reading disability. *Journal of Learning Disabilities, 36,* 4–14.

Shaywitz, S. E. (2003). *Overcoming dyslexia: A new and complete science-based program for reading problems at any level.* New York: Alfred A. Knopf.

Shaywitz, S. E., Escobar, M. D., Shaywitz, B. A., Fletcher, J. M., & Makuch, R. (1992). Evidence that dyslexia may represent the lower tail of a normal distribution of reading ability. *The New England Journal of Medicine, 326,* 145–193.

Shaywitz, B. A., Fletcher, J. M., Holahan, J. M., & Shaywitz, S. E. (1992). Discrepancy compared to low achievement definitions of reading disability: Results from the Connecticut Longitudinal Study. *Journal of Learning Disabilities, 25,* 639–648.

Shaywitz, S. E., Shaywitz, B. A., Fletcher, J. M., & Escobar, M. D. (1990). Prevalence of reading disability in boys and girls. *Journal of the American Medical Association, 264,* 998–1002.

Siegel, L. S. (1984). A longitudinal study of a hyperlexic child: Hyperlexia as a language disorder. *Neuropsychologia, 22,* 577–585.

Siegel, L. S. (1989). IQ is irrelevant to the definition of learning disabilities. *Journal of Learning Disabilities, 22,* 469–478.

Siegel, L. S. (1992). An evaluation of the discrepancy definition of dyslexia. *Journal of Learning Disabilities, 25,* 618–629.

Siegel, L. S., & Smythe, I. S. (2005). Reading disability with special attention to gender issues. *Journal of Learning Disabilities, 38,* 473–477.

Silberberg, N. E., & Silberberg, M. C. (1967). Hyperlexia: Specific word recognition skills in young children. *Exceptional Children, 34,* 41–42.

Snowling, M. (1981). Phonemic deficits in developmental dyslexia. *Psychological Research, 43,* 219–234.

Snowling, M. J., Gallagher, A., & Frith, U. (2003). Family risk of dyslexia is continuous: Individual differences in precursors of reading skill. *Child Development, 74,* 358–373.

Spear-Swerling, L., & Sternberg, R. J. (1996). *Off track: When poor readers become "learning disabled."* Boulder, CO: Westview Press.

Stage, S., Abbott, R. D., Jenkins, J., & Berninger, V. (2003). Predicting response to early reading intervention using verbal IQ-word reading related language abilities, attention ratings, and verbal-IQ-word reading discrepancy: Failure to validate discrepancy. *Journal of Learning Disabilities, 36,* 24–33.

Stanovich, K. E. (1988). The right and wrong places to look for the cognitive locus of reading disability. *Annals of Dyslexia, 38,* 154–177.

Stanovich, K. E. (1991). Discrepancy definitions of reading disability: Has intelligence led us astray? *Reading Research Quarterly, 26,* 7–29.

Stanovich, K. E. (1997). Toward a more inclusive definition of dyslexia. *Dyslexia: An International Journal of Theory and Practice, 2,* 154–166.

Stanovich, K. E. (2005). The future of a mistake: Will discrepancy measurement continue to make the learning disabilities field a pseudoscience? *Learning Disabilities Quarterly, 28,* 103–106.

Stanovich, K. E., Nathan, R. G., & Zolman, J. E. (1988). The developmental lag hypothesis in reading: Longitudinal and matched reading-level comparisons. *Child Development, 59,* 71–86.

Stanovich, K. E., & Siegel, L. S. (1994). The phenotypic performance profile of reading-disabled children: A regression-based test of the phonological-core variable-difference model. *Journal of Educational Psychology, 86,* 24–53.

Stanovich, K. E., Siegel, L. S., & Gottardo, A. (1997). Converging evidence for phonological and surface subtypes of reading disability. *Journal of Educational Psychology, 89,* 114–127.

Stark, J. (1975). Reading failure: A language-based problem. *ASHA, 17,* 832–834.

Steveson, J., Graham, P., Fredman, G., & McLoughlin, V. (1987). A twin study of genetic influences on reading and spelling ability and disability. *Journal of Child Psychology and Psychiatry, 28,* 229–247.

Stuebing, K. K., Fletcher, J. M., LeDoux, J. M., Lyon, G. R., Shaywitz, S. E., & Shaywitz, B. A. (2002). Validity of IQ-discrepancy classifications of reading disabilities: A meta-analysis. *American Educational Research Journal, 39,* 469–518.

Thomson, M. (1984). *Developmental dyslexia: Its nature, assessment and remediation.* London: Edward Arnold.

Tomblin, J. B., Records, N. L., & Zhang, X. (1996). A system for the diagnosis of specific language impairment in kindergarten children. *Journal of Speech and Hearing Research, 39,* 1284–1294.

Torgesen, J. K. (1991). Learning disabilities: Historical and conceptual issues. In B. Wong (Ed.), *Learning about learning disabilities* (pp. 3–37). Orlando, FL: Academic Press.

Torgesen, J. K., Wagner, R. K., & Rashotte, C. A. (1997). *Preventing reading disabilities: Results from 2 1/2 years of intervention.* Paper presented at the Society for the Scientific Study of Reading, Chicago.

van der Wissel, A., & Zegers, F. E. (1985). Reading retardation revisited. *British Journal of Developmental Psychology, 3,* 3–9.

Vellutino, F. (1979). *Dyslexia: Theory and research.* Cambridge, MA: MIT Press.

Vellutino, F. R., Scanlon, D. M., & Lyon, G. R. (2000). Differentiating between difficult-to-remediate and readily remediated poor readers: More evidence against the IQ-achievement discrepancy definition of reading disability. *Journal of Learning Disabilities, 33,* 223–238.

Vellutino, F. R., Scanlon, D. M., Sipay, E. R., Small, S. G., Chen, R., Pratt, A., & Denckla, M. B. (1996). Cognitive profiles of difficult-to-remediate and readily remediated poor readers: Early intervention as a vehicle for distinguishing between cognitive and experiential deficits as basic causes of specific reading disabilities. *Journal of Educational Psychology, 88,* 601–638.

Wadsworth, S. J., Olson, R. K., Pennington, B. F., & DeFries, J. C. (2000). Differential genetic etiology of reading disability as a function of IQ. *Journal of Learning Disabilities, 33,* 192–199.

Wagner, R. K., & Torgesen, J. K. (1987). The nature of phonological processing and its causal role in the acquisition of reading skills. *Psychological Bulletin, 101,* 1–21.

Wallach, G. P., & Butler, K. G. (Eds.). (1994). *Language learning disabilities in school-age children and adolescents.* Boston: Allyn & Bacon.

Wechsler, D. (2009). *Wechsler Individual Achievement Test-Third Edition.* San Antonio, TX: PsychCorp.

Willcutt, E. G., & Pennington, B. F. (2000). Comorbidity of reading disability and attention-deficit/hyperactivity disorder. *Journal of Learning Disabilities, 33,* 179–191.

Wilson, A. M., & Lesaux, N. K. (2001). Persistence of phonological processing deficits in college students with dyslexia who have age-appropriate reading skills. *Journal of Learning Disabilities, 34,* 394–400.

Wimmer, H. (1993). Characteristics of developmental dyslexia in a regular writing system. *Applied Psycholinguistics, 14,* 1–33.

Wolf, M., & Bowers, P. G. (1999). The double-deficit hypothesis for the development dyslexias. *Journal of Educational Psychology, 91,* 415–438.

Wolf, M., Bowers, P., & Biddle, K. (2000). Naming-speed processes, timing, and reading: A conceptual review. *Journal of Learning Disabilities, 33,* 387–407.

Wolf, M., & Obregon, M. (1989). *88 children in search of a name: A 5-year investigation of rate, word-retrieval, and vocabulary in reading development and dyslexia.* Paper presented at the Society for Research in Child Development, Kansas City, MO.

Woodcock, R. (1991). *Woodcock Language Proficiency Battery-Revised.* Chicago: Riverside.

Woodcock, R. W. (1998). *Woodcock Reading Mastery Tests-Revised Normative Update.* Circle Pines, MN: American Guidance Service.

Yule, W., Rutter, M., Berger, M., & Thompson, J. (1974). Over and under achievement in reading: Distribution in the general population. *British Journal of Educational Psychology, 44,* 1–12.

Chapter 4

Causes of Reading Disabilities

Hugh W. Catts, Alan G. Kamhi, and Suzanne M. Adlof

When a parent or teacher learns that a child has a reading disability, he or she inevitably wants to know what has caused the disability. Providing answers about the causes of reading disabilities can be a difficult task. Reading is a complex ability, and breakdowns in the acquisition of this ability can be difficult to understand. Research, however, has provided some answers concerning the causes of reading disabilities. This work indicates that reading disabilities are the result of an interplay of intrinsic and extrinsic factors. Intrinsic factors refer to internal or child-based processes, whereas extrinsic factors concern environmental variables. Definitions have emphasized the intrinsic or constitutional nature of reading disabilities, and the majority of the research has been driven by the quest to find the intrinsic cause of reading problems. As a result, a large body of evidence now indicates the significance of biological factors in reading development and disorders.

Extrinsic factors also appear to play a role in reading disabilities. Although definitions generally exclude factors such as a lack of literacy experience or inadequate instruction from being a cause of reading disabilities, many children diagnosed with reading disabilities have experiential or instructional deficits. These deficits may be the initial cause of reading problems, or they may occur secondary to intrinsic factors.

EXTRINSIC CAUSES OF READING DISABILITIES

To learn to read, children need exposure to print, explicit instruction in how print works, and opportunity to practice their reading skills (Adams, 1990). Without opportunity and instruction, children will not learn to be skilled readers. Although literacy experience is critical for reading acquisition, it generally has been neglected in causal explanations of reading disabilities. Most definitions exclude extrinsic factors such as lack of opportunity or inadequate instruction as causes of reading disabilities. However, in many cases practitioners and researchers have paid only limited attention to whether poor readers have met this exclusionary criterion. Variability in literacy experience often goes unnoticed and can potentially influence reading disabilities.

Unfortunately, the full extent of the contribution of limited literacy experiences to reading disabilities is not known. Because environmental factors have been excluded from definitions of reading disabilities, most researchers in the field have not examined literacy experience in relationship to reading disabilities. Spear-Swerling and Sternberg (1996) noted that, for the most part, the study of the influence of environmental factors on reading disabilities has come from outside the field of reading disabilities. One body of research that is relevant to the role of literacy experience in reading disabilities concerns the impact of early joint book reading on subsequent reading development.

Early Literacy Experience

In Chapter 2, we noted that it is quite common in many homes to find parents reading to their children from an early age. Whereas such practice occurs frequently in mainstream homes, some children enter school without this experience. It seems reasonable to ask about the possible causal role a lack of early joint book reading might play in later reading problems. Although there are many anecdotal claims of children with limited exposure to print having difficulty learning to read (e.g., Spear-Swerling & Sternberg, 1996), few studies have actually examined the influence of a lack of early literacy experience on reading disabilities. As discussed in Chapter 2, research has focused primarily on the relationship between joint book reading and reading development in the general population. Overall, this research has shown only a weak association between early joint book reading and subsequent reading development. Meta-analyses of this literature (Bus, van Ijzendoorn, & Pellegrini, 1995; Mol & Bus, 2010; Scarborough & Dobrich, 1994) indicate that on the average, joint book reading accounts for only about 8 percent of the variance in reading outcome measures. Furthermore, this effect appears to decrease with age, suggesting that school instruction in reading may compensate for a lack of home literacy experience.

Although an absence of joint book reading during the preschool years does not seem to be a primary cause of reading disabilities, it may still play some role in reading problems. For example, a lack of early literacy experience may be particularly detrimental to children with other risk factors. Children from low socioeconomic status backgrounds and/or those with language impairments may be at increased risk for reading disabilities if they have not had home literacy experiences.

Reading Instruction

Because reading is a skill that, for the most part, must be taught, differences in the quality and/or quantity of instruction clearly affect reading development. However, the role instructional factors play in reading disabilities is not well understood. Traditionally, it was thought that instructional factors had little causal impact on reading disabilities. By definition, children with reading disabilities (RD) do not have instructional deficits. However, as noted in Chapter 3, this exclusionary criterion was seldom carefully assessed. Typically, if poor readers were in a grade that was appropriate for their age and they attended school regularly, they were assumed to have had the necessary instruction to learn to read. Such procedures, however, allowed for considerable variability in the quality and quantity of instruction that poor readers may have received.

The response to intervention (RTI) framework introduced in Chapter 3 is a further attempt to rule out lack of appropriate reading instruction as a cause of reading disabilities (Fuchs & Fuchs, 1998; Fuchs, Fuchs, & Speece, 2002). Recall, that in an RTI framework, children are provided with high-quality classroom-based reading instruction and are assessed periodically to evaluate their progress. Children who fail to progress adequately are further provided with supplemental reading instruction. It is only after children fail to make adequate progress with this additional instruction that they may be evaluated for reading disabilities. Thus, the RTI approach may be able to reduce or eliminate instructional inadequacies as a cause of reading disabilities.

Some of the initial support for the usefulness of the RTI framework in ruling out instructional deficits came from work by Vellutino and his colleagues (Scanlon & Vellutino, 1996, 1997; Vellutino et al., 1996). In a large longitudinal investigation, they examined the role of instructional deficits in reading disabilities. From a total sample of 1,400 kindergarten children attending middle- to upper-middle-class schools, they identified 151 children who were at risk for reading disabilities based on poor performance on a letter identification test (Scanlon & Vellutino, 1996, 1997). These children also met exclusionary criteria that included no sensory or intellectual handicaps. Researchers conducted classroom observations in which they evaluated the nature of reading/literacy instruction these children were receiving. They noted, for example, the materials being used (e.g., books, letters, spoken language), the activities in which the children were engaged (e.g., reading text, phoneme awareness, letter naming), and the expected responses of the children (e.g., reading, writing, looking). The participants were subsequently followed into first grade and were divided into those who were good, average, or poor readers based on teacher ratings and tests of reading achievement. Comparisons between outcome groups indicated that the at-risk children who became good readers received more instruction in analyzing the structural (sound and spelling) aspects of spoken and written language than did the other outcome groups. Reader groups did not differ, however, on variables such as time spent in reading connected text or in discussions of word meanings. The researchers concluded that differences in instruction do make a difference in whether at-risk children become reading disabled.

More direct evidence of the role instructional variables play in reading disabilities comes from another component of this longitudinal investigation (Vellutino et al., 1996). As part of their study, Vellutino and his colleagues provided remedial instruction to those children in their sample who had significant reading problems at mid-first grade. These children performed at or below the 15th percentile on tests of reading achievement and met typical exclusionary criteria for reading disabilities. During the second semester of first grade, the children received daily one-to-one tutoring (30 minutes per session) for a minimum of 16 weeks (typically 70 to 80 sessions). It was thought that this remedial instruction might be sufficient to eliminate reading problems in those children who suffered from instructional or experiential deficits, rather than intrinsic problems. Vellutino and his colleagues found that after remedial instruction, 67 percent of the poor readers scored in the average or above-average range on tests of reading achievement. They concluded that among children meeting typical exclusionary criteria for reading disabilities, there will be many who have no intrinsic problems, but who have had inadequate instruction or opportunity to learn to read.

Vellutino and colleagues recently replicated these findings in another study, which identified children at risk in kindergarten (Vellutino, Scanlon, Small, & Fanuele, 2006). In this study, at-risk kindergarten students received small-group instruction two to three days per week for the kindergarten year, and by the beginning of the first grade year, 50 percent of them were determined to be no longer at risk. Those who were still at risk received supplemental one-on-one instruction throughout the first grade year. Over half the children who received supplemental instruction in first grade were performing in the average range in third grade. Again, the authors concluded that providing supplemental instruction (in kindergarten alone or in kindergarten and first grade) helped distinguish experiential deficits, which they suggest may be more easily remediated, from biological deficits, which may be more difficult to remediate.

Although these studies point to the significance of extrinsic factors in reading disabilities, strong conclusions would be premature. Data showing that instruction can improve reading does not necessarily mean that instructional or experiential deficits were the cause of the reading problem in the first place. Children with phonological processing deficits or other intrinsic deficiencies may also benefit from instruction. In support of their conclusions, Vellutino and coworkers (1996, 2006) did show that the "readily remediated" poor readers had fewer problems in phonological processing than poor readers who were difficult to remediate. However, some of the former poor readers could have had mild phonological processing deficits or other intrinsic problems that were amenable to instruction. Also, it is not yet known whether the children who responded to supplemental instruction maintained their skills over the long term. Clearly, more research is needed to understand the role of instructional variables in reading disabilities.

Matthew Effects

Although studies have not yet clearly shown that extrinsic factors play a primary role in reading disabilities, these factors could function to maintain, and in some instances increase, the severity of reading problems. In fact, some have argued that merely considering children to be reading disabled can set into motion a host of negative consequences that can influence reading development (Cole, 1987; Spear-Swerling & Sternberg, 1996). Spear-Swerling and Sternberg (1996) maintain that placing children in low-ability or remedial reading groups or in special education classes can itself bring on further reading problems. Children in low-ability or special reading groups often have low expectations placed on them by their teachers and parents. Their low-ability peers offer them little support, and their teachers provide them with little challenge. These children become less motivated to read and may have other attentional or behavior problems. Spear-Swerling and Sternberg argued that these factors can actually lead to children receiving less instruction and practice in reading. In turn, these children may fall farther and farther behind their peers.

Stanovich (1986, 1988) used the term *Matthew effects* to describe the negative consequences associated with failure in reading. The term comes from a biblical passage in the book of Matthew that comments on how the rich get richer and the poor get poorer. Stanovich argued that because of factors such as low expectations, limited practice, and poor motivation, those who get off to a slow start in reading often get caught in a downward spiral of failure. Spear-Swerling and Sternberg (1994) described these factors as a kind of swamp. They stated that "once children have entered the 'swamp' of negative expectations, lowered motivation, and limited practice, it may be very difficult for them to get back on the right road" (p. 99).

One particularly relevant consequence of Matthew effects is language problems. Because reading is a key source for new vocabulary and advanced grammatical and discourse knowledge, children who do not read much will often begin to fall behind their peers in language development (e.g., Stothard, Snowling, Bishop, Chipchase, & Kaplan, 1998). Thus, as a result of their limited reading experience, poor readers who do not necessarily have a developmental language disorder will soon develop language problems.

INTRINSIC CAUSES OF READING DISABILITIES

Factors intrinsic to the child have traditionally played a prominent role in causal explanations of reading disabilities. Consequently, considerable research attention has been devoted to the study of these factors. This research has examined the genetic and neurological bases of reading disabilities, as well as the cognitive-perceptual deficits that are believed to result from these bases.

Genetic Basis

From the earliest reports, it was recognized that reading disabilities often ran in families (Hallgren, 1950; Hinshelwood, 1917). For example, Hinshelwood (1917) noted that reading disabilities were often found in siblings and/or multiple generations of a family. Later investigations confirmed the familial basis of reading disabilities (Finucci, Gutherie, Childs, Abbey, & Childs, 1976; Gilger, Pennington, & DeFries, 1991; Vogler, DeFries, & Decker, 1985). Taken together, these studies have shown that a brother or sister of an child with RD has an approximately 40 percent chance of having a reading disability, and a parent of an child with RD has a 30 to 40 percent likelihood of having a history of a reading disability. Some studies have further suggested that familial risk for reading disabilities may be continuous as opposed to discrete (Boets et al., 2010; Pennington & Lefly, 2001; Snowling, Gallagher, & Frith, 2003). That is, not only do many high-risk family members have reading disabilities, but also many of those who do not, nevertheless show some deficits in reading and reading-related abilities.

Although reading disabilities are clearly familial, this does not mean that they are necessarily heritable. Bad table manners and cake recipes are among the common examples of things that run in families, but are not genetically transmitted. To determine the heritability of a complex behavior such as reading disability, researchers often examine identical and fraternal twins (DeFries & Alarcon, 1996; Light & DeFries, 1995). Identical or monozygotic twins share all the same genes, whereas fraternal or dizygotic twins only share half their genes on average. If a reading disability is heritable, it should co-occurrence in identical twins more often than it does in fraternal twins. This is essentially what researchers have found. In a representative study, Light and DeFries (1995) reported that in 68 percent of identical twins, when one twin had a reading disability, the other twin also had a reading problem. The corresponding rate in fraternal twins was 40 percent. Although these results support the heritability of reading disabilities, they also indicate that genes do not act alone. The co-occurence of reading problems in identical twins is far from 100 percent, suggesting that factors other than genetics also contribute to reading development. Thus, just because an individual has the gene(s) for reading disabilities, does not mean he or she will develop reading problems; rather, it indicates that the likelihood of having the disorder is much higher.

Recent twin studies have provided interesting insights into the interactions between genetic factors and environmental factors such as schooling in explaining literacy outcomes. For example, Samuelsson and colleagues examined emergent literacy and early reading skills in a two-year longitudinal study of preschool twins from the United States, Australia, and Scandinavia (Samuelsson et al., 2007). In Scandinavia children do not begin formal education until age 7 (first grade), whereas in the United States and Australia, children begin school in kindergarten. In Australia, the kindergarten curriculum is nationally standardized, and all children attend school for 7 hours per day. In the United States, the kindergarten curriculum is locally determined and more variable, and most children in the sample attended half-day kindergarten. Analyses of genetic and environmental contributions to emergent literacy skills in preschool revealed very similar patterns across the three samples. Genetic factors contributed largely to phonological awareness, rapid naming, and verbal memory, whereas shared environment contributed strongly to vocabulary and print knowledge. However, analyses of literacy skills at the end of kindergarten revealed differences between the U.S. and Australian samples (the Scandinavian children were not analyzed because they had not yet started school). In the Australian sample, there was a higher genetic and lower shared environmental influence relative to the U.S. samples. The authors suggested that this was explained by the greater amount of literacy experience and more consistent instructional practices for the Australian children compared to the U.S. children.

Another study by Petrill and colleagues examined the role of genes and environment on growth in reading skills between kindergarten and second grade in a sample of twins based in Ohio (Petrill et al., 2010). Although the estimates of influence varied between different measures of literacy skills, the general pattern of results across all measures suggests that genes influence initial level of performance at kindergarten, whereas shared environment influences growth between kindergarten and second grade. These results underscore the role of environment and instruction in the developmental trajectories of individuals with genetic risk for reading difficulties.

Researchers have also examined data from family studies to determine if reading disabilities are the result of a single gene or a combination of multiple genes (Pennington et al., 1991). Current thinking is that a number of genes work together in an additive manner to influence reading ability (Pennington & Gilger, 1996; Plomin & Kovas, 2005). The genes that work together are referred to as *quantitative trait loci* (QTLs). Each QTL by itself may have a very small effect on reading, but in combination with others the cumulative effects become more significant. Unlike single-gene disorders, in which having the gene guarantees the outcome of the disorder, QTLs influence the probability of reading difficulties. Furthermore, QTLs influence the full distribution of reading ability in general, not just reading disability. Individuals with favorable forms of these genes are believed to have a biological advantage for learning to read, whereas those with unfavorable forms of these genes are at risk for reading disabilities. Of course, these genes are not specific to reading (Plomin & Kovas, 2005). Reading is a relatively new human ability and not one specifically coded in our genes. However, some research suggests that the genes associated with reading are ones that code phonological processing abilities, abilities known to underlie word decoding (Byrne et al., 2002). Other research suggests that the genes that underlie word reading and phonological difficulties could differ from those that underlie nonphonological oral language and comprehension skills (Bishop, Adams, & Norbury, 2006; Keenan, Betjemann, Wadsworth, DeFries, & Olson, 2006).

Finally, studies have sought to determine which chromosomes contain genes associated with reading ability/disability (e.g., Grigorenko et al., 2001; Morris et al., 2000). This work has identified regions on chromosomes 1, 6, and 15 as possible locations for important genes related to reading (see Raskind, 2001; Wood & Grigorenko, 2001), and four candidate genes have been identified in these regions as susceptibility candidates for reading disabilities: *DYX1C1, DCDC2, KIAA0319,* and *ROBO1* (see Paracchini, Scerri, & Monaco, 2007). Recently, Meaburn and colleagues scanned over 100,000 possible DNA markers (or QTLs) to examine their correlation with reading disability. Results suggested that 10 DNA markers are significantly related to reading ability, although each one explained less than 1 percent of the variance in reading outcomes (Meaburn, Harlaar, Craig, Schalkwyk, & Plomin, 2008). In the coming years, we will surely learn more about the genetic basis of reading disabilities, which in turn should affect early identification and prevention of these disabilities.

Neurological Basis

Considerable attention has been devoted to the study of the brain and its role in reading disabilities. Early accounts suggested that children with RD lacked cerebral dominance for language (Orton, 1937). In most individuals, the left cortical hemisphere plays a more dominant role in language processing than does the right. Orton (1937) and other early investigators proposed that in children with RD, the right hemisphere shared language dominance with the left (i.e., mixed dominance) or was the dominant hemisphere for language. To test this proposal, researchers initially had to rely on behavioral data, such as handedness. Because left-handedness is some-times associated with mixed or right dominance, the study of handedness was seen as a way to examine brain laterality in individuals with RD. This work, however, has found no consistent association between handedness and reading disabilities (see Bishop, 1990; Bryden, 1982).

Other behavioral techniques have also been used to study laterality differences in reading disabilities. These have included dichotic listening (Obrzat, 1979; Satz & Sparrow, 1970), visual split-field (Olson, 1973), and time-sharing studies (Obrzat, 1979; Stellern, Collins, & Bayne, 1987). This research has been fraught with mixed results and methodological shortcomings (Obrzat, Hynd, & Boliek, 1986; Satz, 1977). However, most reviews of this work (e.g., Bryden, 1982; Gerber, 1993) have concluded that the evidence seems to support the view that individuals with RD, as a group, show less left dominance for language than normal readers.

Researchers have also directly examined the brains of individuals with RD for evidence of abnormalities. For example, Galaburda and his colleagues conducted postmortem examinations of the brains of a small number of individuals who had previously been diagnosed as dyslexic (Galaburda, 1988; Galaburda, Corsiglia, Rosen, & Sherman, 1987; Galaburda, Sherman, Rosen, Aboitiz, & Geschwind, 1985). One frequently cited finding from these studies concerned the planum temporale, a structure in the temporal lobe thought to be involved in language processing (Foundas, Leonard, Gilmore, Fennell, & Heilman, 1994). Galaburda reported that in nondisabled individuals the planum is generally larger in the left hemisphere than in the right, but in the brains of individuals with dyslexia, the temporal plana were symmetrical. This symmetry was accounted for, not by a smaller than normal left planum, but rather a larger than expected right planum.

Galaburda and his team also identified microscopic anomalies in the brains of dyslexics. These involved focal dysplasias that are nests of neurons in areas of the cortex where they are seldom found. Galaburda (1991) suggested that in dyslexics, neuronal pruning necessary to re-fine neuron networks and correct developmental errors may be disrupted. This disruption could account for the larger than normal right planum as well as the focal dysplasias.

Advancements in technology have provided additional ways to examine the brain structure of individuals with RD in vivo. Of primary significance is *magnetic resonance imaging* (MRI), a noninvasive technique that uses a strong magnetic field and high-frequency radio waves to pro-duce precise two- or three-dimensional images of the brain. These images are much superior to those available by x-ray technology. A number of studies have employed MRI techniques to examine the relationship between planum temporale symmetry and reading disabilities (Eckert et al., 2003; Hynd, Semrud-Clikeman, Lorys, Novey, & Eliopulos, 1990; Leonard et al., 2002; Leonard & Eckert, 2008; Robichon, Levrier, Farnarier, & Habib, 2000; Rumsey, Donahue, et al., 1997). These studies have indicated that the relationship might be more complex than previously thought based on postmortem examinations. Leonard and Eckert (2008) traced this complexity back to the language and cognitive profiles of participants with RD. They noted that the atypical pattern of planum temporale symmetry was found most often in individuals who would fit the mixed deficit or "garden-variety" poor reader profile, with word reading deficits accompanied by deficits in several other aspects of oral language. Individuals with specific word-reading and phonological deficits tend to show normal, or even exaggerated, leftward asymmetry (Leonard & Eckert, 2008).

Studies have reported a host of other structural differences between normal individuals and those with RD in other regions of the temporal lobe (Brown et al., 2001; Hynd et al., 1990; Jernigan, Hesselink, Sowell, & Tallal, 1991), in the corpus callosum (Duara et al., 1991; Hynd et al., 1995; Lubs et al., 1991; but see Pennington et al., 1999), in the inferior parietal lobe (Brown et al., 2001; Lubs et al., 1991; Robichon et al., 2000), and in the cerebellum (Eckert et al., 2003;

Rae et al., 2002). However, it is still not clear whether these anatomical differences are the cause of reading problems or a result of them.

Functional aspects of the brain have also been examined in individuals with RD using neuroimaging techniques (e.g., Flowers, Wood, & Naylor, 1991; Pauleau et al., 2001). Hemodynamic techniques measure contrast in blood flow across various regions of the brain as an indication of the level of activity of these areas during specific tasks. One such technique is functional MRI (fMRI). Because differences in blood oxygenation correspond to differences in magnetic resonance, fMRI can provide a noninvasive measure of blood flow and regional brain activity. Another technique is *positron emission tomography* (PET), in which regional blood flow is monitored by recording the distribution of cerebral radioactivity following the intravenous injection of a radioactive isotope. A third, nonhemodynamic imaging technique known as *magnetic source imaging* (MSI) has also been employed to examine sources of brain activation differences. MSI combines MRI with *magnetoencephalography* (MEG) techniques, which records magnetic fields produced by electrical activity in the brain. MEG is traditionally known for its excellent temporal resolution, but when combined with MRI, good spatial resolution is possible for examining sources of brain activity during reading and other tasks.

In a review of studies using these imaging technologies, Sandak and colleagues identified three functional neural systems involved in reading (Sandak, Mencl, Frost, & Pugh, 2004). The first two systems are located in the posterior regions of the left hemisphere. The dorsal (temporoparietal) system is thought to be involved with phonological processing and mapping letters to sounds, whereas the ventral (occipitotemporal) system is thought to be involved in the processing of visual word forms in skilled reading. The third (frontal) system, located in the inferior frontal gyrus, is also thought to be involved with effortful phonological decoding.

Several studies have reported significant differences in activation of these systems during reading-related tasks for dyslexics and controls. Most often, studies report significant underactivation for dyslexics versus controls in the dorsal and ventral systems of the left hemisphere. Some studies have also reported that dyslexics show overactivation in the frontal system and in some areas of the right hemisphere relative to controls. For example, an fMRI study by Shaywitz and colleagues reported that children with dyslexia had significantly less activation in the temporoparietal area and significantly more activation in the inferior frontal gyrus than did nonimpaired readers (e.g., Shaywitz et al., 1998). Another fMRI study by Eden and colleagues found that adult dyslexics differed from controls in task-related functional activation of the magnocellular layers of the lateral geniculate nucleus located at the junction of the occipital and temporal lobes (Eden et al., 1996). This area appears to be responsive to visual motion and has also been implicated in behavioral studies of dyslexia (described later in the chapter). Studies using PET scan technology have found that dyslexics show less activation than controls in the mid- to posterior temporal cortex bilaterally and in the left inferior parietal cortex during reading and phonological processing tasks (Paulesu et al., 1995; Paulesu, Frith, & Frackowiak, 1993; Rumsey et al., 1997). Paulesu and colleagues (2001) have further shown that individuals with dyslexia from three countries (each with a different language) had the same pattern of reduced blood flow in these regions during reading and phonetic tasks.

In studies using MSI technology, Salmelin and colleagues found that in a reading task, dyslexic adults, as compared to controls, failed to show appropriate cortical activity in the left occipital and temporal lobes (Salmelin, Service, Kiesila, Uutela, & Salonen, 1996). These findings have been extended by Simos and his group (Simos, Breier, Fletcher, Bergman, & Papanicolaou, 2000; Simos et al., 2000). They found that children with RD demonstrated reduced cortical activity in the posterior superior temporal gyrus and inferior parietal areas of the left hemisphere and increased activity in the corresponding areas of the right hemisphere in word and nonword reading tasks. They argued that these differences might underlie group differences in phonological processing. In a follow-up study, they showed that short-term reading intervention with children with RD resulted in these children having a more normal profile of left temporoparietal activity during reading tasks (Simos, Fletcher, Bergman, et al., 2002).

Other studies have also provided converging evidence for underactivation in left hemisphere occipitotemporal and temporoparietal regions prior to reading intervention and more normal activation patterns following a period of intensive intervention (e.g., Shaywitz et al., 2004; Meyler, Keller, Cherkassky, Gabrieli, & Just, 2008). In addition, Keller and Just (2009) reported that intensive intervention improves the structural organization of the white matter connections between reading-related regions of the brain in poor readers.

In summary, numerous differences have been found in the brain structure and function of individuals with RD as compared to normal readers. Although group differences have been uncovered, considerable individual variation exists. In addition, the abnormalities that have been observed are unlike the focal lesions found in acquired reading disorders; instead, they appear to be more diffuse, involving a variety of structures in the brain. These findings are consistent with the view that individual differences in neurological development, not neurological deficits, are associated with many cases of developmental reading disabilities.

Whereas brain anomalies are present in many individuals with dyslexia, it is still unclear how they are related to reading disabilities and to the cognitive–perceptual abilities associated with them. Many assume that the observed brain differences are causally linked to reading disabilities. Those who find differences in posterior regions (e.g., occipital lobe) of the brain propose that visual impairments cause reading problems, whereas those who identify temporoparietal differences have argued that language impairments underlie reading problems. Alternatively, it may be that dyslexia involves a diffuse pattern of brain abnormalities with diverse cognitive–behavioral consequences, only some of which are the causes of reading disabilities.

It might also be argued that some of the observed brain abnormalities could be the result rather than the cause of reading problems. Learning to read in a different way should result in differences in brain function and structure. Thus, the brain differences seen in some poor readers, especially older poor readers, may reflect years of poor reading rather than the cause of the poor reading. Studies showing that brain structure and functional activation patterns become more normal following intervention can be interpreted as evidence for this hypothesis. On the other hand, there is also emerging evidence that some brain differences may be observed early in the reading acquisition process, or even in infancy. For example, Simos and colleagues (Simos, Fletcher, & Foorman, et al., 2002) have reported brain abnormalities in at-risk 6- to 7-year-old children that are similar to those observed in older poor readers. Other investigators using electroencephalography (EEG) technologies have shown that infants at family risk of dyslexia (Guttorm, Leppänen, Tolvanen, & Lyytinen, 2003) or who later manifest dyslexia at age 8 (Molfese, 2000) show significantly different neural responses to auditory stimuli than typically developing infants. Hopefully, the research conducted in the next few years will answer the question of whether brain abnormalities cause reading problems or whether these abnormalities are primarily correlates or consequences of reading disabilities.

Visually Based Deficits

Because the visual system is an important sensory system for reading, it should not be surprising that visually based explanations of reading disabilities have a long history in the field (Bronner,

1917; Fildes, 1922; Frostig, 1968). Many early reported cases of reading disabilities were seen by ophthalmologists, who explained these problems in terms of visual difficulties. As noted in Chapter 3, the term "word blindness" was frequently used to refer to reading disabilities. Several early clinics for reading difficulties also bore the name "Word Blind" in their title. Since these early accounts, there have been numerous attempts to uncover the visual deficits that might cause reading disabilities. These attempts have considered reversal errors, problems in visual memory, erratic eye movements, light sensitivity, and visual timing deficits.

REVERSAL ERRORS.   Over the years, much attention has been focused on the reversal errors made by children with RD. These errors, which involve, for example, the reading/writing of *b* for *d* or *was* for *saw,* have traditionally been linked closely with dyslexia. Even today, most people still think of dyslexia as a problem reading letters or words backward. Despite this view, surprisingly little research has systematically investigated reversal errors. The few studies that have examined reversal errors have found that these errors do not actually occur that often in children with RD (Fischer, Liberman, & Shankweiler, 1978; Liberman, Shankweiler, Orlando, Harris, & Berti, 1971). Furthermore, when considered in terms of percentage of overall errors, reversal errors may be no more prevalent in young poor readers than they are in young good readers (Holmes & Peper, 1977). In other words, all beginning readers occasionally make reversal errors, just as all children learning to talk make errors involving grammatical morphemes (e.g., past tense *-ed,* third person *-s*). Just as children with language delays continue to have difficulty with grammatical morphemes beyond the developmental period, children with RD often continue to make reversal errors in later grades.

When reversal errors do occur, they generally are not the result of perceptual problems. Children who write *saw* as *was* or *girl* as *gril* typically do not have trouble perceiving letter sequences. Vellutino and his colleagues (Vellutino, Pruzek, Steger, & Meshoulam, 1973; Vellutino, Steger, DeSetto, & Phillips, 1975) found that children with RD could accurately copy what they sometimes failed to read correctly. Rather than having problems perceiving letter sequences, poor readers are more likely to have difficulties remembering the order of letters in words. Because of the spatial orientation of words, a primary way a word can be misspelled/misread is to fail to remember the correct order of its letters.

ERRATIC EYE MOVEMENTS.   When reading, we get the impression that our eyes are moving smoothly and continuously across the printed page. Actually, eye movements for reading (and many other visual activities) involve a series of rapid jerks, called *saccades,* that move from left to right, and occasionally from right to left (i.e., regressions). Each of these saccades is followed by a short fixation period averaging 200 to 250 milliseconds. It is during these fixations that information is obtained for the purpose of recognizing words.

Could problems in eye movements be a cause of reading disabilities? Poor readers have been noted to have more fixations per line, longer fixations, shorter saccades, and more regressions than good readers (Rayner, 1978). Rayner (1985) and others point out, however, that these differences in eye movements may actually be a reflection of cognitive processing difficulties during reading rather than problems in oculomotor control. For example, because poor readers take longer to recognize words and often need to go back to refresh their memory, they may show longer fixations and more regressions. In opposition to such a conclusion, Pavlidis (1981, 1985) has reported that dyslexics demonstrated abnormal eye movements in nonreading tasks (also see Eden, Stein, Wood, & Wood, 1994, 1995). Olson, Conners, and Rack (1991), however, have argued that even such findings could be a consequence of a reading problem and not a cause. They demonstrated that when

poor readers were matched for reading skill with younger normal readers, no differences were observed in eye movements during nonreading tasks (but see Eden et al., 1994).

The belief that erratic eye movements are a cause of reading disabilities has often led to the
popularity of visually oriented treatment approaches that involve "eye movement training" devices (Metzer & Werner, 1984). The assumption is that if poor readers could learn to move their
eyes in a smoother, less erratic fashion, reading would improve. But as we pointed out earlier, the
basic premise that skilled reading involves smooth eye movements is false. Not surprisingly,
these training programs have not proven to be effective. Today, most professionals agree that
oculomotor exercises, and behavioral optometry in general, have little to offer in the treatment of
reading disabilities (Clark & Uhry, 1995; Keogh & Pelland, 1985; Silver, 1995).

SCOTOPIC SENSITIVITY SYNDROME.   In 1983, Irlen introduced a visual-perceptual condition
called *scotopic sensitivity syndrome* (SSS; Irlen, 1983). This condition was argued to result from
an oversensitivity to particular frequencies of light. Individuals with SSS were noted to experience
a variety of problems during reading, including perceptual distortions, reduced visual field, poor
focus, eyestrain, and/or headaches. Irlen reported that colored eyeglass lenses or tinted plastic
overlays could eliminate troublesome wavelengths of light and reduce the symptoms of SSS. The
use of colored lenses/overlays soon became part of a commercial enterprise. Because it was often
claimed in promotional materials that many dyslexics suffer from SSS, colored filters became a
well-known alternative, but controversial, treatment for reading disabilities (Silver, 1995).

Despite heavy press coverage, supportive testimonials, and some research, little is known
about SSS and its role in reading disabilities (Stanley, 1994). As Stanley (1994) pointed out, the
condition is probably misnamed because most reading involves the photopic, rather than the scotopic, visual system. Futhermore, it is unclear what mechanisms may be responsible for the
symptoms associated with SSS and how colored lenses may affect these mechanisms. Deficits in
visual timing (discussed in the next section) have been linked with SSS (Breitmeyer, 1989;
Weiss, 1990), but the relationship between these deficits, SSS, and improvements with the use of
colored filters is far from clear (Stanley, 1994). Of more significance is the fact that there is still
little empirical evidence to show a causal link between SSS and reading disabilities. Despite
what is claimed in promotional materials and publications (Irlen & Lass, 1989), it is unclear if
children with RD have a higher incidence of SSS than nondisabled readers. It is also unresolved
whether SSS, if present, is a cause of reading disabilities or an associated problem.

Notwithstanding the aforementioned concerns, some studies have examined the effectiveness of colored filters. Although some investigations have found significant improvements in vision and/or reading with the use of colored lenses or overlays (Fletcher & Martinez, 1994;
Robinson & Conway, 1990; but see Blaskey et al., 1990; Cotton & Evans, 1989), much of this
improvement could be due to a placebo effect or an arousal effect. Wearing colored glasses or
using tinted overlays could motivate some poor readers to improve or could affect their mood
and, thus, their performance (Cotton & Evans, 1989; Stanley, 1991, 1994). These and other problems make it difficult to recommend the use of colored lens or overlays as a viable treatment alternative for reading disabilities (Parker, 1990; Stanley, 1991). Because scientific evidence does
not support their efficacy, a recent joint position statement by the American Academy of
Pediatrics and American Academy of Ophthalmology firmly discouraged the use of colored
lenses, as well as eye exercises or other forms of behavioral vision therapy for the treatment of
reading difficulties (American Academy of Pediatrics, Section on Ophthalmology, Council on
Children with Disabilities, American Academy of Ophthalmology, American Association for
Pediatric Ophthalmology and Strabismus, American Association of Certified Orthoptists, 2009).

TRANSIENT PROCESSING DEFICITS.   Scotopic sensitivity syndrome and problems in eye movements have both been suggested to be the result of more primary deficits in visual processing. Researchers have identified two basic visual processing systems, the transient and sustained systems (Campbell, 1974; Graham, 1980). Each system appears to specialize in the processing of particular visual information. The transient system seems to be especially sensitive to global visual features and is thought to play an important role in guiding eye movement. The sustained system, on the other hand, responds to fine detail and is used in visual feature identification (e.g., letter/word recognition). Both of these systems must operate efficiently to meet the visual perceptual demands of reading.

Lovegrove and his colleagues (Lovegrove, 1992; Lovegrove, Martin, & Slaghuis, 1986) observed that individuals with RD have significant difficulties on a number of nonverbal visual tasks believed to involve the transient system. They proposed that individuals with RD may have a sluggish transient processing system. The slowed processing of the transient visual system could disrupt parallel operation with the sustained system, which in turn might lead to visual distortions and other visual problems during reading.

Others have also found individuals with RD to have deficits on visual tasks related to transient processing (Cestnick & Coltheart, 1999; Eden et al., 1995; Livingstone, Rosen, Drislane, & Galaburda, 1991; Solman & May, 1990). In addition, these behavioral findings are consistent with reports of anatomical and physiological deficits in dyslexia (Eden et al., 1996; Livingstone et al., 1991). Livingstone and colleagues (1991), for example, found in postmortem examinations that dyslexics may have less organized and smaller neurons in the brain regions associated with transient visual processing than do normal individuals. Also, as noted earlier, Eden and colleagues (1996) reported that dyslexics show less task-related activation in these brain regions.

Although there is some converging support of a transient visual processing deficit in poor readers, more than a few studies have failed to find evidence of these deficits (e.g., Chiappe, Stringer, Siegel, & Stanovich, 2002; Hayduk, Bruck, & Cavanagh, 1993; Hogben, Rodino, Clark, & Pratt, 1995; see also Skottun & Skoyles, 2008). Some of the conflicting findings across group studies could be the result of these deficits being present only in a subset of poor readers. Thus, the subject composition of a given study could influence its outcome. Consistent with this explanation, Ramus (2003) calculated that only 29 percent of poor readers across a number of recent studies (those that presented individual subject data) had visual processing deficits. Conflicting results could also be due to methodological differences in the way visual processing has been measured across studies. Some have further argued that visual processing deficits might in part be explained by problems in attention or motivation (Stuart, McAnally, & Castles, 2001).

Regardless of the issues concerning conflicting results, the question still remains whether visual deficits, if present, are a sufficient cause of reading disabilities. Some have questioned, for example, how transient deficits themselves could lead to the range of problems seen in children with RD (Skottun, 2000). Also, at least some evidence suggests that transient processing deficits often occur in concert with phonological processing deficits (e.g., Eden et al., 1995). A visually based explanation of reading disabilities would be better supported if a group of children with RD could be identified who have a documented history of visual deficits but no impairments in phonological processing or other known causal factors (Share & Stanovich, 1995).

Auditory Processing Deficits

Auditory processing deficits have frequently been proposed as a cause of reading disabilities (Farmer & Klein, 1995; Tallal, 1980). According to traditional accounts, deficits in auditory perception, especially problems perceiving rapidly occurring or changing sounds, leads to poor phonological representations and, in turn, difficulties in phonological awareness and reading. Early support for this view was provided by Tallal (1980). She found that poor readers had deficits in perceptual judgments of rapidly presented nonspeech stimuli and that their perform-ance was closely related to phonological decoding skills. These findings and others have led to assessment protocols (Jerger & Musiek, 2000) and intervention programs (e.g., Tallal, 2000) to address temporal auditory processing problems in poor readers.

Although several other studies provided support for nonspeech perceptual deficits in poor readers (Helenius, Uutela, & Hari, 1999; Menell, McAnally, & Stein, 1996; Reed, 1989), many failed to uncover such deficits (Chiappe et al., 2002; Kronbichler, Hutzler, & Wimmer, 2002; Nittrouer, 1999). Others reported that auditory processing deficits may be limited to speech per-ception and/or may not necessarily be temporal in nature (Adlard & Hazan, 1998; Breier, Gray, Fletcher, Foorman, & Klaas, 2002; Waber, Weiler et al., 2001). For example, Breier and col-leagues (2002) found that good and poor readers differed significantly only in speech perception (not tone perception) and that these differences were not related to temporal factors such as inter-stimulus interval (see also Mody, Studdert-Kennedy, & Brady, 1997).

Numerous factors could account for the inconsistency in this research. McArthur & Bishop (2001) suggested that a lack of reliability and/or validity of auditory processing measures might explain some of the variability in the findings. They also proposed that individual differences within the population of poor readers could lead to varying results. That is, if auditory process-ing deficits were limited to a small portion of poor readers, then differences in subject selection approaches and/or criteria could lead to different findings. Indeed, Ramus (2003), in a review of the research (those studies providing individual data), estimated that only 39 percent of subjects showed evidence of auditory deficits. Others have also reported that processing deficits may be present only in a subgroup of poor readers (Boets, Wouters, van Wieringen, & Ghesquière, 2007; Heath & Hogben, 2004; Rosen, 2003). Some have proposed that these deficits are found prima-rily in poor readers who also have specific language impairments (Joanisse, Manis, Keating, & Seidenberg, 2000; McArthur & Hogben, 2001) or who have accompanying attention deficit dis-orders (Breir, Fletcher, Foorman, Klaas, & Gray, 2003; Kronbichler et al., 2002).

Not only are there inconsistencies in the evidence for the presence and nature of auditory processing deficits in poor readers, but there are also serious questions of whether or not these deficits represent a sufficient cause of reading problems. In general, research indicates that per-formance on most measures of auditory processing is unrelated or, at best, weakly related to measures of phonological awareness and reading (Bretherton & Holmes, 2003; Chiappe et al., 2002; Share, Jorm, Maclean, & Matthews, 2002; Waber et al., 2001). For example, in a popula-tion-based study of over 500 children, Share and colleagues (2002) found no significant relation-ship between auditory temporal processing in kindergarten and phonological awareness and phonological decoding abilities in second grade. Furthermore, they found that a select group of poor readers with temporal processing deficits were no less proficient on later phonological or reading measures than poor readers with no history of temporal processing deficits.

Although the original theory that rapid temporal auditory processing deficits play a causal role in dylsexia has lost favor, an alternative hypothesis has gained attention in recent years (see Zhang & McBride-Chang, 2010, for a recent review). Goswami and colleagues have suggested that a lack of sensitivity to syllable-level prosodic information in speech could negatively affect the development of phonological awareness in children and, in turn, lead to reading difficulties (Goswami et al., 2002; Richardson, Thomson, Scott, & Goswami, 2004). To test this hypothesis, Goswami and colleagues have conducted several studies employing nonspeech "beat detection" tasks, in which participants are asked to discriminate between amplitude-modulated sounds. In such tasks, faster rise times, or sharper increases in amplitude, should lead to the perception of "beats," whereas slower rise times should lead to the perception of a single sound fluctuating in volume. Significant deficits in the perception of rise time have been reported for school-age children with dyslexia (Goswami, 2002; Richardson et al., 2004) and high functioning adults with a history of developmental dyslexia (Pasquini, Corriveau, & Goswami, 2007). Individual differences in rise time perception also correlate with literacy skills in languages other than English (Halmalainen, Leppanen, Torppa, Muller, & Lyytinen, 2005; Muneaux, Ziegler, True, Thomson, & Goswami, 2004). A recent study of preschoolers also found that growth in phonological awareness from ages 4.5 to 5.5 was significantly related to rise time sensitivity at age 4.5 (Corriveau, Goswami, & Thomson, 2010). Taken together, the work on the dection of suprasegmental aspects of speech is intriguing and may hold promise for explaining some problems experienced by children and adults with dyslexia. However, further work is necessary to better understand the role of this aspect of auditory perception in dyslexia and other reading disabilities.

Attention-Based Deficits

Attention problems have often been associated with reading disabilities. *Attention deficit hyperactivity disorder* (ADHD), the clinical classification for problems in inattention, implusivity, and overactivity, has become a prominant clinical diagnosis for children with behavioral and academic problems. Because reading requires considerable attentional resources, many practitioners think that most children with ADHD have reading/learning problems and vice versa. Initial accounts seemed to support the co-occurrence of these disorders (Safer & Allen, 1976; Silver, 1981). However, these reports were largely based on clinic-referred samples of children with RD or ADHD. Such samples often overestimate the co-occurrence of disorders. When more representative samples of children were examined, the association between reading disabilities and ADHD has been shown to be much weaker. Specifically, Shaywitz and colleagues found that in a research-identified sample of children with ADHD, only 36 percent of the children had reading problems (Shaywitz, Fletcher, & Shaywitz, 1994). More significantly, in a similarly identified sample of children with RD, they found that only 15 percent of the subjects had ADHD (see also Gilger, Pennington, & DeFries, 1992). Research also suggests that the overlap between reading disabilities and ADHD is stronger for ADHD symptoms of inattention than for those of hyperactivity/impulsivity (e.g., Willcutt & Pennington, 2000).

In further support of the distinction between ADHD and reading disabilities, some researchers have identified distinct cognitive profiles associated with these disorders. For example, in one study, children with RD were found to perform poorly on phonological processing tests, whereas children with ADHD generally performed well on these tasks, but poorly on visual memory tasks (Shaywitz et al., 1995). Willcutt and colleagues (2001) also reported a double dissociation between reading disabilities and ADHD. They found that children with ADHD had deficits on tasks of inhibition but normal performance on measures of phonological awareness and verbal working memory. Children with RD showed the opposite profile. More recently, however, Willcutt and colleagues failed to find a double dissociation in the cognitive profiles of individuals with ADHD and RD. In this study, phonological processing deficits were unique to individuals with RD, but there was no defining neuropsychological deficit in individuals with ADHD (Willcutt, Pennington, Olson, Chhabildas, & Hulslander, 2005). Although a clear core deficit to ADHD was not found, this finding underscores the role of phonological processing difficulties in reading disabilities.

Researchers have also examined the relative contribution of attentional factors to reading achievement (Shaywitz et al., 1995). In an investigation of children from the Connecticut Longitudinal Study, Shaywitz and colleagues found that measures of attention failed to explain significant variance in word recognition once language measures had been considered (see also Felton & Wood, 1989). Attention variables did, however, account for a small but significant percentage of the variance in silent reading comprehension over and above that explained by language variables.

In summary, research indicates that attentional deficits are not a primary cause of reading disabilities. Although reading disabilities and ADHD may occur together in children, they appear to be distinct developmental disorders, each with its own set of causal factors. In cases where reading disabilities and ADHD co-occur, attentional deficits (especially inattention) may contribute to reading problems.

Language-Based Deficits

In Chapter 3, we argued that reading disabilities are best characterized as a developmental language disorder. From a theoretical perspective, such a claim is well founded. Reading is first and foremost a language activity. Reading relies heavily on one's knowledge of the phonological, semantic, syntactic, and pragmatic aspects of language. As such, deficiencies in one or more of these aspects of language could significantly disrupt one's ability to read. Not only is a language-based account of reading disabilities theoretically sound, but considerable evidence has also accumulated over the last thirty years to support this view.

LONGITUDINAL STUDY OF LANGUAGE-IMPAIRED CHILDREN. The relationship between language deficits and reading disabilities has been examined from several different perspectives. One approach has been the longitudinal study of children with early spoken language impairments (Aram, Ekelman, & Nation, 1984; Bishop & Adams, 1990; Catts, 1993; Catts, Adlof, Hogan, & Ellis Weismer, 2005; Catts, Bridges, Little, & Tomblin, 2008; Catts, Fey, Tomblin, & Zhang, 2002; Conti-Ramsden & Durkin, 2007; Silva, McGree, & Williams, 1987; Stothard et al., 1998; Tallal, Curtiss, & Kaplan, 1989). In this work, children displaying significant impairments in language (generally in semantic-syntactic aspects) have been identified in preschool or kindergarten and tested for reading and academic achievement in the later grades. Evidence that children with language impairments (LI) are more likely than typically developing children to have subsequent reading disabilities indicates that language deficits precede and play a causal role in reading disabilities.

The results of longitudinal studies have consistently shown that children with LI often have reading disabilities. In general, research indicates that 50 percent or more of children with LI in preschool or kindergarten go on to have reading disabilities in primary or secondary grades. In the most comprehensive study to date, the first author and colleagues (Catts, Fey, Tomblin, & Zhang, 2002) investigated the reading outcomes of 208 kindergarten children with LI. These children were a subsample of children who participated in an epidemiological study of developmental language impairments in children (Tomblin' et al., 1997).

Results indicated that the group of children with LI in kindergarten read well below expected levels in second and fourth grades. Approximately 50 percent of the children with LI performed one or more standard deviations (SDs) below the mean on a composite measure of reading comprehension. Although the remaining children with LI did not meet this criterion, many were, nevertheless, poor readers. When the criterion for a reading disability was changed to below the 25th percentile, nearly 70 percent of children with LI were classified as poor readers. Furthermore, analyses showed that children with low nonverbal abilities in addition to language problems performed significantly less well in reading than those with normal nonverbal IQs. Those children who continued to have language deficits in second and fourth grades were also at a much higher risk for reading disabilities than those whose language abilities had improved by the early school grades. A subsequent study that followed these children through 10th grade found that the children with kindergarten language impairments continued to perform more poorly than typically developing children on measures of reading (Catts et al., 2008).

LANGUAGE PROBLEMS IN POOR READERS.   The fact that many children with LI exhibit reading disabilities does not necessarily mean that most children with RD have a history of language impairments. To better investigate such a claim, studies have directly examined the language abilities of children with RD. In one body of research, investigators have selected school-age children identified as reading disabled (or in some cases, learning disabled) and studied their performance on traditional measures of language development. This work has shown that children with RD often have problems in receptive and/or expressive vocabulary (e.g., Fry, Johnson, & Muehl, 1970; Wiig & Semel, 1975; Wise, Sevcik, Morris, Lovett, & Wolf, 2007) or in the use and/or comprehension of morphology and syntax (e.g., Doehring, Trites, Patel, & Fiedorowitcz, 1981; Fletcher, 1981; Rispens, Roeleven, & Koster, 2004; Stanovich & Siegel, 1994; Vogel, 1974). Deficits have also been reported in the production and/or comprehension of text-level language (e.g., Hagtvet, 2003; Roth & Spekman, 1986; Stothard & Hulme, 1992; Yuill & Oakhill, 1991).

Although this research clearly shows that children with RD have language deficits, it does not necessarily indicate that these deficits are causally related to reading disabilities. A major problem for the interpretation of this work is that in most cases language abilities were examined in children who had reading problems for several years. This makes it difficult to determine if the observed language deficits were the cause or the consequence of a reading problem. Recall that earlier in the chapter we argued that Matthew effects can lead to language deficits in children with RD. Thus, at least some of the language problems observed in children with RD will be a consequence rather than the initial cause of their reading difficulties.

Not all studies of language problems in children with RD have examined reading and language abilities concurrently. Some studies have investigated language deficits in children with RD prior to their learning to read. Scarborough (1990, 1991), for example, investigated the early language development of children who later developed reading disabilities. In this study, the language abilities of children with a family history of dyslexia ($N = 34$) and children without a family history ($N = 44$) were assessed at age 2½ years, and at 6- or 12-month intervals through age 5. Language assessments included measurements of receptive and expressive vocabulary, sentence comprehension, and grammatical production (not all measurements were administered at each age). In second grade, children's reading abilities were assessed. Of the 34 children with a family history of dyslexia, 22 were themselves diagnosed as dyslexic in second grade. The early language abilities of these dyslexic children through 4 years of age were found to be significantly poorer than those of the children without a family history of dyslexia. By age 5, however, only expressive vocabulary differentiated the two groups. Several other studies employing the same design have reported early language deficits in children at risk for reading disabilities (Boets et al., 2010; Lyytinen, Poikkeus, Laakso, Eklund, & Lyytinen, 2001; Snowling et al., 2003).

In another study, the first author and colleagues (Catts, Fey, Zhang, & Tomblin, 1999) investigated the language abilities of a large group of poor readers. The study identified 183 second-grade children who performed at least one SD below normal on a composite measure of reading comprehension. We did not exclude children on the basis of low IQ (except for those with mental retardation), as others have done in the past. The latter practice may bias results concerning language deficits in poor readers because IQ tests often measure verbal abilities. We compared the poor readers' performance on a battery of kindergarten language tests to that of a normal control group. We also used weighted scores based on epidemiological data (Tomblin et al., 1997) to better ensure that our results were representative of poor readers from the population at large. Our findings indicated that the poor readers performed significantly less well than the good readers on tests of oral language. In addition, a large percentage of poor readers performed at least one SD below the mean on tests of vocabulary (39 percent), grammar (56 percent), and narration (44 percent).

Our results further indicated that the poor reader's early language deficits extended beyond vocabulary, grammar, and narration. Poor readers were also found to have difficulties in phonological awareness and phonological retrieval in the kindergarten assessment. Specifically, 56 percent of the poor readers performed at least one SD below that of the normative sample on a measure of phonological awareness (syllable/phoneme deletion), and 45 percent performed below that level on a test of phonological retrieval (rapid naming). These deficits, however, rarely occurred in isolation from problems in vocabulary, grammar, and narration.

In the sections that follow, we review research that more specifically investigated phonological awareness, phonological retrieval (as well as other aspects of what has come to be known as phonological and processing) deficits in children with RD. However, before moving to that discussion, it is important to review a further body of research that has examined nonphonological language deficits in children with RD. Whereas the aforementioned work investigating the language basis of RD has included children with broadly defined problems in reading including deficits in both word reading and comprehension, other research has examined children with specific deficits in comprehension. These children are often referred to as "poor comprehenders" (e.g. Catts, Adlof, & Weismer, 2006; Nation, Clarke, Marshall, & Durand, 2004). Poor comprehenders tend to perform as well as good readers on tasks assessing the phonological domains of language that are reviewed later, including phonological awareness (e.g., Cain, Oakhill, & Bryant, 2000; Nation et al., 2004; Stothard & Hulme, 1995) and phonological memory (Catts et al., 2006; Nation, Adams, Bowyer-Crane, & Snowling, 1999; Nation et al., 2004). However, compared to their same-age typical peers, they show deficits in expressive and receptive vocabulary knowledge (Catts et al., 2006; Nation et al., 2004; Nation & Snowling, 1998; Nation, Snowling, & Clarke, 2005). In addition to knowing fewer words overall, poor comprehenders also appear to have less well-specified semantic representations of the words they do know (Landi & Perfetti, 2007; Nation & Snowling, 1998, 1999). Poor comprehenders also show difficulties relative to good readers on tasks measuring grammar and syntax skills (Adlof, 2010; Cragg & Nation, 2006; Marshall & Nation, 2003; Nation et al., 2004; Nation et al., 2005; Oakhill, Cain, & Bryant, 2003; Stothard & Hulme, 1992) and text-level language (Cain, 2003; Cragg & Nation, 2006).

The existence of poor comprehenders is predicted by the simple view of reading model we reviewed in Chapter 3, in which oral language skills are considered an independent contributor to reading comprehension in addition to word reading skills. Most of the research investigating nonphonological language deficits in poor comprehenders has investigated language and reading skills concurrently, making it difficult to determine the direction of causality. However, recent evidence from longitudinal studies has revealed that deficits in nonphonological aspects of language can be observed prior to the onset of reading instruction in children who will later become poor comprehenders (Ewer & Samuelsson, 2010; Catts et al., 2006; Nation, Cocksey, Taylor, & Bishop, 2010; Torppa et al., 2007). So far, findings suggest that these nonphonological language deficits are heterogeneous and not always severe enough to qualify for a diagnosis of language impairment. More research is needed, however, to clarify the role of nonphonological language deficits in poor comprehenders. This work needs to be conducted in conjunction with the examination of deficits outside the language domain. Emerging research suggests that poor comprehenders also may have deficits in other cognitive abilities such as executive functioning and/or attention (Locascio, Mahone, Eason, & Cutting, 2010; McInnes, Humphries, Hogg-Johnson, & Tannock, 2003; Sesma, Mahone, Levine, Eason, & Cutting, 2009).

Phonological Awareness.   As reported earlier, children with RD often have deficits in phonological processing. The largest body of research in this area has focused on problems in phonological awareness. Phonological awareness is the explicit awareness of, or sensitivity to, the sound structure of speech (Stanovich, 1988; Torgesen, 1996). It is one's ability to attend to, reflect on, or manipulate the speech sounds in words. Children who are aware of the sounds of speech appear to more quickly and accurately acquire sound–letter correspondence knowledge and learn to use this knowledge to decode printed words. Evidence of a relationship between phonological awareness and reading has been demonstrated across a wide range of ages (Calfee & Lindamood, 1973; Gallagher, Laxon, Armstrong, & Frith, 1996; Storch & Whitehurst, 2002; Swanson & Hsieh, 2009; Torgesen, Wagner, Rashotte, Burgess, & Hecht, 1997), experimental tasks (Catts, Wilcox, Wood-Jackson, Larrivee, & Scott, 1997), and languages (Cossu, Shankweiler, Liberman, Katz, & Tolar, 1988; Denton, Hasbrouck, Weaver, & Riccio, 2000; Hu & Catts, 1997; Lundberg, Olofsson, & Wall, 1980; Treutlein, Zoller, Roos, & Scholer, 2008).

Numerous studies have shown that children with RD have deficits in phonological awareness (Bradley & Bryant, 1983; Fletcher et al., 1994; Fox & Routh, 1980; Katz, 1986; Olson, Wise, Conners, Rack, & Fulker, 1989). In fact, Torgesen (1996) argued that "dyslexic children are consistently more impaired in phonological awareness than any other single ability" (p. 6). It is possible that the deficits in phonological awareness observed in children with RD are due, at least in part, to their reading problems (Morais, 1991). Because of the abstract nature of phonology, children are often unaware of some phonological aspects of language until their attention is directly drawn to these features of language. For example, the fact that words are composed of individual phonemes does not become apparent to most language users until these units are explicitly highlighted through instruction and practice in an alphabetic orthography. Support for this view comes from studies that show that preschoolers, as well as illiterate adults, are generally unable to perform tasks that require the explicit segmentation of words into individual phonemes (Anthony et al., 2002; Lundberg & Hoien, 1991; Morais, Bertelson, Cary, & Alegria, 1986; Morais, Cary, Alegria, & Bertelson, 1979; Read & Ruyter, 1985).

Findings such as these suggest that children with RD might be expected to have some deficits in phonological awareness as a result of their poor reading abilities. Because children with RD have less experience and skill in using the alphabet, they may not acquire the same level of speech–sound awareness as their normal reading peers. Not all deficits in phonological awareness, however, are a consequence of reading problems. Research clearly demonstrates that some phonological awareness deficits are apparent in at-risk children prior to beginning reading instruction, and that these deficits are related to subsequent problems in learning to read. As reported earlier, we found that over half of a group of second-grade poor readers had deficits in phonological awareness in kindergarten (Catts et al., 1999). In further analyses, we found that phonological awareness was the best predictor among our kindergarten language and cognitive measures of word recognition abilities in second-grade children in general. Our results also showed that phonological awareness was significantly related to reading even after kindergarten letter-naming ability, a measure of alphabetic experience, was taken into consideration. Thus, it is not simply limited exposure to the alphabet during the preschool years that causes phonological awareness and subsequent reading problems. Studies of familial risk for reading disabilities provides additional evidence that problems in phonological awareness are a precursor of reading disabilities (Pennington & Lefly, 2001; Snowling et al., 2003). For example, Pennington and Lefly reported that high-risk preschool children who developed reading disabilities performed less well on measures of phonological awareness (as well as other aspects of phonological processing) than did low-risk preschoolers and high-risk preschoolers who did not later show reading disabilities.

The best evidence of the causal role of phonological awareness in reading comes from training studies (see Ehri et al., 2001; Bus & Van Ijzendoorn, 1999; & Troia, 1999; for reviews). In these studies, children are provided with instruction in phonological awareness and are subsequently evaluated for phonological awareness ability and reading achievement. In general, this work has found that phonological awareness training can increase speech–sound awareness and, in turn, improve reading achievement. Because the greatest gains are made when phonological awareness training is combined with explicit phonics instruction, Share and Stanovich (1995) argue that phonological awareness is better described as a corequisite to learning to read. In Chapter 5, Al Otaiba and colleagues provide further discussion concerning the relationship between phonological awareness training and reading achievement.

Phonological Retrieval.   Clinical observations have shown that children with RD frequently have word-finding difficulties and are sometimes described as dysnomic (Rudel, 1985). Word-finding problems include substitutions (e.g., "knife" for "fork"), circumlocutions (e.g., "you know, what you eat with"), and overuse of words lacking specificity (e.g., "stuff," "thing"). It is often assumed that because individuals with RD seem to know the words they are looking for, that these naming problems are due to difficulties in remembering phonological information.

The word-finding difficulties observed clinically in individuals with RD have also been borne out in research. Studies have consistently found that poor readers perform less well than good readers on tasks involving confrontation picture naming (Catts, 1986; Denckla & Rudel, 1976; Hanly & Vandenberg, 2010; Scarborough, 1989; Wolf, 1984). For example, Denckla and Rudel (1976) administered the Oldfield–Wingfield Picture-Naming Test to dyslexic, nondyslexic learning disabled (LD), and normal achieving children. Dyslexic children were slower and made more errors on this naming task than nondyslexic LD and normal children. Because the dyslexic and normal children performed similarly on a test of receptive vocabulary, the naming deficits observed in dyslexic children were most likely due to retrieval problems (see also Swan & Goswami, 1997; Wolf & Goodglass, 1986). However, equating reading groups on receptive vocabulary may control for semantic knowledge and name recognition, but it does not ensure that reading groups are comparable in expressive lexical knowledge. Hanly and Vandenberg (2010) investigated this by using a "tip-of-the-tongue" task. During a picture-naming activity, when participants reported that they knew the target word but could not remember its name, they were asked to provide semantic information about the word. Dyslexic children experienced more tip-of-the-tongue episodes than controls, but they were equally able to provide semantic infomration about the target word. This supported the hypothesis that their difficulty was not in lexical knowledge, but rather phonological retrieval. In fact, differences in the quality of phonological memory codes (see next section) probably explain a portion of the reading group differences in naming abilities (Kamhi, Catts, & Mauer, 1990; Katz, 1986).

Perhaps the best evidence of phonological retrieval deficits in children with RD comes from studies using continuous naming tasks. These tasks, often referred to as *rapid naming* or *rapid automatic naming* tasks, require the individual to quickly and automatically say the name of a series of letters, numbers, familiar objects, or colors. Because the names of the items are quite common, it is assumed that storage factors play little role in these tasks. As a result, rapid naming tasks may be thought of as a "purer" measure of naming retrieval than other confrontation naming tasks.

Children with RD have been found to be slower on rapid naming tasks than normal children (Denckla & Rudel, 1976; Vellutino, Scanlon, & Spearing, 1995; Wolf, 1991).[1] Studies also indicate that variability in rapid naming during the preschool years is predictive of reading achievement during the school years (Badian, 1994; Catts, 1993; Wolf, Bally, & Morris, 1986). Research further indicates that rapid naming explains unique variance in reading achievement beyond that accounted for by phonological awareness (Badian, 1994; Bowers & Swanson, 1991; Catts et al., 1999; Kirby, Parilla, & Pfeiffer, 2003; Pennington, Cardoso-Martins, Green, & Lefly, 2001; Wolf' et al., 2002). Although this contribution is often small and relatively modest compared to that of phonological awareness, it seems to be greatest for measures of orthographic processing and fluency.

The latter findings have led in part to the proposal of a *double deficit* in some poor readers (Wolf & Bowers, 1999). Wolf and Bowers have argued that children with RD may have a "core deficit" in phonological awareness alone, rapid naming alone, or deficits in both areas. The latter is referred to as a *double deficit*. Wolf and colleagues (2002) found that within a group of second- and third-grade poor readers, 60 percent had a double deficit, and 15 to 20 percent had problems in a single area. Wolf and colleagues have also argued that, because children with double deficits often have reading problems that go beyond phonological decoding, including deficits in orthographic processing and fluency, they will have more severe reading disabilities than children with single deficits. Although most studies have shown that children with double deficits do have poorer reading achievement (Doi & Manis, 1996; Sundeth & Bowers, 1997), at least a part of this difference is explained by the fact that as a group these children have more severe problems in each deficit area than children with single deficits (Compton, DeFries, & Olson, 2001; Schatschneider, Carlson, Francis, Foorman, & Fletcher, 2002). There is disagreement on whether rapid naming is a separate core deficit from phonological awareness (e.g., Vaessen, Gerretsen, & Blomert, 2009; Vukovic & Siegel, 2006); nonetheless, the presence of difficulties in both phonological awareness and naming speed seems to place a child at greater risk for reading failure.

Wolf, Bowers, and Biddle (2000) raised the possibility that the problems many poor readers have in rapid naming may go beyond deficits in phonological retrieval. They stated that rapid naming not only involves accessing a phonological code, but it also includes a demanding array of attentional, perceptual, memory, lexical, and articulatory processes. Catts, Gillispie, Leonard, Kail, and Miller (2002) further suggested that naming speed may also be a reflection of a domain-general speed of processing. Thus, rapid naming may not be a pure measure of phonological retrieval (but see Vaessen et al., 2009), but it is a good approximation of the reading process and a useful tool for early identification and assessment.

Phonological Memory.   Children with RD also demonstrate problems in phonological memory (Hulme, 1988; Jorm & Share, 1983; Torgesen, 1985). Phonological memory, or what

---

[1]Reading group differences in speed of retrieval in discrete trial tasks have been less consistent. For a discussion of this work and its implications for conclusions concerning retrieval problems, see Bowers, Golden, Kennedy, and Young (1994), Catts (1989a), or Share (1995).

some call phonological coding, refers to the encoding and storage of phonological information in memory. Phonological memory has typically been assessed by memory-span tasks involving meaningful or nonmeaningful strings of verbal items (e.g., digits, letters, words). Poor readers have been found to perform more poorly than good readers on these tasks (Cohen & Netley, 1981; Mann & Ditunno, 1990; Mann, Liberman, & Shankweiler, 1980; Rapala & Brady, 1990; Shankweiler, Liberman, Mark, Fowler, & Fischer, 1979; Stone & Brady, 1995; Vellutino & Scanlon, 1982). Reading group differences have been observed for verbal stimuli even when they are presented visually. As noted earlier in this chapter, studies typically have failed to find differences between good and poor readers when stimuli are nonverbal and cannot be phonologically labeled (Brady, 1986; Holmes & McKeever, 1979; Katz, Shankweiler, & Liberman, 1981; Liberman, Mann, Shankweiler, & Werfelman, 1982; Rapala & Brady, 1990; Vellutino, Steger, Harding, & Phillips, 1975).

These findings suggest that poor readers have particular problems using phonological memory codes to store verbal information. Speech–sound based memory codes are the most efficient way to hold verbal information in memory (Baddeley, 1986). These codes are automatically activated in listening and in skilled reading. Further evidence of poor readers' difficulties using phonological memory codes comes from comparisons of good and poor readers' memory for lists of rhyming and nonrhyming words. Good readers generally have been found to perform more poorly in recalling rhyming than nonrhyming words. This difficulty is presumed to be the result of interference or confusion caused by similar phonological memory codes being activated in the rhyming condition. Poor readers typically have not shown a performance difference on rhyming and nonrhyming word lists, suggesting that they utilize phonological memory codes to a lesser extent than good readers (Brady, Shankweiler, & Mann, 1983; Shankweiler et al., 1979; but see Holligan & Johnston, 1988).

Good and poor readers have also been compared on tasks involving memory of single items rather than strings of items (Catts, 1986; Catts et al., 2005; Kamhi & Catts, 1986; Kamhi, Catts, Mauer, Apel, & Gentry, 1988; Rispens & Parigger, 2010; Snowling, 1981; Stone & Brady, 1995). These tasks have usually required participants to repeat multisyllablic nonwords spoken by the examiner. Because nonword repetition is less influenced by attentional factors and rehearsal strategies, it may be a more direct measure of the ability to use phonogical codes in memory. In an early investigation, Snowling (1981) reported that dyslexic children made more errors than reading-age-matched children in the repetition of nonwords such as *bagmivishent*. In a follow-up study, Snowling and colleagues (Snowling, Goulandris, Bowlby, & Howell, 1986) had dyslexic, age-matched, and reading-age-matched children repeat high- and low-frequency real words and nonwords. They found that high-frequency words were repeated equally well by the three groups. However, dyslexic children performed worse in the repetition of low-frequency real words and nonwords than both the other groups. Subsequent studies have further confirmed these results (Catts, 1986; Kamhi et al., 1988, 1990; Stone & Brady, 1995).

Deficits in phonological memory do not seem to be a consequence of reading problems because performance on memory tasks in kindergarten is predictive of reading achievement in the primary grades (Catts, Fey, Zhang, & Tomblin, 2001; Elbro, Borstrøm, & Petersen, 1998; Ellis & Large, 1987; Mann & Liberman, 1984; Puolakanaho et al., 2007; Torgesen, Wagner, & Rashotte, 1994). Measures of phonological memory, however, do not account for variability in reading achievement independent of measures of phonological awareness (Torgesen et al., 1994; Wagner et al., 1987; Wagner, Torgesen, & Rashotte, 1994). These findings have Wagner and Torgesen to speculate that the problems children with RD have on tasks of phonological memory and phonological awareness stem from a common cause, namely, deficiencies in the quality of phonological representations. Elbro and colleagues also proposed a "distinctness hypothesis" to explain the problems poor readers have in phonological awareness and memory (Elbro et al., 1998; Elbro, Nielsen, & Petersen, 1994). They argued that children with RD have access to phonological representations that are underspecified and lack phonological detail. It is still unclear at this point, however, what may account for this underspecification.

Phonological Production. A final area of phonological processing that has been empirically linked to reading achievement is speech production abilities. Clinical accounts of poor readers' difficulty producing complex speech–sound sequences (Blalock, 1982; Johnson & Myklebust, 1967; Miles, 1983) have been confirmed by a number of empirical studies (Apthorp, 1995; Catts, 1986; Catts, 1989b; Kamhi et al., 1988; Rapala & Brady, 1990; Snowling, 1981). Catts (1986), for example, found that adolescents with RD made significantly more speech production errors than age-matched peers in naming pictured objects with complex names (e.g., ambulance, thermometer) and repeating phonologically complex words (e.g., specific, aluminum) and phrases (e.g., brown and blue plaid pants). In a follow-up study, Catts (1989b) examined the ability of college students with and without a history of RD to rapidly repeat simple (e.g., small wristband) and complex phrases (e.g., Swiss wristwatch). Students with a history of RD repeated the complex phrases at a significantly slower rate and made more errors than students without a history of RD.

The difficulty individuals with RD have in producing complex phonological sequences may be due, in part, to problems in phonological memory. In fact, some of this work converges well with research involving nonword repetition. That is, in the former studies, individuals with RD are asked to produce real but novel words. Like nonword production tasks, the repetition of these stimuli rests heavily on the formation and storage of accurate phonological memory codes. However, individuals with RD have also been shown to have problems producing words/phrases with which they were clearly familiar. For example, Catts (1989b) showed that college students with a history of RD had little difficulty correctly producing complex phrases in isolation (thus demonstrating accurate memory for the words), but had significant problems in the rapid repetition of these sequences. These findings suggest that deficits in speech planning may contribute to the speech production problems in individuals with RD, a suggestion that has been supported by work showing that the relationship between production of complex stimuli and reading remains after statistically controlling for memory factors (Apthorp, 1995).

The link between complex speech production (and phonology in general) and reading has led some researchers to consider a possible association between expressive phonological disorders and reading disabilities. Children with expressive phonological disorders display difficulties in the development of the speech sound system. Unlike the problems noted earlier, these children have difficulties with sound segments in both complex and simple contexts. In these contexts, they delete or substitute speech sounds that are produced correctly by most children of a comparable age.

A large body of research has found both behavioral and genetic links between expressive phonological disorders and reading disabilities (Gillon, 2004; Larrivee & Catts, 1999; Rvachew, 2007; Tunick & Pennington, 2002). However, not all children with expressive phonological disorders have been shown to have reading disabilities. Reading outcomes in these children appear to be most closely related to the severity of the phonological disorder, other language abilities, and level of phonological awareness (Bird, Bishop, & Freeman, 1995; Larrivee & Catts, 1999; Peterson, Pennington, Shriberg, & Boada, 2009; Preston & Edwards, 2010; Snowling, Bishop, & Stothard, 2000). Children with more severe phonological disorders who have broad-based language impairments and who perform poorly on tests of phonological awareness are most at risk for reading disabilities.

LANGUAGE DEFICITS: CAUSES OR CONSEQUENCES.   The research reviewed in these studies clearly demonstrates that language deficits are closely associated with reading disabilities. In many cases, these language deficits precede and are causally linked to reading problems. Reading is a linguistic behavior, and as such, it depends on adequate language development. Many children with RD have developmental language disorders that become manifested as reading problems on entering school. Although language problems often play a causal role in reading disabilities, they may also be a consequence of reading difficulties. As noted in the section on Matthew effects, poor readers do not read as much as good readers and, as a result, gain less language experience. Over time this limited experience can lead to less-well-developed language abilities. For example, poor readers would be expected to fall behind their peers in knowledge and use of vocabulary, advanced grammar, and text-level structures (e.g., story grammar). These and other aspects of language are dependent on rich literacy experiences that poor readers seldom encounter during the school years.

The fact that language deficits are both a cause and consequence of reading disabilities ensures that language problems will be a major component of almost all cases of reading disabilities. In some instances, it may be possible to differentiate between those language problems that are causal and those that are consequences of reading disabilities. However, in other cases, intrinsic and extrinsic factors will interact to such an extent that causes and consequences become indistinguishable, especially in older poor readers. Regardless of whether language problems are causes or consequences, they will need to be addressed in intervention. Early problems in both phonological and nonphonological language skills will need to be considered to ensure that at-risk children get off to a good start in reading. Practitioners will also have to address problems in vocabulary, grammar, and discourse that can arise as a lack of reading experience. Although these problems may emerge as a consequence of reading difficulties, once present, they will interfere with further reading development. In the following chapters, specific suggestions will be provided to improve language knowledge and skills for poor readers.

References

Adams, M. J. (1990). *Beginning to read: Thinking and learning about print.* Cambridge, MA: MIT Press.

Adlard, A., & Hazan, V. (1998). Speech perception in children with specific reading difficulties (dyslexia). *The Quarterly Journal of Experimental Psychology, 51A,* 153–177.

Adler, L., & Atwood, M. (1987). *Poor readers: What do they really see on the page?* West Covina, CA: East San Gabriel Valley Regional Occupational Program.

Adlof, S. M. (2010). Morphosyntactic skills in poor comprehenders. *Dissertation Abstracts International-B, 70*(8). (UMI Dissertation Service, Document ID 3369543).

American Academy of Pediatrics, Section on Ophthalmology, Council on Children with Disabilities, American Academy of Ophthalmology, American

Association for Pediatric Ophthalmology and Strabismus, American Association of Certified Orthoptists. (2009). Joint statement: Learning disabilities, dyslexia, and vision. *Pediatrics, 124,* 837–844.

Anthony, J. L., Lonigan, C. J., Burgess, S. R., Driscoll, K., Phillips, B. M., & Cantor, B. G. (2002). Structure of preschool phonological sensitivity: Overlapping sensitivity to rhyme, words, syllables, and phonemes. *Journal of Experimental Child Psychology, 82,* 65–92.

Apthorp, H. S. (1995). Phonetic coding and reading in college students with and without learning disabilities. *Journal of Learning Disabilities, 28,* 342–352.

Aram, D. M., Ekelman, B. L., & Nation, J. E. (1984). Preschoolers with language disorders: 10 years later. *Journal of Speech and Hearing Research, 27,* 232–244.

Baddeley, A. (1986). Working memory, reading and dyslexia. In E. Hjelmquist & L. Nilsson (Eds.), *Communication and handicap: Aspects of psychological compensation and technical aids* (pp. 141–152). New York: Elsevier.

Badian, N. A. (1994). Barker Preschool prediction: Orthographic and phonological skills, and reading. *Annals of Dyslexia, 44,* 3–25.

Bird, J., Bishop, D. V. M., & Freeman, N. H. (1995). Phonological awareness and literacy development in children with expressive phonological impairments. *Journal of Speech and Hearing Research, 38,* 446–462.

Bishop, D. V. M. (1990). *Handedness and developmental disorder.* Oxford: Blackwell Scientific.

Bishop, D. V. M., & Adams, C. (1990). A prospective study of the relationship between specific language impairment, phonological disorders and reading retardation. *Journal of Child Psychology and Psychiatry, 31,* 1027–1050.

Bishop, D. V. M., Adams, C. V., & Norbury, C. F. (2006). Distinct genetic influences on grammar and phonological short-term memory deficits: Evidence from 6-year-old twins. *Genes, Brain and Behavior, 5*(2), 158–169.

Blalock, J. W. (1982). Persistent auditory language deficits in adults with learning disabilities. *Journal of Learning Disabilities, 15,* 604–609.

Blaskey, P., Scheiman, M., Parisi, M., Ciner, E. B., Gallaway, M., & Selznick, R. (1990). The effectiveness of Irlen filters for improving reading performance: A pilot study. *Journal of Learning Disabilities, 23,* 604–610.

Boets, B., De Smedt, B., Cleuren, L., Vandewalle, E., Wouters, J., & Ghesquière, P. (2010). Towards a further characterization of phonological and literacy problems in Dutch-speaking children with dyslexia. *British Journal of Developmental Psychology, 28,* 5–31.

Boets, B., Wouters, J., van Wieringen, A., & Ghesquière, P. (2007). Auditory processing, speech perception and phonological ability in pre-school children at high-risk for dyslexia: A longitudinal study of the auditory temporal processing theory, *Neuropsychologia, 45*(8), 1608–1620.

Bowers, P. G., Golden, J., Kennedy, A., & Young, A. (1994). Limits upon orthographic knowledge due to processes indexed by naming speed. In V. Berninger (Ed.), *The varieties of orthographic knowledge. I: Theoretical and developmental issues* (pp. 173–218). Dordecht: Klüwer.

Bowers, P. G., & Swanson, L. B. (1991). Naming speed deficits in reading disability: Multiple measures of a singular process. *Journal of Experimental Child Psychology, 51,* 195–219.

Bradley, L., & Bryant, P. (1983). Categorizing sounds and learning to read: A causal connection. *Nature, 301,* 419–421.

Brady, S. (1986). Short-term memory, phonological processing, and reading ability. *Annals of Dyslexia, 36,* 138–153.

Brady, S., Shankweiler, D., & Mann, V. (1983). Speech perception and memory coding in relation to reading ability. *Journal of Experimental Child Psychology, 35,* 345–367.

Breier, J. I., Fletcher, J. M., Foorman, B. R., Klaas, P., & Gray, L. C. (2003). Auditory temporal processing in children with specific reading disability with and without attention deficit/hyperactivity disorder. *Journal of Speech, Language, and Hearing Research, 46,* 31–42.

Breier, J. I., Gray, L. C., Fletcher, J. M., Foorman, B., & Klaas, P. (2002). Perception of speech and nonspeech stimuli by children with and without reading disability and attention deficit hyperactivity disorder. *Journal of Experimental Child Psychology, 82,* 226–250.

Breitmeyer, B. (1989). A visually based deficit in specific reading disability. *The Irish Journal of Psychology, 10,* 534–541.

Bretherton, L., & Holmes, V. M. (2003). The relationship between auditory temporal processing, phonemic awareness, and reading disability. *Journal of Experimental Child Psychology, 84,* 218–243.

Bronner, A. (1917). *The psychology of special abilities and disabilities.* Boston: Little, Brown.

Brown, W. E., Eliez, S., Menon, V., Rumsey, J. M., White, C. D., & Reiss, A. L. (2001). Preliminary evidence of widespread morphological variations of the brain in dyslexia. *Neurology, 56,* 781–783.

Bryden, M. P. (1982). *Laterality: Functional asymmetry in the intact brain.* New York: Academic Press.

Bus, A. G., & van Ijzendoorn, M. H. (1999). Phonological awareness and early reading: A meta-analysis of experimental training programs. *Journal of Educational Psychology, 91,* 403–414.

Bus, A. G., van Ijzendoorn, M., & Pellegrini, A. (1995). Joint book reading makes success in learning to read: A meta-analysis on intergenerational transmission of literacy. *Review of Educational Research, 65,* 1–21.

Byrne, B., Delaland, C., Fielding-Barnsley, R., Quain, P., Samuelsson, S., Hoien, T., Corley, R., DeFries, J., Wadsworth, S., Willcutt, E., & Olson, R. K. (2002). Longitudinal twin study of early reading development in three countries: Preliminary results. *Annals of Dyslexia, 52,* 49–74.

Cain, K. (2003). Text comprehension and its relation to coherence and cohesion in children's fictional narratives. *British Journal of Developmental Psychology, 21*, 335–351.

Cain, K., Oakhill, J., & Bryant, P. (2000). Phonological skills and comprehension failure: A test of the phonological processing deficit hypothesis. *Reading and Writing: An Interdisciplinary Journal, 13*, 31–56.

Calfee, R. C., & Lindamood, P. (1973). Acoustic-phonetic skills and reading—kindergarten through twelfth grade. *Journal of Educational Psychology, 64*, 293–298.

Campbell, F. W. (1974). The transmission of spatial information through the visual system. In F. O. Schmidt & F. S. Worden (Eds.), *The neurosciences third study program* (pp. 95–103). Cambridge, MA: MIT Press.

Catts, H. W. (1986). Speech production/phonological deficits in reading-disordered children. *Journal of Learning Disabilities, 19*, 504–508.

Catts, H. W. (1989a). Phonological processing deficits and reading disabilities. In A. Kamhi & H. Catts (Eds.), *Reading disabilities: A developmental language perspective.* Boston: Allyn & Bacon.

Catts, H. W. (1989b). Speech production deficits in developmental dyslexia. *Journal of Speech and Hearing Research, 54*, 422–428.

Catts, H. W. (1993). The relationship between speech-language impairments and reading disabilities. *Journal of Speech and Hearing Research, 36*, 948–958.

Catts, H. W., Adlof, S. M., Hogan, T. P., & Ellis Weismer, S. (2005). Are specific language impairment and dyslexia distinct disorders? *Journal of Speech, Language, and Hearing Research, 48*(6), 1378–1396.

Catts, H. W., Adlof, S. M., & Ellis Weismer, S. (2006). Language deficits in poor comprehenders: A case for the simple view of reading. *Journal of Speech, Language, and Hearing Research, 49*, 278–293.

Catts, H. W., Bridges, M. S., Little, T. D., & Tomblin, J. B. (2008). Reading achievement growth in children with language impairments. *Journal of Speech, Language, and Hearing Research, 51*(6), 1569–1579.

Catts, H. W., Fey, M. E., Tomblin, J. B., & Zhang, Z. (2002). A longitudinal investigation of reading outcomes in children with language impairments. *Journal of Speech, Language, and Hearing Research, 45*, 1142–1157.

Catts, H. W., Fey, M. E., Zhang, X., & Tomblin, J. B. (1999). Language basis of reading and reading disabilities: Evidence from a longitudinal investigation. *Scientific Studies in Reading, 3*, 331–361.

Catts, H. W., Fey, M. E., Zhang, X., & Tomblin, J. B. (2001). Estimating risk for future reading difficulties in kindergarten children: A research-based model and its clinical implications. *Language, Speech, and Hearing Services in Schools, 32*, 38–50.

Catts, H., Gillispie, M., Leonard, L., Kail, R., & Miller, C. (2002). The role of speed of processing, rapid naming, and phonological awareness in reading achievement. *Journal of Learning Disabilities, 35*, 509–524.

Catts, H. W., Wilcox, K. A., Wood-Jackson, C., Larrivee, L., & Scott, V. G. (1997). Toward an understanding of phonological awareness. In C. K. Leong & R. M. Joshi (Eds.), *Cross-language studies of learning to read and spell: Phonologic and orthographic processing* (pp. 31–52). Dordrecht: Klüwer.

Cestnick, L., & Coltheart, M. (1999). The relationship between language processing and visual processing deficits in developmental dyslexia. *Cognition, 7*, 231–255.

Chiappe, P., Stringer, R., Siegel, L., Stanovich, K. (2002). Why the timing deficit hypothesis does not explain reading disability in adults. *Reading and Writing: An Interdisciplinary Journal, 15*, 73–107.

Clark, D. B., & Uhry, J. K. (1995). *Dyslexia: Theory and practice of remedial instruction.* Baltimore: York Press.

Cohen, R. L., & Netley, C. (1981). Short-term memory deficits in reading disabled children in the absence of opportunity for rehearsal strategies. *Intelligence, 5*, 69–76.

Cole, G. (1987). *The learning mystique.* New York: Pantheon.

Compton, D. L., DeFries, J. C., & Olson, R. K. (2001). Are RAN- and phonological awareness-deficits additive in children with reading disabilities? *Dyslexia: An International Journal of Research and Practice, 7*, 125–149.

Conti-Ramsden, G., & Durkin, K. (2007). Phonological short-term memory, language and literacy: Developmental relationships in early adolescence in young people with SLI. *Journal of Child Psychology and Psychiatry, 48*(2), 147–156.

Corriveau, K., Goswami, U., & Thomson, J. M. (2010). Auditory processing and early literacy skills in a preschool and kindergarten population. *Journal of Learning Disabilities, 43*, 369–382.

Cossu, G., Shankweiler, D., Liberman, I. Y., Katz, L., & Tolar, G. (1988). Awareness of phonological segments and reading ability in Italian children. *Applied Psycholinguistics, 9*, 1–16.

Cotton, M. M., & Evans, K. M. (1989). *An evaluation of the Irlen lenses as a treatment for specific learning disorders. Australian Journal of Psychology, 42*, 1–12.

Cragg, L., & Nation, K. (2006). Exploring written narrative in children with poor reading comprehension. *Educational Psychology, 26*, 55–72.

DeFries, J. C., & Alarcon, M. (1996). Genetics of specific reading disability. *Mental Retardation and Development Disabilities, 2,* 39–47.

Denckla, M. B., & Rudel, R. G. (1976). Rapid automatized naming (RAN): Dyslexia differentiated from other learning disabilities. *Neuropsychologia, 14,* 471–479.

Denton, C. D., Hasbrouck, J. E., Weaver, L. R., & Riccio, C. A. (2000). What do we know about phonological awareness in Spanish? *Reading Psychology, 21,* 335–352.

Doehring, D., Trites, R., Patel, P., & Fiedorowitcz, C. (1981). *Reading difficulties: The interaction of reading, language, and neuropsychological deficits.* New York: Academic Press.

Doi, L. M., & Manis, F. R. (1996). *The impact of speeded naming ability on reading performance.* Paper presented at the Society for the Scientific Study of Reading, New York.

Duara, R., Kushch, A., Gross-Gleen, K., Barker, W. W., Jallad, B., Pascal, S., Loewenstein, D. A., Sheldon, J., Rabin, M., Levin, B., & Lubs, H. (1991). Neuroanatomic differences between dyslexic and normal readers on magnetic resonance imaging scans. *Archives of Neurology, 48,* 410–416.

Eckert, M. A., Leonard, C. M., Richards, T. L., Aylward, E. H., Thomson, J., & Berninger, V. W. (2003). Anatomical correlates of dyslexia: frontal and cerebellar findings. *Brain, 126,* 482–494.

Eden, G. F., Stein, J. F., Wood, M. H., & Wood, F. B. (1994). Differences in eye movements and reading problems in reading disabled and normal children. *Vision Research, 34,* 1345–1358.

Eden, G. F., Stein, J. F., Wood, M. H., & Wood, F. B. (1995). Verbal and visual problems in reading disability. *Journal of Learning Disabilities, 28,* 272–290.

Eden, G. F., VanMeter, J., Rumsey, J., Maisog, J., Woods, R., & Zeffiro, T. (1996). Abnormal processing of visual motion in dyslexia revealed by functional brain imaging. *Nature, 382,* 66–69.

Ehri, L., Nunes, S., Willows, D., Schuster, B., Yaghoub-Zadeh, Z., & Shanahan, T. (2001). Phonemic awareness instruction helps children learn to read: Evidence from the National Reading Panel's meta-analysis. *Reading Research Quarterly, 36,* 250–287.

Elbro, C., Borstrøm, I., & Petersen, D. (1998). Predicting dyslexia from kindergarten: The importance of distinctness of phonological representations of lexical items. *Reading Research Quarterly, 33*(1), 36–60.

Elbro, C., Nielsen, I., & Petersen, D. K. (1994). Dyslexia in adults: Evidence for deficits in nonword reading and in the phonological representation of lexical items. *Annals of Dyslexia, 44,* 205–226.

Ellis, N., & Large, B. (1987). The development of reading: As you seek so shall you find. *British Journal of Psychology, 78,* 1–28.

Ewer, A., & Sameulsson, S. (2010, July). *Developmental trajectories distinguishing between dyslexics and poor comprehenders.* Poster presented at the annual conference of the Society for the Scientific Study of Reading, Berlin, Germany.

Farmer, M. E., & Klein, R. M. (1995). The evidence for a temporal processing deficit linked to dyslexia: A review. *Psychonomic Bulletin & Review, 2,* 460–493.

Felton, R. H., & Wood, F. B. (1989). Cognitive deficits in reading disability and attention deficit disorder. *Journal of Learning Disabilities, 22,* 3–13.

Fildes, L. (1922). A psychological inquiry into the nature of the condition known as congenital word blindness. *Brain, 44,* 286–307.

Finucci, J. M., Gutherie, J. T., Childs, A. L., Abbey, H., & Childs, B. (1976). The genetics of specific reading disability. *Annual Review of Human Genetics, 40,* 1–23.

Fischer, F. W., Liberman, I. Y., & Shankweiler, D. (1978). Reading reversals and developmental dyslexia: A further study. *Cortex, 14,* 496–510.

Fletcher, J. M. (1981). Linguistic factors in reading acquisition: Evidence for developmental changes. In *Neuropsychological and Cognitive Processes in Reading* (pp. 261–294). New York: Academic Press.

Fletcher, J. M., & Martinez, G. (1994). An eye-movement analysis of the effects of scotopic sensitivity correction on parsing and comprehension. *Journal of Learning Disabilities, 27*(94/01), 67–70.

Fletcher, J. M., Shaywitz, S. E., Shankweiler, D. P., Katz, L., Liberman, I. Y., Stuebing, K. K., Francis, D. J., Fowler, A. E., & Shaywitz, B. A. (1994). Cognitive profiles of reading disability: Comparisons of discrepancy and low achievement definitions. *Journal of Educational Psychology, 86,* 6–23.

Flowers, D. L., Wood, F. B., & Naylor, C. E. (1991). Regional cerebral blood flow correlates of language processes in reading disability. *Archives of Neurology, 48,* 637–643.

Foundas, A. L., Leonard, C. M., Gilmore, R., Fennell, E., & Heilman, K. M. (1994). Planum temporal asymmetry and language dominance. *Neuropsychologia, 32,* 1225–1231.

Fox, B., & Routh, D. K. (1980). Phonemic analysis and severe reading disability in children. *Journal of Psycholinguistic Research, 9,* 115–119.

Frostig, M. (1968). Education for children with learning disabilities. In H. Myklebust (Ed.), *Progress in learning disabilities* (pp. 234–266). New York: Grune & Stratton.

Fry, M. A., Johnson, C. S., & Muehl, S. (1970). Oral language production in relation to reading achievement among select second graders. In D. Baker & P. Satz (Eds.), *Specific reading disability: Advances in theory and method* (pp. 123–159). Rotterdam: Rotterdam University Press.

Fuchs, L. S., & Fuchs, D. (1998). Treatment validity: A unifying concept for the identification of learning disabilities. *Learning Disability Research and Practice, 14,* 204–219.

Fuchs, L. S., Fuchs, D., & Speece, D. L. (2002). Treatment validity as a unified construct for identifying learning disabilities. *Learning Disabilities Quarterly, 25,* 33–46.

Galaburda, A. M. (1988). The pathogenesis of childhood dyslexia. In F. Plum (Ed.), *Language, communication, and the brain.* New York: Raven Press.

Galaburda, A. M. (1991). Anatomy of dyslexia: Argument against phrenology. In D. D. Duane & D. B. Gray (Eds.), *The reading brain: The biological basis of dyslexia* (pp. 119–131). Parkton, MD: York Press.

Galaburda, A. M., Corsiglia, J., Rosen, G. D., & Sherman, G. F. (1987). Planum temporale asymmetry: Reappraisal since Geschwind and Levitsky. *Neuropsychologia, 28,* 314–318.

Galaburda, A. M., Sherman, G. F., Rosen, G. D., Aboitiz, F., & Geschwind, N. (1985). Developmental dyslexia: Four consecutive patients with cortical anomalies. *Annals of Neurology, 18*(85), 222–233.

Gallagher, A. M., Laxon, V., Armstrong, E., & Frith, U. (1996). Phonological difficulties in high-functioning dyslexics. *Reading and Writing, 8,* 499–509.

Gerber, A. (1993). *Language-related learning disabilities: Their nature and treatment.* Baltimore: Brookes.

Gilger, J. W., Pennington, B. F., & DeFries, J. C. (1991). Risk for reading disability as a function of parental history in three family studies. *Reading and Writing: An Interdisciplinary Journal, 3,* 205–217.

Gilger, J. W., Pennington, B. F., & DeFries, J. C. (1992). A twin study of the etiology of comorbidity: Attention-deficit hyperactivity disorder and dyslexia. *Journal of the American Academy of Child and Adolescent Psychiatry, 31,* 343–348.

Gillon, G. (2004). *Phonological awareness: From research to practice.* New York: Guilford.

Goswami, U., Thomson, J., Richardson, U., Stainthorp, R., Hughes, D., Rosen, S., et al. (2002). Amplitude envelope onsets and developmental dyslexia: A new hypothesis. *Proceedings of the National Academy of Sciences of the USA, 99,* 10911–10916.

Goswami, U. (2002). Phonology, reading development, and dyslexia: A cross-linguistic perspective. *Annals of Dyslexia, 52,* 142–163.

Graham, N. (1980). Spatial frequency channels in human vision. Detecting edges without edge detectors. In C. S. Harris (Ed.), *Visual coding and adaptability* (pp. 215–262). Hillsdale, NJ: Erlbaum.

Grigorenko, E. L., Wood, F. B., Meyer, M. S., Pauls, J., Hart, L. A., & Pauls, D. L. (2001). Linkage studies suggest a possible locus for developmental dyslexia on chromosome 1p. *American Journal of Medical Genetics, 105,* 120–129.

Guttorm, T. K., Leppänen, P. H. T., Tolvanen, A., & Lyytinen, H. (2003). Event-related potentials in newborns with and without familial risk for dyslexia: Principal component analysis reveals differences between the groups. *Journal of Neural Transmission, 110*(9), 1059–1074.

Hagtvet, B. E. (2003). Listening comprehension and reading comprehension in poor decoders: Evidence for the importance of syntactic and semantic skills as well as phonological skills. *Reading and Writing: An Interdisciplinary Journal, 16,* 505–539.

Hallgren, B. (1950). Specific dyslexia (congenital word blindness): A clinical and genetic study. *Acta Psychiatrica et Neurologica Supplement, 65,* 1–287.

Hamalainen, J., Leppanen, P. H. T., Torppa, M., Muller, K., & Lyytinen, H. (2005). Detection of sound rise time by adults with dyslexia. *Brain and Language, 94*(1), 32–42.

Hanly, S., & Vandenberg, B. (2010). Tip-of-the-tongue and word retrieval deficits in dyslexia. *Journal of Learning Disabilities, 43*(1), 15–23.

Hayduk, S., Bruck, M., & Cavanagh, P. (1993). *Do adult dyslexics show low level visual processing deficits? Annals of the New York Academy of Sciences, 682,* 351–353.

Heath, S. M., & Hogben, J. H. (2004). Cost-effective prediction of reading difficulties. *Journal of Speech, Language, and Hearing Research, 47,* 751–765.

Helenius, P., Uutela, L., & Hari, R. (1999). Auditory stream segregation in dyslexic adults. *Brain, 122,* 907–913.

Hinshelwood, J. (1917). *Congenital word blindness.* London: H.K. Lewis.

Hogben, J., Rodino, I., Clark, C., & Pratt, C. (1995). A comparison of temporal integration in children with specific reading disability and normal reading. *Vision Research, 35,* 2067–2074.

Holligan, C., & Johnston, R. S. (1988). The use of phonological information by good and poor readers in memory and reading tasks. *Memory & Cognition, 16,* 522–532.

Holmes, D., & McKeever, W. (1979). Material-specific serial memory deficit in adolescent dyslexics. *Cortex, 15,* 51–62.

Holmes, D., & Peper, R. (1977). An evaluation of the use of spelling error analysis in the diagnosis of reading disabilities. *Child Development, 48,* 1708–1711.

Hu, C., & Catts, H. W. (1997). The role of phonological processing in early reading ability: What we can learn from Chinese. *Scientific Studies in Reading, 2,* 55–79.

Hulme, C. (1988). Short-term memory development and learning to read. In M. Gruneberg, P. Morris, & R. Sykes (Eds.), *Practical aspects of memory: Current research and issues. Vol. 2: Clinical and educational implications* (pp. 234–271). Chichester, England: Wiley.

Hynd, G. W., Hall, J., Novey, E. S., Eliopulos, D., Black, K., Gonzalez, J. J., Edmonds, J. E., Riccio, C., & Cohen, M. (1995). Dyslexia and corpus callosum morphology. *Archives of Neurology, 52,* 32–38.

Hynd, G. W., Semrud-Clikeman, M., Lorys, A. R., Novey, E. S., & Eliopulos, D. (1990). Brain morphology in developmental dyslexia and attention deficit disorder/hyperactivity. *Archives of Neurology, 47,* 919–926.

Irlen, H. (1983). *Successful treatment of learning disabilities.* Paper presented at the 91st Annual Convention of the American Psychological Association, Anaheim, CA.

Irlen, H., & Lass, M. J. (1989). Improving reading problems due to symptoms of scotopic sensitivity using Irlen lenses and overlays. *Education, 109,* 413–417.

Jerger, J., & Musiek, F. (2000). Report of the consensus conference on the diagnosis of auditory processing disorders in school-age children. *Journal of the American Academy of Audiology, 11,* 467–474.

Jernigan, T. L., Hesselink, J. R., Sowell, E., & Tallal, P. A. (1991). Cerebral structure on magnetic resonance imaging in language- and learning-impaired children. *Archives of Neurology, 48,* 539–545.

Joanisse, M. F., Manis, F. R., Keating, P., & Seidenberg, M. S. (2000). Language deficits in dyslexic children: Speech perception, phonology, and morphology. *Journal of Experimental Child Psychology, 77,* 30–60.

Johnson, D., & Myklebust, H. (1967). *Learning disabilities: Educational principles and practice.* New York: Grune & Stratton.

Jorm, A. F., & Share, D. L. (1983). Phonological recoding and reading acquisition. *Applied Psycholinguistics, 4,* 103–147.

Kamhi, A. G., & Catts, H. W. (1986). Toward an understanding of developmental language and reading disorders. *Journal of Speech and Hearing Disorders, 51,* 337–348.

Kamhi, A. G., Catts, H. W., & Mauer, D. (1990). Explaining speech production deficits in poor readers. *Journal of Learning Disabilities, 23,* 632–636.

Kamhi, A. G., Catts, H. W., Mauer, D., Apel, K., & Gentry, B. (1988). Phonological and spatial processing abilities in language and reading impaired children. *Journal of Speech and Hearing Disorders, 3,* 316–327.

Katz, R. B. (1986). Phonological deficiencies in children with reading disability: Evidence from an object-naming task. *Cognition, 22,* 225–257.

Katz, R. B., Shankweiler, D., & Liberman, I. (1981). Memory for item order and phonetic recoding in the beginning reader. *Journal of Experimental Child Psychology, 32,* 474–484.

Keenan, J. M., Betjemann, R. S., Wadsworth, S. J., DeFries, J. C., & Olson, R. K. (2006). Genetic and environmental influences on reading and listening comprehension. *Journal of Research in Reading, 29,* 75–91.

Keller, T. A., & Just, M.A. (2009). Altering cortical connectivity: Remediation-induced changes in the white matter of poor readers. *Neuron, 64,* 624–631.

Keogh, B. K., & Pelland, M. (1985). Vision training revisited. *Journal of Learning Disabilities, 18,* 228–236.

Kirby, J. R., Parrila, R., & Pfeiffer, S. (2003). Naming speed and phonological awareness as predictors of reading development. *Journal of Educational Psychology, 95,* 453–464.

Kronbichler, M., Hutzler, F., & Wimmer, H. (2002). Dyslexia: Verbal impairments in the absence of magnocellular impairments. *Neuroreport, 13,* 617–620.

Landi, N., & Perfetti, C. A. (2007). An electrophysiological investigation of semantic and phonological processing in skilled and less-skilled comprehenders. *Brain and Language, 102,* 30–45.

Larrivee, L. S., & Catts, H. W. (1999). Early reading achievement in children with expressive phonological disorders. *American Journal of Speech-Language Pathology, 8,* 118–128.

Leonard, C. M., & Eckert, M. A. (2008). Asymmetry and dyslexia. *Developmental Neuropsychology, 33*(6), 663–681.

Leonard, C. M., Lombardino, L. J., Walsh, K., Eckert, M. A., Mockler, J. L., & Rowe, L. A. (2002). Anatomical risk factors that distinguish dyslexia from SLI predict reading skill in normal children. *Journal of Communication Disorders, 35,* 501–531.

Liberman, I. Y., Mann, V. A., Shankweiler, D., & Werfelman, M. (1982). Children's memory for recurring linguistic and nonlinguistic material in relation to reading ability. *Cortex, 18,* 367–375.

Liberman, I. Y., Shankweiler, D., Orlando, C., Harris, K., & Berti, F. (1971). Letter confusion and reversal of sequence in the beginning reader: Implications for Orton's theory of developmental dyslexia. *Cortex, 7*, 127–142.

Light, J. G., & DeFries, J. C. (1995). Comorbidity of reading and mathematics disabilities: Genetic and environmental etiologies. *Journal of Learning Disabilities, 28*, 96–106.

Livingstone, M., Rosen, G., Drislane, F., & Galaburda, A. (1991). Physiological and anatomical evidence for a magnocellular defect in developmental dyslexia. *Proceedings of the National Academy of Science, 88*, 7943–7947.

Locascio, G., Mahone, M., Eason, S., & Cutting, L. (2010). Executive dysfunction among children with reading comprehension deficits. *Journal of Learning Disabilities, 43*, 441–454.

Lovegrove, W. (1992). The visual deficit hypothesis. In N. Singh & I. Beale (Eds.), *Learning disabilities: Nature, theory, and treatment* (pp. 246–269). New York: Springer-Verlag.

Lovegrove, W., Martin, F., & Slaghuis, W. (1986). The theoretical and experimental case for a visual deficit in specific reading disability. *Cognitive Neuropsychology, 3*, 225–267.

Lubs, H., Duara, R., Levin, B., Jallad, B., Lubs, M., Rabin, M., Kushch, A., & Gross-Glenn, K. (1991). Dyslexia subtypes: Genetics, behavior, and brain imaging. In D. D. Drake & D. B. Gray (Eds.), *The reading brain: The biological basis of dyslexia* (pp. 89–117). Parkton, MD: York Press.

Lundberg, I., & Hoien, T. (1991). Initial enabling knowledge and skills in reading acquisition: Print awareness and phonological segmentation. In D. J. Sawyer & B. J. Fox (Eds.), *Phonological awareness in reading: The evolution of current perspectives* (pp. 74–95). New York: Springer-Verlag.

Lundberg, I., Olofsson, A., & Wall, S. (1980). Reading and spelling skills in the first school years predicted from phonemic awareness skills in kindergarten. *Scandinavian Journal of Psychology, 21*, 159–173.

Lyytinen, P., Poikkeus, A. M., Laakso, M. L., Eklund, K., & Lyytinen, H. (2001). Language development and symbolic play in children with and without familial risk for dyslexia. *Journal of Speech, Language, and Hearing Research, 44*, 873–885.

Mann, V. A., & Ditunno, P. (1990). Phonological deficiencies: Effective predictors of future reading. In G. T. Pavlidis (Ed.), *Perspectives on dyslexia: Cognition, language and treatment* (Vol. 2, pp. 105–131). New York: Wiley.

Mann, V. A., & Liberman, I. Y. (1984). Phonological awareness and verbal short-term memory. *Journal of Learning Disabilities, 17*, 592–599.

Mann, V. A., Liberman, I. Y., & Shankweiler, D. (1980). Children's memory for sentences and word strings in relation to reading ability. *Memory & Cognition, 8*, 329–335.

Marshall, C. M., & Nation, K. (2003). Individual differences in semantic and structural errors in children's memory for sentences. *Educational and Child Psychology, 20*, 7–18.

McArthur, G. M., & Bishop, D. V. M. (2001). Auditory perceptual processing in people with reading and oral language impairments: Current issues and recommendations. *Dyslexia, 7*, 150–170.

McArthur, G. M., & Hogben, J. H. (2001). Auditory backward recognition masking in children with a specific language impairment and children with a specific reading disability. *Journal of the Acoustical Society of America, 109*, 1092–1100.

McInnes, A., Humphries, T., Hogg-Johnson, S., & Tannock, R. (2003). Listening comprehension and working memory are impaired in attention-deficit hyperactivity disorder irrespective of language impairment. *Journal of Abnormal Child Psychology, 31*, 427–443

Meaburn, E. L., Harlaar, N., Craig, I. W., Schalkwyk, L. C., & Plomin, R. 2008. Quantitative trait locus association scan of early reading disability and ability using pooled DNA and 100K SNP microarrays in a sample of 5,760 children. *Molecular Psychiatry, 13*(7), 729–740.

Menell, P., McAnally, K. I., & Stein, J. F. (1999). Psychophysical sensitivity and physiological response to amplitude modulation in adult dyslexic listeners. *Journal of Speech, Language, and Hearing Research, 42*, 797–803.

Metzer, R. I., & Werner, D. B. (1984). Use of visual training for reading disabilities: A review. *Pediatrics, 73*, 824–829.

Meyler, A., Keller, T. A., Cherkassky, V. L., Gabrieli, J. D. E., & Just, M. A. (2008). Modifying the brain activation of poor readers during sentence comprehension with extended remedial instruction: A longitudinal study of neuroplasticity. *Neuropsychologia, 46*, 2580–2592.

Miles, T. (1983). *Dyslexia: The pattern of difficulties*. Springfield, IL: Charles C Thomas.

Mody, M., Studdert-Kennedy, M., & Brady, S. (1997). Speech perception deficits in poor readers: Auditory processing or phonological coding. *Journal of Experimental Child Psychology, 64*, 199–231.

Mol, S., & Bus, A. G. (2010, July). *A meta-analysis on young children's home literacy environment; An update and replication of Bus et al. (1995)*. Poster presented at the annual convention of the Society for the Scientific Study of Reading, Berlin, Germany.

Molfese, D. L. (2000). Predicting dyslexia at 8 years of age using neonatal brain responses. *Brain and Language, 72*, 238–245.

Morais, J. (1991). Phonological awareness: A bridge between language and literacy. In D. Sawyer & B. Fox (Eds.), *Phonological awareness and reading acquisition* (pp. 31–71). New York: Springer-Verlag.

Morais, J., Bertelson, P., Cary, L., & Alegria, J. (1986). Literacy training and speech segmentation. *Cognition, 24*, 45–64.

Morais, J., Cary, L., Alegria, J., & Bertelson, P. (1979). Does awareness of speech as a sequence of phones arise spontaneously? *Cognition, 7*, 323–331.

Morris, D., Robinson, L., Turic, D., Duke, M., Webb, V., Milham, C., et al. (2000). Family-based association mapping provides evidence for a gene for reading disability on Chromosome 15q. *Human Molecular Genetics, 9*, 843–848.

Muneaux, M., Ziegler, J. C., True, C., Thomson, J., & Goswami, U. (2004). Deficits in beat perception and dyslexia: Evidence from French. *Neuroreport, 15*(8), 1255–1259.

Nation, K., Adams, J. W., Bowyer-Crane, C. A., & Snowling, M. J. (1999). Working memory deficits in poor comprehenders reflect underlying language impairments. *Journal of Experimental Child Psychology, 73*, 139–158.

Nation, K., Clarke, P., Marshall, C. M., & Durand, M. (2004). Hidden language impairments in children: Parallels between poor reading comprehension and specific language impairment? *Journal of Speech, Language, and Hearing Research, 47*(1), 199–211.

Nation, K., Cocksey, J., Taylor, J. S., & Bishop, D. V. (2010). A longitudinal investigation of early reading and language skills in children with poor reading comprehension. *Journal of Child Psychology and Psychiatry, 51*(9), 1031–1039.

Nation, K., & Snowling, M. J. (1998). Semantic processing and the development of word-recognition skills: Evidence from children with reading comprehension difficulties. *Journal of Memory and Language, 39*, 85–101.

Nation, K., & Snowling, M. J. (1999). Developmental differences in sensitivity to semantic relations among good and poor comprehenders: Evidence from semantic priming. *Cognition, 70*, B1–B13.

Nation, K., Snowling, M. J., & Clarke, P. (2005). Production of the English past tense by children with language comprehension impairments. *Journal of Child Language, 32*, 117–137.

Nittrouer, S. (1999). Do temporal processing deficits cause phonological processing problems? *Journal of Speech, Language, and Hearing Research, 42*, 925–942.

Oakhill, J. V., Cain, K., & Bryant, P. E. (2003). The dissociation of word reading and text comprehension: Evidence from component skills. *Language and Cognitive Processes, 18*, 443–468.

Obrzat, J. E. (1979). Dichotic listening and bisensory memory in qualitatively dyslexic readers. *Journal of Learning Disabilities, 12*, 304–313.

Obrzat, J. E., Hynd, G. W., & Boliek, C. A. (1986). Lateral asymmetries in learning disabled children: A review. In S. J. Ceci (Ed.), *Handbook of cognitive, social, and neuropsychological aspects of learning disabilities* (Vol. 1, pp. 441–473). Hillsdale, NJ: Erlbaum.

Olson, R. K., Conners, F. A., & Rack, J. P. (1991). Eye movements in normal and dyslexic readers. In J. F. Stein (Ed.), *Vision and visual dyslexia* (pp. 243–250). London: Macmillan.

Olson, R. K., Wise, B., Conners, F., Rack, J., & Fulker, D. (1989). Specific deficits in component reading and language skills: Genetic and environmental influences. *Journal of Learning Disabilities, 22*, 339–348.

Orton, S. (1937). *Reading, writing and speech problems in children*. London: Chapman Hall.

Paracchini, S., Scerri, T., & Monaco, A. P. (2007). The genetic lexicon of dyslexia. *Annual Review of Genomics and Human Genetics, 8*, 57–79.

Parker, R. M. (1990). Power, control, and validity in research. *Journal of Learning Disabilities, 23*, 613–620.

Pasquini, E. S., Corriveau, K. H., & Goswami, U. (2007). Auditory processing of amplitude envelope rise time in adults diagnosed with developmental dyslexia. *Scientific Studies of Reading, 11*(3), 259–286.

Paulesu, E., Connelly, A., Frith, C. D., Friston, K. J., Heather, J., & Myers, R. (1995). Functional MR imaging correlations with positron emission tomography: Initial experience using a cognitive activation paradigm on verbal working memory. *Neuroimaging Clinics of North America, 5*, 207–212.

Paulesu, E., Demonet, J., Fazio, F., McCrory, E., Charoine, V., Brunswick, N., Cappa, S., Cossu, G., Habib, M., Frith, C., & Frith, U. (2001). Dyslexia: Cultural diversity and biological unity. *Science, 291*, 2165–2167.

Paulesu, E., Frith, C. D., & Frackowiak, R. S. (1993). The neural correlates of the verbal component of working memory. *Nature, 362*, 342–345.

Pavlidis, G. T. (1981). Do eye movements hold the key to dyslexia? *Neuropsychologia, 19,* 57–64.

Pavlidis, G. T. (1985). Eye movement differences between dyslexics, normal and slow readers while sequentially fixating digits. *American Journal of Optometry and Physiological Optics, 62,* 820–822.

Pennington, B. F., Cardoso-Martins, C., Green, P. A., & Lefly, D. L. (2001). Comparing the phonological and double deficit hypotheses for developmental dyslexia. *Reading and Writing: An Interdisciplinary Journal, 14,* 707–755.

Pennington, B. F., & Gilger, J. W. (1996). How is dyslexia transmitted? In C. H. Chase, G. D. Rosen, & G. F. Sherman (Eds.), *Developmental dyslexia: Neural, cognitive, and genetic mechanisms* (pp. 41–62). Baltimore: York Press.

Pennington, B. F., Gilger, J. W., Pauls, D., Smith, S. A., Smith, S. D., & DeFries, J. C. (1991). Evidence for major gene transmission of developmental dyslexia. *Journal of American Medical Association, 266,* 1527–1534.

Pennington, B. F., Filipek, P. A., Lefly, D. L., Churchwell, J., Kennedy, D. N., Simon, J. H., et al. (1999). Brain morphometry in reading-disabled twins. *Neurology, 53,* 723–739.

Pennington, B. F., & Lefly, D. L. (2001). Early reading development in children at family risk for dyslexia. *Child Development, 72,* 816–833.

Peterson, R. L., Pennington, B. F., Shriberg, L. D., & Boada, R. (2009). What influences literacy outcome in children with speech sound disorder? *Journal of Speech, Language, and Hearing Research, 52*(5), 1175–1188.

Petrill, S. A., Hart, S. A., Harlaar, N., Logan, J., Justice, L. M., Schatschneider, C., et al. (2010). Genetic and environmental influences on the growth of early reading skills. *Journal of Child Psychology and Psychiatry, 51*(6), 660–667.

Plomin, R., & Kovas, Y. (2005). Generalist genes and learning disabilities. *Psychological Bulletin, 131,* 592–617.

Poeppel, D., & Rowley, H. A. (1996). Magnetic source imaging and the neural basis of dyslexia. *Annals of Neurology, 40,* 137–138.

Preston, J. E., & Edwards, M. L. (2010). Phonological awareness and types of sound errors in preschoolers with speech sound disorders. *Journal of Speech, Language, and Hearing Research, 53,* 44–60.

Puolakanaho, A., Ahonen, T., Aro, M., Eklund, K., Leppanen, P. H., Poikkeus, A. M., et al., (2007). Very early phonological and language skills: Estimating individual risk of reading disability. *Journal of Child Psychology and Psychiatry, 48,* 923–931.

Rae, C., Harasty, J. A., Dzendrowskyj, T. E., Talcott, J. B., Simpson, J. M., Blamire, A. M., et al. (2002). Cerebellar morphology in developmental dyslexia. *Neuropsychologia, 40*(8), 1285–1292.

Ramus, F. (2003). Developmental dyslexia: Specific phonological deficit or general sensorimotor dysfunction? *Current Opinion in Neurobiology, 13,* 212–218.

Rapala, M. M., & Brady, S. (1990). Reading ability and short-term memory: The role of phonological processing. *Reading and Writing: An Interdisciplinary Journal, 2,* 1–25.

Raskind, W. H. (2001). Current understanding of genetic basis of reading and spelling disability. *Learning Disability Quarterly, 24,* 141–157.

Rayner, K. (1978). Eye movements in reading and information processing. *Psychological Bulletin, 85,* 618–660.

Rayner, K. (1985). Do faulty eye movements cause dyslexia? *Developmental Neuropsychology, 1,* 3–15.

Read, C., & Ruyter, L. (1985). Reading and spelling skills in adults of low literacy. *Remedial and Special Education, 6,* 43–52.

Reed, M. A. (1989). Speech perception and the discrimination of brief auditory cues in reading disabled children. *Journal of Experimental Child Psychology, 48,* 270–292.

Richardson, U., Thomson, J., Scott, S. K., & Goswami, U. (2004). Auditory processing skills and phonological representation in dyslexic children. *Dyslexia, 10,* 215–233.

Rispens, J., & Parigger, E. (2010). Non-word repetition in Dutch-speaking children with specific language impairment with and without reading problems. *British Journal of Developmental Psychology, 28,* 177–188.

Rispens, J., Roeleven, S., & Koster, C. (2004). Sensitivity to subject-verb agreement in spoken language in children with developmental dyslexia. *Journal of Neurolinguistics, 17,* 333–347.

Robichon, F., Levrier, O., Farnarier, P., & Habib, M. (2000). Developmental dyslexia: Atypical cortical asymmetries and functional significance. *European Journal of Neurology, 7*(1), 35–46.

Robinson, G. L. W., & Conway, R. N. F. (1990). The effects of Irlen colored lenses on students' specific reading skills and their perception of ability: A 12-month validity study. *Journal of Learning Disabilities, 23,* 589–596.

Rosen, S. R. (2003). Auditory processing in dyslexia and specific language impairment: Is there a deficit? What is its nature? Does it explain anything? *Journal of Phonetics, 31,* 509–527.

Roth, P., & Spekman, N. J. (1986). Narrative discourse: Spontaneously generated stories of learning-disabled and normally achieving students. *Journal of Speech and Hearing Disorders, 51*, 8–23.

Rudel, R. (1985). The definition of dyslexia: Language and motor deficits. In F. H. Duffy & N. Geschwind (Eds.), *Dyslexia: A neuroscientific approach to clinical evaluation* (pp. 33–53). Boston: Little, Brown.

Rumsey, J. M., Donohue, B. C., Brady, D. R., Nace, K., Giedd, J. N., & Andreason, P. (1997). A magnetic resonance imaging study of planum temporale asymmetry in men with developmental dyslexia. *Archives of Neurology, 54*(12), 1481–1489.

Rumsey, J. M., Nace, K., Donohue, B., Wise, D., Maisog, J., & Andreason, P. (1997). A positron emission tomographic study of impaired word recognition and phonological processing in dyslexic men. *Archives of Neurology, 54*, 562–573.

Rvachew, S. (2007). Phonological processing and reading in children with speech sound disorders. *American Journal of Speech-Language Pathology, 16*, 260–270.

Safer, D. J., & Allen, R. D. (1976). *Hyperactive children: Diagnosis and management.* Baltimore: University Park Press.

Salmelin, R., Service, E., Kiesila, P., Uutela, K., & Salonen, O. (1996). Impaired visual word processing in dyslexia revealed with magnetoencephalography. *Annals of Neurology, 40*, 157–162.

Samuelsson, S., Olson, R., Wadsworth, S. J., Corley, R., DeFries, J. C., Willcutt, E. G., et al. (2007). Genetic and environmental influences on pre-reading skills and early reading and spelling development: A comparison among United States, Australia, and Scandinavia. *Reading and Writing: An Interdisciplinary Journal, 20*(1), 51–75.

Sandak, R., Mencl, W. E., Frost, S. J., & Pugh, K. R. (2004). The neurobiological basis of skilled and impaired reading: Recent findings and new directions. *Scientific Studies of Reading, 8*(3), 273–292.

Satz, P. (1977). Laterality tests: An inferential problem. *Cortex, 13*, 208–212.

Satz, P., & Sparrow, S. S. (1970). Specific developmental dyslexia: A theoretical formulation. In D. J. Bakker & P. Satz (Eds.), *Specific reading disability: Advances in theory and method* (pp. 41–60). Rotterdam: Rotterdam University Press.

Scanlon, D. M., & Vellutino, F. R. (1996). Prerequisite skills, early instruction and success in first grade reading: Selected results from a longitudinal study. *Mental Retardation and Developmental Disabilities, 2*, 54–63.

Scanlon, D. M., & Vellutino, F. R. (1997). A comparison of the instructional backgrounds and cognitive profiles of poor, average, and good readers who were initially identified as at risk for reading failure. *Scientific Studies of Reading, 1*, 191–216.

Scarborough, H. S. (1989). Prediction of reading disability from familial and individual differences. *Journal of Educational Psychology, 81*, 101–108.

Scarborough, H. S. (1990). Very early language deficits in dyslexic children. *Child Development, 61*, 1728–1743.

Scarborough, H. S. (1991). Early syntactic development of dyslexic children. *Annals of Dyslexia, 41*, 207–220.

Scarborough, H. S., & Dobrich, W. (1994). On the efficacy of reading to preschoolers. *Developmental Review, 14*, 245–302.

Schatschneider, C., Carlson, C. D., Francis, D. J., Foorman, B. R., & Fletcher, J. M. (2002). Relationship of rapid naming and phonological awareness in early reading achievement: Implications for the double deficit hypothesis. *Journal of Learning Disabilities, 35*, 245–256.

Sesma, H., Mahone, M., Levine, T., Eason, S., & Cutting, L. (2009). The contribution of executive skills to reading comprehension. *Child Neuropsychology, 15*, 232–246.

Shankweiler, D., Liberman, I. Y., Mark, L. S., Fowler, C. A., & Fischer, F. W. (1979). The speech code and learning to read. *Journal of Experimental Psychology: Human Learning and Memory, 5*, 531–545.

Share, D. L. (1995). Phonological recoding and self-teaching: Sine qua non of reading acquisition. *Cognition, 55*, 151–218.

Share, D. L., Jorm, A. F., Maclean, R., & Matthews, R. (2002). Temporal processing and reading disability. *Reading and Writing: An Interdisciplinary Journal, 15*, 151–178.

Share, D. L., & Stanovich, K. E. (1995). Cognitive processes in early reading development: Accommodating individual differences into a model of acquisition. *Issues in Education, 1*, 1–57.

Shaywitz, B. A., Fletcher, J. M., Holahan, J. M., Shneider, A. E., Marchione, K. E., Stuebing, K. K., Francis, D. J., Shankweiler, D. P., Katz, L., Liberman, I. Y., & Shaywitz, S. E. (1995). Interrelationships between reading disability and attention-deficit/hyperactivity disorder. *Cognitive Neuropsychology, 1*, 170–186.

Shaywitz, S. E., Fletcher, J. M., & Shaywitz, B. A. (1994). Issues in the definition and classification of attention deficit disorder. *Topics in Language Disorders, 14*, 1–25.

Shaywitz, B. A, Shaywitz, S. E, Blachman, B,. Pugh, K. R., Fulbright, R., Skudlarski, P., et al. (2004). Development of left occipito-termporal systems for skilled reading following a phonologically-based intervention in children. *Biological Psychiatry, 55*, 926–933.

Shaywitz, S., Shaywitz, B. A., Pugh, K. R., Fulbright, R. K., Constable, R. T., Mencl, W. E., Shankweiler, D. P., Liberman, A. M., Skudlarski, P., Fletcher, J. M., Katz, L., Marchione, K. E., Lacadie, C., Gatenby, C., & Gore, J. C. (1998). Functional disruption in the organization of the brain for reading in dyslexia. *Proceedings of the National Academy of Sciences USA, 95,* 2636–2641.

Silva, P. A., McGree, R., Williams, S. M. (1987). Developmental language delay from three to seven and its significance for low intelligence and reading difficulties at age seven. *Developmental Medicine and Clinical Neurology, 25,* 783–793.

Silver, L. B. (1981). The relationship between learning disabilities, hyperactivity, distractibility, and behavioral problems. *Journal of the American Academy of Child Psychiatry, 20,* 385–397.

Silver, L. B. (1995). Controversial therapies. *Journal of Child Neurology, 10,* S96–S100.

Simos, P. G., Brier, J. L., Fletcher, J. M., Bergman, E., & Papanicolauo, A. C. (2002). Cerebral mechanisms involved in word reading in dyslexic children: A magnetic source imaging approach. *Cerebral Cortex, 10,* 809–816.

Simos, P. G., Fletcher, J. M., Bergman, M. D., Brier, J. I., Foorman, B. R., Castillo, E. M., Davis, R. N., Fitzgerald, M., & Papanicolaou, A. C. (2002). Dyslexia-specific brain activation profile becomes normal following successful remedial training. *Neurology, 58,* 1203–1213.

Simos, P. G., Fletcher, J. M., Foorman, B. R., Frances, D. J., Castillo, E. M., Davis, R. N., Fitzgerald, M., Mathes, P. G., Denton, C., & Papanicolaou, A. C. (2002). Brain activation profiles during the early stages of reading acquisition. *Journal of Child Neurology, 17,* 159–163.

Simos, P. G., Papanicolaou, A. C., Brier, J. L., et al. (2000). Brain activation profiles in dyslexic children during non-word reading: A magnetic source imaging study. *Neuroscience Letter, 290,* 61–65.

Skottun, B. C. (2000). The magnocellular deficit theory of dyslexia: The evidence from contrast sensitivity. *Vision Research, 40,* 111–127.

Skottun, B. C., & Skoyles, J. R. (2008). Dyslexia and rapid visual processing: A commentary. *Journal of Clinical and Experimental Neuropsychology, 30*(6), 666–673.

Snowling, M. (1981). Phonemic deficits in developmental dyslexia. *Psychological Research, 43,* 219–234.

Snowling, M. J., Bishop, D. V. M., & Stothard, S. E. (2000). Is preschool language impairment a risk factor for dyslexia in adolescence? *Journal of Child Psychology and Psychiatry, 41,* 587–600.

Snowling, M. J., Gallagher, A., & Frith, U. (2003). Family risk of dyslexia is continuous: Individual differences in precursors of reading skill. *Child Development, 74,* 358–373.

Snowling, M. J., Goulandris, N., Bowlby, M., & Howell, P. (1986). Segmentation and speech perception in relation to reading skill: A developmental analysis. *Journal of Experimental Child Psychology, 41,* 489–507.

Solman, R. T., & May, J. G. (1990). Spatial localization discrepancies: A visual deficiency in poor readers. *American Journal of Psychology, 103,* 243–263.

Spear-Swerling, L., & Sternberg, R. J. (1994). The road not taken: An integrative theoretical model of reading disability. *Journal of Learning Disabilities, 27,* 91–103, 122.

Spear-Swerling, L., & Sternberg, R. J. (1996). *Off track: When poor readers become "learning disabled."* Boulder, CO: Westview Press.

Stanley, G. (1991). Glare, scotopic sensitivity and colour therapy. In J. F. Stein (Ed.), *Vision and visual dyslexia.* London: Macmillan.

Stanley, G. (1994). Visual deficit models of dyslexia. In G. Hales (Ed.), *Dyslexia matters.* San Diego, CA: Singular.

Stanovich, K. E. (1986). Matthew effects in reading: Some consequences of individual differences in the acquisition of literacy. *Reading Research Quarterly, 86,* 360–406.

Stanovich, K. E. (1988). *Children's reading and the development of phonological awareness.* Detroit, MI: Wayne State University Press.

Stanovich, K. E., & Siegel, L. S. (1994). The phenotypic performance profile of reading-disabled children: A regression-based test of the phonological-core variable-difference model. *Journal of Educational Psychology, 86,* 24–53.

Stellern, J., Collins, J., & Bayne, M. (1987). A dual-task investigation of language-spatial lateralization. *Journal of Learning Disabilities, 20,* 551–556.

Stone, B., & Brady, S. (1995). Evidence for phonological processing deficits in less-skilled readers. *Annals of Dyslexia, 95,* 51–78.

Storch, S. A., & Whitehurst, G. J. (2002). Oral language and code-related precursors to reading: Evidence from a longitudinal structural model. *Developmental Psychology, 38*(6), 934–947.

Stothard, S. E., & Hulme, C. (1992). Reading comprehension difficulties in children: The role of language comprehension and working memory skills. *Reading and Writing: An Interdisciplinary Journal, 4,* 245–256.

Stothard, S. E., & Hulme, C. (1995). A comparison of phonological skills in children with reading comprehension difficulties and children with decoding difficulties. *Journal of Child Psychology and Psychiatry, 36*, 399–408.

Stothard, S. E., Snowling, M. J., Bishop, D. V. M., Chipcase, B., & Kaplan, C. A. (1998). Language-impaired preschoolers: A follow-up into adolescence. *Journal of Speech, Language, and Hearing Research, 41*, 407–418.

Stuart, G. W., McAnally, K. I., & Castles, A. (2001). Can contrast sensitivity functions in dyslexia be explained by inattention rather than a magnocellar deficit? *Vision Research, 41*, 3205–3211.

Sundeth, K., & Bowers, P. G. (1997). *The relationship between digit naming speed and orthography in children with and without phonological deficits.* Paper presented at the Society for the Scientific Study of Reading, Chicago, IL.

Swan, D. M., & Goswami, U. (1997). Picture naming deficits in developmental dyslexia: The phonological representations hypothesis. *Brain and Language, 56*, 334–353.

Swanson, H. L., & Hsieh, C. J. (2009). Reading disabilities in adults: A selective meta-analysis of the literature. *Review of Educational Research, 79*(4), 1362–1390.

Tallal, P. (1980). Auditory temporal perception, phonics, and reading disabilities in children. *Brain and Language, 9*, 182–198.

Tallal, P. (2000). Experimental studies of language learning impairments: From research to remediation. In D. V. M. Bishop & L. B. Leonard (Eds.), *Speech and language impairments in children: Causes, characteristics, intervention and outcome* (pp. 131–155). Hove, UK: Psychology Press.

Tallal, P., Curtiss, S., & Kaplan, R. (1989). *The San Diego longitudinal study: Evaluating the outcomes of preschool impairments in language development.* Bethesda, MD: NINCDS.

Tomblin, J. B., Records, N. L., Buckwalter, P., Zhang, X., Smith, E., & O'Brien, M. (1997). The prevalence of specific language impairment in kindergarten children. *Journal of Speech, Language, and Hearing Research, 40*, 1245–1260.

Torgesen, J. K. (1985). Memory processes in reading disabled children. *Journal of Learning Disabilities, 18*, 350–357.

Torgesen, J. K. (1996). *Phonological awareness: A critical factor in dyslexia.* Baltimore: Orton Dyslexia Society.

Torgesen, J. K., Wagner, R. K., & Rashotte, C. A. (1994). Longitudinal studies of phonological processing and reading. *Journal of Learning Disabilities, 27*, 276–286.

Torgesen, J. K., Wagner, R. K., Rashotte, C. A., Burgess, S., & Hecht, S. (1997). Contributions of phonological awareness and rapid naming to the growth of word-reading skills in second- and fifth-grade children. *Scientific Studies in Reading, 1*, 161–185.

Torppa, M., Tolvanen, A., Poikkeus, A., Eklund, K., Lerkkanen, M., Leskinen, E., & Lyytinen, H. (2007). Reading development subtypes and their early characteristics. *Annals of Dyslexia, 57*, 3–32.

Troia, G. A. (1999). Phonological awareness intervention research: A critical review of the experimental methodology. *Reading Research Quarterly, 34*, 28–52.

Treutlein, A., Zoller, I., Roos, J., & Scholer, H. (2008). Effects of phonological awareness training on reading achievement. *Written Language & Literacy, 11*(2), 147–166.

Tunick, R. A., & Pennington, B. F. (2002). The etiological relationship between reading disability and phonological disorder. *Annals of Dyslexia, 52*, 75–98.

Vaessen, A., Gerretsen, P., & Blomert, L. (2009). Naming problems do not reflect a second independent core deficit in dyslexia: Double deficits explored. *Journal of Experimental Child Psychology, 103*(2), 202–221.

Vellutino, F. R., Pruzek, R., Steger, J. A., & Meshoulam, U. (1973). Immediate visual recall in poor and normal readers as a function of orthographic-linguistic familiarity. *Cortex, 9*, 368–384.

Vellutino, F. R., & Scanlon, D. M. (Eds.). (1982). *Verbal processing in poor and normal readers.* New York: Springer-Verlag.

Vellutino, F. R., Scanlon, D. M., Sipay, E. R., Small, S. G., Chen, R., Pratt, A., & Denckla, M. B. (1996). Cognitive profiles of difficult-to-remediate and readily remediated poor readers: Early intervention as a vehicle for distinguishing between cognitive and experiential deficits as basic causes of specific reading disabilities. *Journal of Educational Psychology, 88*, 601–638.

Vellutino, F. R., Scanlon, D. M., Small, S., & Fanuele, D. P. (2006). Response to intervention as a vehicle for distinguishing between children with and without reading disabilities: Evidence for the role of kindergarten and first grade interventions. *Journal of Learning Disabilities, 39*, 157–169.

Vellutino, F. R., Scanlon, D. M., & Spearing, D. (1995). Semantic and phonological coding in poor and normal readers. *Journal of Experimental Child Psychology, 59*, 76–123.

Vellutino, F. R., Steger, J. A., DeSetto, L., & Phillips, F. (1975). Immediate and delayed recognition of visual stimuli in poor and normal readers. *Journal of Experimental Child Psychology, 19*, 223–232.

Vellutino, F. R., Steger, J. A., Harding, C. J., & Phillips, F. (1975). Verbal vs. non-verbal paired-associate learning in poor and normal readers. *Neuropsychologia, 13,* 75–82.

Vogel, S. A. (1974). Syntactic abilities in normal and dyslexic children. *Journal of Learning Disabilities, 7,* 47–53.

Vogler, G. P., DeFries, J. C., & Decker, S. N. (1985). Family history as an indicator of risk for reading disability. *Journal of Learning Disabilities, 18,* 419–421.

Vukovic, R. K., & Siegel, L. S. (2006). The double-deficit hypothesis. *Journal of Learning Disabilities, 39*(1), 25–47.

Waber, D. P., Weiler, M. D., Wolff, P. H., Bellinger, D., Marcus, D. J., Ariel, R., Forbes, P., & Wypij, D. (2001). Processing of rapid auditory stimuli in school-age children referred for evaluation of learning disorders. *Child Development, 72,* 37–49.

Wagner, R. K., Balthazor, M., Hurley, S., Morgan, S., Rachotte, C., Shaner, R., Simmons, K., & Stage, S. (1987). The nature of prereaders' phonological processing abilities. *Cognitive Development, 2,* 355–373.

Wagner, R. K., Torgesen, J. K., & Rashotte, C. A. (1994). Development of reading-related phonological processing abilities: New evidence of bidirectional causality from a latent variable longitudinal study. *Developmental Psychology, 30,* 73–87.

Weiss, R. (1990). Dyslexics read better with blues. *Science News, 138,* 196.

Wiig, E. H., & Semel, E. M. (1975). Productive language abilities in learning disabled adolescents. *Journal of Learning Disabilities, 8*(9), 578–586.

Willcutt, E. G., & Pennington, B. F. (2000). Comorbidity of reading disability and attention-deficit/hyperactivity disorder. *Journal of Learning Disabilities, 33,* 179–191.

Willcutt, E. G., Pennington, B. F., Boada, R., Ogline, J. S., Tunick, R. A., Chhabildas, N. A., & Olson, R. K. (2001). A comparison of the cognitive deficits in reading disability and attention-deficit/hyperactivity disorder. *Journal of Abnormal Psychology, 170,* 157–172.

Willcutt, E. G., Pennington, B. F., Olson, R. K., Chhabildas, N., & Hulslander, J. (2005). Neuropsychological analyses of comorbidity between reading disability and attention deficit hyperactivity disorder: In search of the common deficit. *Developmental Neuropsychology, 27*(1), 35–75.

Wise, J. C., Sevcik, R. A., Morris, R. D., Lovett, M. W., & Wolf, M. (2007). The relationship among receptive and expressive vocabulary, listening comprehension, pre-reading skills, word identification skills, and reading comprehension by children with reading disabilities. *Journal of Speech, Language and Hearing Research, 50*(4), 1093–1109.

Wolf, M. (1984). Naming, reading, and the dyslexias: A longitudinal overview. *Annals of Dyslexia, 34,* 87–136.

Wolf, M. (1991). Naming speed and reading: The contribution of the cognitive neurosciences. *Reading Research Quarterly, 26,* 123–141.

Wolf, M., Bally, H., & Morris, R. (1986). Automaticity, retrieval processes, and reading: A longitudinal study in average and impaired readers. *Child Development, 57,* 988–1000.

Wolf, M., & Bowers, P. (1999). The "double-deficit hypothesis" for the development dyslexias. *Journal of Educational Psychology, 91,* 1–24.

Wolf, M., Bowers, P., & Biddle, K. (2000). Naming-speed processes, timing, and reading: A conceptual review. *Journal of Learning Disabilities, 33,* 387–407.

Wolf, M., & Goodglass, H. (1986). Dyslexia, dysnomia, and lexical retrieval: A longitudinal investigation. *Brain and Language, 28,* 154–168.

Wolf, M., O'Rourke, A. G., Gidney, C., Lovett, M., Cirino, P., & Morris, R. (2002). The second deficit: An investigation of the independence of phonological and naming-speed deficits in developmental dyslexia. *Reading and Writing: An Interdisciplinary Journal, 15,* 43–72.

Wood, F. B., & Grigorenko, E. L. (2001). Emerging issues in genetics of dyslexia: Methodological preview. *Journal of Learning Disabilities, 34,* 503–511.

Yuill, N., & Oakhill, J. (1991). *Children's problems in test comprehension.* Cambridge, England: Cambridge University Press.

Zhang, J., & McBride-Chang, C. (2010). Auditory sensitivity, speech perception, and reading development and impairment. *Educational Psychology Review, 22*(3), 323–338.

Chapter 5

Assessment and Instruction for Phonemic Awareness and Word Recognition Skills

Stephanie Al Otaiba, Marcia L. Kosanovich, and Joseph K. Torgesen

A number of factors influence how readily young school-age children become proficient readers, including exposure to print, letter knowledge, phonemic awareness (PA), and general language (particularly vocabulary; e.g., National Early Literacy Panel, Lonigan, Schatschneider, & Westberg, 2008). Previous chapters have discussed the importance of these skills and how they develop. The focus of this chapter is the assessment and instruction of phonemic awareness and word recognition skills in the early elementary school years. By third grade, all but the most struggling students would be well on their way toward mastery of these skills. By necessity, we have made a number of assumptions about readers of the book and, hence, this chapter. We assume that the reader has already learned from other chapters about the nature of reading disabilities and reading acquisition processes and will understand the language disabilities that directly interfere with the acquisition of good word recognition skills. The reader should also understand that the ultimate goal of reading instruction and intervention is to help children acquire all the skills required to comprehend the meaning of text, and that the acquisition of effective word-level reading skills is critical to the attainment of that goal. Finally, we assume that the reader has some knowledge about Response to Intervention (RTI), which is a prevention-oriented approach that provides early literacy intervention to children who are struggling with learning to read.

Because the development of phonemic awareness is critical to the subsequent acquisition of good word recognition skills, it seems logical to organize this chapter by an initial discussion about development and assessment in this area, and then to continue the discussion to the more complex issues involved in the assessment of word identification skills. Next, we use the RTI framework to organize a discussion of instruction and interventions for phonemic awareness and word recognition skills. We discuss both Tier 1, or classroom instruction that all children receive, and additional

This work was supported by a Multidisciplinary Learning Disabilities Center Grant P50HD052120 from the National Institute of Child Health and Human Development. Requests for reprints should be sent to: Stephanie Al Otaiba, Florida Center for Reading Research, e-mail: salotaiba@fcrr.org interventions, which are provided only to students who are not making adequate progress within Tier 1. Because there is currently such variation in how RTI is implemented, including the number of instructional tiers available and when special education actually begins, we will simply describe interventions and their suggested intensity, rather than assigning them to specific tiers.

DEVELOPMENT AND ASSESSMENT OF PHONEMIC AWARENESS

Several general issues related to assessment of phonological awareness must be considered before information about specific tests is presented. Perhaps the most central of these issues is the matter of definition. Before any construct can be assessed, it should be defined, and phonemic awareness is a construct that is not easy to pin down to a simple definition. One issue is whether we should consider phonemic awareness to be a kind of conceptual understanding about language or whether it should be considered a skill. What do we mean, precisely, when we say that a child's phonemic awareness has increased from the last time we measured it?

On the one hand, part of what we mean by phonemic awareness is that it involves an understanding that a single-syllable word such as *cat*, which is experienced by the listener as a single beat of sound, actually can be subdivided into beginning, middle, and ending sounds. Similarly, it involves the understanding that individual segments of sound at the phonemic level can be combined together to form words. Otherwise, the child would not be able to make sense of the request to blend the sounds represented by the letters *c - a - t* to make a word.

On the other hand, a complete understanding of phonemic awareness must also account for the fact that it behaves like a skill that develops across time in fairly predictable ways. That is, children seem to acquire an increasing ability to notice, think about, and manipulate the phonemes in words as they move from preschool through elementary school. For example, in the first few weeks of preschool, a student might express surprise about a classmate whose name starts "the same as mine." At the beginning of kindergarten, one child we asked to tell us the sounds in *dog* answered "woof-woof," indicating he either was unfamiliar with the task, or was unaware of sounds in words. But, by the middle of kindergarten the same child was able to isolate and pronounce the first sound and the onset of *dog*, and by the end of kindergarten, like most children, he could segment all the sounds in three- and four-phoneme words (Good, Wallin, Simmons, Kame'enui, & Kaminski, 2002). Children also show regular improvements during this same period of time in their ability to blend individually presented sounds together to form words (Torgesen & Morgan, 1990).

To account for both the conceptual and skill components of the construct, we need a definition of phonemic awareness such as the following: It involves a more or less explicit understanding that words are composed of segments of sound smaller than a syllable, as well as knowledge, or awareness, of the distinctive features of individual phonemes themselves. It is this latter knowledge of the identity of individual phonemes themselves that continues to increase after an initial understanding of the phonemic structure of words is acquired. For example, children must acquire a knowledge of the distinctive features of a phoneme such as /l/ so they can recognize it when it occurs with slightly varied pronunciation at the beginning of a word such as *last*, as the second sound in a consonant blend as in *flat*, in the middle of a word, such as *shelving*, at the end, as in *fall*, or when it occurs in a final blend such as in *fault*.

Sometimes, the term *phonological awareness* is used to refer to the construct we are discussing here, but this more global term actually implies a more general level of awareness than the words *phonemic awareness*. For example, awareness of the syllabic structure of words would qualify as a form of phonological awareness because it involves awareness of part of the sound structure in words. In addition, rhyme awareness is a beginning form of phonological awareness because it involves an ability to analyze words at the level of the onset and rime (*c-at, m-at*). The distinction between these more general forms of phonological awareness and the more specific, discrete, form of phonemic awareness is supported by factor analyses of groups of these tasks, and it is important because measures of phonemic awareness appear to be more predictive of individual differences in reading and spelling growth (Høien, Lundberg, Stanovich, & Bjaalid, 1995; Lonigan, Schatschneider, & Westberg, 2008).

Thus, researchers have cautioned that preschool children with speech or language impairments (SI and LI, respectively) appear slower to develop phonological and phonemic awareness compared to their typically developing peers (Bird, Bishop, & Freeman, 1995; Boudreau & Hedberg, 1999), elevating their risk for reading difficulties (Aram & Hall, 1989; Bishop & Adams, 1990; Catts, 1991, 1993; Scarborough & Dobrich, 1990). This risk appears substantially higher for children with LI; according to the American Speech-Language-Hearing Association (2001), young children with LI are four to five times more likely than their peers to have reading problems later in elementary school and beyond. Catts and colleagues (2002) reported that roughly half of kindergarteners with LI developed reading disabilities by second grade. Similarly, when Puranik, Petscher, Al Otaiba, Catts, and Lonigan (2008) examined oral reading fluency scores of over 1,900 students with SI and LI across first through third grade, they found that significant differences in growth trajectories could be seen by January of first grade. Although reading growth was generally better for students with SI than those with LI, a large proportion of students with either impairment did not meet grade-level reading fluency benchmarks. Those students with persistent impairments grew slower than students whose impairments were resolved. These results highlight the need to identify, monitor, and address the phonological and word reading difficulties early among students with SI or LI.

The Importance of Phonemic Awareness in Learning to Read

In addition to understanding the concept of phonemic awareness, assessment must also be informed by an understanding of why phonemic awareness is important to the growth of word-reading ability. Phonemic awareness contributes to the growth of early reading skills in at least three ways:

1. *It helps children understand the alphabetic principle and develop alphabetic knowledge.* To take advantage of the fact that English is an alphabetic language, a child must be aware that words have sound segments that are represented by the letters in print. Without at least emergent levels of phonemic awareness, the rationale for learning individual letter sounds and "sounding out" words is not understandable.
2. *It helps children notice the regular ways that letters represent sounds in words.* If children can "hear" four sounds in the word *clap*, it helps them to notice the way the letters correspond to the sounds. The ability to notice the correspondence between the sounds in a word and the way it is spelled has two potential benefits. First, it reinforces knowledge of individual sound–letter correspondences, and second, it helps in forming mental representations of words that involve a close amalgamation of their written and spoken forms. Linnea Ehri (1998, 2002) has shown how developing readers use their awareness of the phonemes in words as a mnemonic to help them remember the words' spellings so they can eventually recognize many thousands of words "by sight."

3. *It helps children become flexible decoders to decode even irregular words, and it makes it possible to generate possibilities for words in context that are only partially "sounded out."* For example, consider a first grader who comes to a sentence such as, "The boy and his friends ride th_ _ _ bikes to the store," and cannot recognize the high-frequency but irregular word *their*, but knows the sound represented by the first digraph. An early level of phonemic awareness supports the ability to search the lexicon for words that begin with similar sounds. That is, in addition to being categorized by their meanings, words can be categorized by their beginning, middle, or ending sounds. If children are able to use information about the phonemes in an unknown word that they obtain from even a partial phonemic analysis to constrain their search for words that also fit the meaning of the sentence or paragraph, they will significantly increase the accuracy of their first guesses about the identity of unknown words in text. It is important for young children to become accurate readers as quickly as possible because words must be read accurately a number of times before they can become part of a child's sight vocabulary (Share & Stanovich, 1995).

This analysis suggests that phonemic awareness has its primary impact on early reading growth through its contribution to children's ability to use sound–letter correspondences to decode words in text. The ability to phonemically decode words is not an end in itself because phonemic decoding is too slow and effortful to support fluent reading and good comprehension. However, accumulating knowledge about reading trajectories indicates that phonemic reading skills play a critical role in supporting overall reading growth, particularly the growth of a rich vocabulary of words that can be recognized orthographically, or "by sight" (Ehri, 2002; Share & Stanovich, 1995). Further, the National Early Literacy Panel (NELP; Lonigan et al., 2008) synthesized existing correlational studies that examined the prediction of decoding ability and comprehension from children's preschool phonological skills. The Panel examined 69 studies and, on average, found a moderate relation ($r = .40$) between phonological awareness during preschool and later decoding once reading instruction began in school. A similar relation ($r = .44$) was found when the panel analyzed findings from 20 studies that examined the prediction of reading comprehension from early phonological awareness.

We now have compelling scientific evidence that phonemic awareness is an important prerequisite for learning to read. The most important evidence comes from well-designed experiments, or training studies, in which instruction in phonemic awareness has been shown to facilitate the acquisition of beginning word-reading skills, particularly phonemic decoding skills. In a seminal analysis of the results from 52 carefully selected experimental studies, Ehri and her colleagues (2001) reported a highly consistent effect for training in phonemic awareness on the development of reading skills. Not surprisingly, these studies showed that the effect of training in phonemic awareness was strongest for phonemic decoding skills in reading, and less strong, but still statistically significant, for measures of reading comprehension.

The NELP (Lonigan et al., 2008), in a synthesis of intervention studies with children age 5 and younger, showed it is possible to improve phonological awareness in preschool children through direct instruction. They reviewed studies that trained children in phonological awareness and in the alphabetic principle. In 51 studies that assessed phonological awareness as an outcome measure, the average effect size was .82, indicating a large impact. "This result means that, on average, children who received a code-focused intervention scored 0.82 of a standard deviation higher on measures of PA than did children who did not receive a code-focused intervention. To put this in context, if the average children not receiving a code-focused intervention scored 100 on a standardized test of PA that had a mean of 100 and a standard deviation of 15, the average children receiving a code-focused intervention scored 112 on the test (i.e., the difference between scoring at the 50th and 79th percentiles)" (p. 109). Furthermore, in secondary analyses, the NELP authors found even stronger effects of code-focused interventions for children who had weaker knowledge about the alphabet (ES = .99). They also compared the effect sizes of interventions that provided only phonological training (ES = .91), phonological and alphabetic knowledge training (ES = .70), only alphabetic knowledge training (ES = .48), and phonological awareness and phonics training (ES =.74).

Purposes for Assessment of Phonemic Awareness

The significant correlations between emerging phonemic awareness and later growth of reading skills (see Blachman, 2000; Lonigan et al., 2008 for a more recent reviews) suggests one of three reasons why we should be concerned about assessment of this construct. At present, phonemic awareness is being assessed to identify children at risk for reading failure before reading instruction actually begins, to monitor children's progress in acquiring critical reading skills, and to help describe the level of phonological impairment in children being diagnosed with reading disabilities (RD). Although these are all promising areas for the development of useful assessment procedures, we are still some distance away from being able to precisely identify children with RD on the basis of their performance on single measures of phonemic awareness in preschool or kindergarten, particularly for children with speech and language impairments and children with impoverished language and reading readiness. The most important problem is that these measures produce too high a number of false positives (children who are predicted to be poor readers, but turn out to be good readers; Blachman, 2000; Torgesen, Burgess, & Rashotte, 1996).

One solution to the problems inherent in single-screening assessments of phonemic awareness is to monitor progress in the growth of phonemic awareness skills several times across preschool through first grade. The advantage of multiple assessments of phonemic awareness is that they can provide an indication of children's response to the instruction they are receiving, and they can be used to identify children who are not keeping pace with expected levels of growth before the learning failure has become too severe (Good, Simmons, & Kame'enui, 2001; Good, Simmons, Kame'enui, Kaminski, & Wallin, 2002).

As an aid in the diagnosis of reading disabilities, measures of phonemic awareness are consistently more useful than any other measure of nonreading skills (Fletcher et al., 1994). However, the issue here is whether they actually add any precision to the diagnosis of reading disability beyond the information that is provided by direct measures of phonemic decoding ability. In one study that addressed this question (Torgesen, Wagner, Rashotte, Burgess, & Hecht, 1997), it was found that measures of phonemic awareness in second- and third-grade children provided a small amount of useful information beyond that provided by reading measures. However, the amount of additional information may not have been large enough to warrant the additional time it took to administer the phonemic awareness tests. Catts and Hogan (2002) reported very similar findings in a longitudinal study of kindergarten, second-, and fourth-grade-level students. Measures of phonemic awareness administered in kindergarten provided important unique information (beyond that provided by measures of phonemic decoding given in kindergarten) in explaining individual differences in word reading accuracy in second grade. However, when measures of phonemic awareness were given along with measures of phonemic decoding in second grade, level of phonemic awareness added very little to the prediction of problems in word reading accuracy once individual differences on measures of phonemic decoding were taken into account.

The principal reason why assessment of phonemic awareness may not add to the diagnosis of reading disability once children have begun to learn to read is that phonemic decoding skills and phonemic awareness are very highly correlated with one another. However, it is far too early to rule out the use of phonemic awareness measures as part of a diagnostic battery for older children or adolescents with RD. In individual cases, these measures may have clinical or educational implications that go substantially beyond those derived from measures of nonword reading.

Procedures and Measures Used to Assess Phonemic Awareness

More than a decade ago, Catts and his colleagues (Catts, Wilcox, Wood-Jackson, Larrivee, & Scott, 1997) reviewed methods used to assess phonemic awareness and found over 20 different tasks that have been used by researchers to measure awareness of phonemes in words. In their analysis, they grouped these measures into three broad categories: (1) phoneme segmentation, (2) phoneme synthesis, and (3) sound comparison. *Phoneme segmentation* tasks require a relatively explicit level of awareness of phonemes because they involve counting, pronouncing, deleting, adding, or reversing the individual phonemes in words. Common examples of this type of task require pronouncing the individual phonemes in words ("Say the sounds in *cat* one at a time."), deleting sounds from words ("Say *card* without saying the /d/ sound."), or counting sounds ("Put one marker on the line for each sound you hear in the word *fast*.")

There is really only one kind of task that can be used to measure *phoneme synthesis*. This is the sound-blending task in which the tester attempts to pronounce a series of phonemes in isolation and asks the child to blend them together to form a word (i.e., "What word do these sounds make, /f/ - /a/ - /t/?). Easier variants of the sound-blending task can be produced by allowing the child to choose from two or three pictures of a word that is represented by a series of phonemes (Torgesen & Bryant, 1993).

Sound comparison tasks use a number of different formats that have a common requirement to make comparisons between the sounds in different words. For example, a child might be asked to indicate which of several words begins or ends with the same sound as a target word. In addition, tasks that require children to generate words that have the same first, last, or middle sound as a target word would fall in this category.

An important point about these different kinds of tasks is that they all appear to be measuring essentially the same construct. Although some research (Yopp, 1988) has indicated that the tasks may vary in the complexity of their overall cognitive requirements, and there may be some differences between analysis and synthesis tasks at certain ages (Wagner, Torgesen, & Rashotte, 1994), for the most part, they all seem to be measuring different levels of growth in the same general ability (Ehri et al., 2001; Høien et al., 1995; Stanovich, Cunningham, & Cramer, 1984). Differences among these tasks in their level of difficulty seem primarily related to the extent to which they require explicit manipulation of individual phonemes. For example, many kindergarten children have difficulty with certain kinds of phoneme segmentation tasks, but most can perform sound comparison tasks successfully.

A number of readily available measures can be used to assess phonemic awareness, and more are currently under development. It is beyond the scope of this chapter to critically evaluate each of the available tests; so in Table 5.1 we provide a list of 16 measures and summarize important information about each. Table 5.1 summarizes for each test the appropriate age range,

TABLE 5.1 Measures of Phonological and Phonemic Awareness

Measure	Appropriate Grade Range	Skills Tested and Use		Test Design and Administration	
	K–3	Skills Tested	Most Common Use	Individual vs. Group	Criterion or Norm Referenced
Comprehensive Test of Phonological Processing	K–12	Blending, Segmenting, Elision, Phoneme identity	Diagnostic	I	Norm
Preschool Test of Phonological and Print Processes	Pre-K	Blending, Elision	Preschool diagnostic	I	Norm
Dynamic Indicators of Basic Early Literacy Skills	K–1	Phoneme identity, Initial sound fluency, Segmenting	Screening, Progress monitoring	I	Criterion
Early Reading Diagnostic Assessment	K–3	Blending, Rhyming, Segmenting	Diagnostic	I	Norm
Fox in a Box	K–2	Blending, Rhyming, Segmenting	Diagnostic	I	Criterion
Lindamood Auditory Conceptualization Test	K–12	Segmenting and Substitution	Diagnostic	I	Criterion
The Phonological Awareness Test	K–5	Rhyme, Blending, Segmenting, Elision	Diagnostic	I	Norm
Rosner Test of Auditory Analysis	K–3	Elision	Diagnostic	I	Criterion

Test	Grade/Age	Skill	Purpose	G/I	Type
Test of Invented Spelling	K–1	Letter–sound correspondence	Informal	G	Criterion
Test of Phonological Awareness–2+	K–2	Sound comparison	Screening, Outcome	G	Norm
Yopp-Singer Test of Phoneme Segmentation	K–1	Segmenting	Informal	I	Criterion
Woodcock Diagnostic Reading Battery	Pre-K–adult	Blending, Segmenting	Diagnostic	I	Norm
Texas Primary Reading Inventory	K–3	Blending, Segmenting	Screening, Progress monitoring, Outcome	I	Criterion
Test of Phonemic Awareness 2 Plus (TOPA–2+)	K–2	Initial and final sound and letter–sound correspondence	Screening	G	Norm
AIMSweb	K–1	Phoneme segmentation	Progress monitoring	I	Criterion
Get it Got it Go!	Pre-K	Alliteration, Rhyming	Progress monitoring	I	Criterion

skills tested, appropriate usage, administration, and design. Although the tests may be norm referenced or criterion based, they all have well-established predictive relationships with the growth of word recognition skills.

DEVELOPMENT AND ASSESSMENT OF WORD RECOGNITION

Assessment of word recognition skills is considerably more complex than assessment of phonemic awareness because readers can identify words in a number of different ways as they process text. To understand how children develop reading skills, it is important to understand how children learn to recognize written words accurately and automatically. Words in text can be identified in at least five different ways (Ehri, 2002):

1. By identifying and blending together the individual phonemes in words
2. By noticing and blending together familiar spelling patterns, which is a more advanced form of decoding
3. By recognizing words as whole units, or reading them "by sight"
4. By making analogies to other words that are already known
5. By using clues from the context to guess a word's identity

Researchers have also emphasized that morphological awareness, or the conscious knowledge of the individual units of meaning in language, including prefixes and suffixes, assists children in identifying unknown words in text (Apel, Wilson-Fowler, & Masterson, in press; Carlisle, 2004). For example, if the child can read *hope*, then knowing the inflected ending *ing*, could facilitate recognition of *hoping*. Older students also use morphological awareness to read derived words that share meaning (e.g., structure, construction). Different processes and knowledge are required to use each of these word identification methods, and these methods play roles of varying importance during different stages of learning to read.

A method that is of primary importance during early stages of learning to read is *phonemic decoding*. To use this method, readers must know the sounds that are usually represented by letters in words, then they must blend together the individual sounds that are identified in each word. This method is important to early reading success because it provides a relatively reliable way to identify words that have not been seen before. As children become more experienced readers, they begin to *process letters in larger chunks called spelling patterns.*

This improves decoding speed because it allows children to process groups of letters as units, rather than having to decode each graphophonic unit individually. Some common spelling patterns found at the ends of single syllable words in English are *-ack, -ight, -unk, -eat, -ay, -ash, -ip, -ore,* and *-ell.* Common affixes for longer words include *-able, -ing, -ous, -ize, pro-, con-, pre-,* and *un-.* A number of studies have shown that words that contain common spelling patterns like those listed are easier to decode if children are familiar with the patterns (Bowey & Hansen, 1994; Trieman, Goswami, & Bruck, 1990).

As children repeatedly read the same word several times, it eventually becomes stored in memory as a "sight word." No analysis is required to read sight words. A single glance at these words is sufficient to activate information about their pronunciation and meaning. Sight words are read rapidly (within one second) with no pauses between different parts of the word. Sight words are not recognized on the basis of shape or just some of the letters, but rather information about all the letters in a word is used to accurately identify it as a sight word (Raynor, Foorman, Perfetti, Pesetsky, & Seidenberg, 2001).

Those who conduct research on word recognition use the term *orthographic processing* (Ehri, 2002) to refer to the way that words are recognized "by sight." The orthography of a language refers to the way it is represented visually. Hence, when researchers indicate that words are processed as *orthographic units*, they are implying that they are recognized on the basis of a visual representation that has been integrated with the word's phonemic structure and its meaning.

When sight words are well practiced (and hence orthographic representations are well established), they can be identified automatically, with almost no expenditure of attention or effort (LaBerge & Samuels, 1974). Having a large vocabulary of "sight words" that can be recognized automatically is the key to fluent text reading (Torgesen, Rashotte, & Alexander, 2001). Because so little effort is required to identify sight words, the reader is able to concentrate effectively on the complex processes involved in constructing the meaning of text (Perfetti, 1985).

Words can also be read by *analogy to known words* (Glushko, 1981; Laxon, Coltheart, & Keating, 1988). For example, the word *cart* might be read by noticing the word *car* and then adding to it the /t/ sound at the end. A longer word like *fountain* might be initially read by noticing its similarity to a known word like *mountain* and making the slight adjustment to pronunciation required for the different initial phoneme. Research has shown that children need to have at least a beginning level of phonemic decoding skill before they can effectively use an analogy strategy to identify unknown words (Ehri & Robbins, 1992).

A very different, and less effective, way to identify words in text is to *guess their identity from the context* in which they occur. This context may include pictures on the page or the meaning of the passage. When children make errors in their oral reading, the errors are often consistent with the context, which indicates that this is one source of information they are using to help them identify the words (Biemiller, 1970).

Research has shown that skilled readers do not rely on context as a major source of information about words in text, but that poor readers do (Share & Stanovich, 1995). Guessing words from context, by itself, is not a very accurate way to identify words in text, as is clear from work by Gough and Walsh (1991), which showed that only about 10 percent of the words that are critical to the meaning of passages can be guessed correctly from context alone. Nevertheless, when children phonemically decode words, often they do not arrive at the fully correct pronunciation unless they can use contextual constraints to suggest a real word that sounds like their decoding and makes sense within that context and unless they self-correct after reading words that do not make sense (Adams, 1990; Share & Stanovich, 1995).

Issues in the Assessment of Word Recognition

Children with RD, and many children with SI and LI, lack the ability to apply alphabetic strategies in reading new words (phonemic decoding) and the ability to retrieve sight words from memory (orthographic processing). They not only have difficulty becoming accurate in the application of these processes, but they frequently also have additional special difficulties with becoming fluent in their application. Before discussing specific methods for the diagnostic assessment of these word recognition skills, two general issues require discussion.

First, it is important for teachers and clinicians to have precise and reliable information about level of performance on important subskills in reading. The goal of the kind of assessments that will be discussed in this chapter is to quantify the degree of skill a child possesses in word identification processes that have been shown in many research studies to be critical contributors to overall reading success. This information is vital for learning who is on grade level, for grouping children with similar instructional needs, for differentiating intervention, and for monitoring progress within RTI implementation.

The second issue is that the type of diagnostic assessments described here are also different from the more informal assessments of word recognition skills that are frequently used by teachers to help guide instruction. The kinds of assessments used by many teachers to help them plan instruction involve the use of placement tests and informal inventories designed to indicate the specific knowledge or skill a child has within several broad domains of word-reading skill. For example, such inventories might be used to indicate which letter–sound correspondences are already known to the child, whether the child can blend the sounds in words that contain final consonant blends, what is known about common prefixes and suffixes, whether syllabification strategies are understood, and precisely what words are known from a list of high-frequency words. Or, teachers may use mastery tests that accompany a core reading program to learn which students have mastered a critical skill taught within the curriculum. Therefore, we emphasize that these informal measures are neither designed nor intended to meet acceptable standards of reliability and validity for use within an RTI framework to determine who needs extra intervention. In other words, these informal measures are not suitable candidates for screening, progress monitoring, diagnostic, or outcome assessments.

Commonly Used Measures of Word Recognition Ability

It is beyond the scope of this chapter to identify all the available tests of word-level reading skills. Rather, in Table 5.2, we provide examples of tests that can be used to assess the major dimensions of word-reading ability. An adequate diagnostic assessment of children's word recognition abilities should include an assessment of: (1) word-reading accuracy (both in and out of context); (2) phonemic decoding skill; and (3) reading fluency. Fluency measures become more important after about second to third grade, after children have acquired foundational word recognition skills they can apply with reasonable accuracy. Measures that involve out-of-context word reading more directly assess the kinds of word recognition skills that are particularly problematic for children with RD because they eliminate the contextual support on which these children rely heavily. However, it may be useful diagnostically to determine the difference for a specific child between "in context" and "out of context" reading accuracy to determine how well the child can use context to support the word recognition processes. In addition to formal assessments in these domains, it is usually useful to observe the way a child reads text at varying levels of difficulty. Careful observations of oral reading behavior can provide useful information about the way that the child integrates all sources of information about words in text.

CODE-FOCUSED CLASSROOM INSTRUCTION AND MORE INTENSIVE SMALL-GROUP SUPPLEMENTAL INTERVENTION

There is now a very strong consensus among professionals who study reading and reading disabilities that instruction in phonological awareness, alphabetic knowledge, and word reading strategies is an important part of any good reading curriculum (Adams, 1990; Blachman, 1989; Bus & Van Ijzendoorn, 1999; Ehri et al., 2001; Lonigan et al., 2008; National Reading Panel [NRP], 2000; Snow, Burns, & Griffin, 1998). Because it is so important for all students to acquire sound word-level reading skills in the early grades, policy makers have passed

TABLE 5.2 Commonly Used Measures of Word Recognition Ability

Measure	Grade Range	Word Reading Skills Tested	Most Common Use	Individual vs. Group Administration	Criterion or Norm Referenced
Diagnostic Assessment of Reading	1–3	PD, TRA, TRF	Diagnostic	I	Criterion
Early Reading Diagnostic Assessment	K–3	PD, WRA	Diagnostic	I	Normed
Fox in a Box	K–2	PDA, TRA, TRF, WRA	Diagnostic, Progress Monitoring	I	Criterion
Dynamic Indicators of Basic Early Literacy Skills	K–3	PDF, TRF	Screening, Progress Monitoring,	I	Normed Benchmarks
Test of Word Reading Efficiency	1–12	PDF, WRF	Screening, Progress Monitoring, Diagnostic	I	Normed
Gates-MacGinitie Reading Test, 3rd ed.	K–12	PDA, WRA	Diagnostic, Outcome	I/G	Normed
Gray Oral Reading Test–4	1–12	TRA, TRF	Diagnostic, Outcome	I	Normed
Group Reading Assessment & Diagnostic Evaluation	K–12	PDA, WRA	Diagnostic, Outcome	I/G	Normed
Texas Primary Reading Inventory	K–2	PDA, WRA, TRF	Diagnostic, Progress Monitoring	I	Criterion
Wide Range Achievement Test	K–12	WRA	Diagnostic, Outcome	I	Normed
Woodcock Reading Mastery Test–R	K–3	PDA, WRA	Diagnostic, Outcome	I	Normed
Woodcock-Johnson Psychoeducational Battery	K–12	PDA, WRA	Diagnostic, Outcome	I	Normed
Test of Silent Word Reading Fluency	1–12	SWRF	Progress Monitoring	G	Normed
AIMSweb	K–8	LNF, LSF, NWF, ORF	Progress Monitoring	I	Criterion

Note: PDA = Phonemic Decoding Accuracy, PDF = Phonemic Decoding Fluency, WRA = Word Reading Accuracy, WRF = Word Reading Fluency, TRA = Text Reading Accuracy, TRF = Text Reading Fluency, SWRF = Silent Word Reading Fluency, ORF = Oral Reading Fluency, LNF = Letter Naming Fluency, LSF = Letter–Sound Fluency, NWF = Nonsense Word Fluency legislation (i.e., NCLB, IDEA) encouraging the use of *multitiered* models of instruction and assessment to ensure that all students receive the instruction they need (President's Commission on Special Education, 2002). Multitiered models appear necessary because some children, including children with speech or language impairments and children at risk for reading disabilities, will need more intensive instruction than is delivered in general education classrooms (Fuchs & Fuchs, 1998; Fuchs, Fuchs, McMaster, & Al Otaiba, 2003; Torgesen, 2002b; Vellutino et al., 1996). Multitiered models are also preferable to traditional service delivery because intervention is provided sooner (Vaughn & Linan-Thompson, 2003). In the past, special services were not available for many children until they fell far behind their expected reading achievement in third or fourth grade (President's Commission on Special Education, 2002).

The foundation of a multitiered approach, or Tier 1, calls for the classroom teacher to faithfully implement explicit and systematic *classroom* instruction with the expectation that the teacher will accelerate most children's learning. At this level, it is expected that teachers ensure each child is given a combination of whole-class and small-group instruction on tasks that are at the appropriate level for his or her literacy development until they understand and master early word-reading skills (Ehri, 2002; Snider, 1995). To ensure that such instruction is benefiting most children and to identify, or screen for, children who are not mastering skills taught, progress on essential word-reading skills is monitored in all students.

For small numbers of students who do not respond well to Tier 1 instruction, subsequent supplemental tiers of *intervention* that increase in intensity are provided. Intervention may involve more practice on certain instructional components, may be delivered more frequently and with greater duration, and ideally will be provided by a more expert teacher or clinician. Because of its comparative complexity and intensity, intervention may eventually be conducted by someone other than the classroom teacher who works with small student groups or individual tutorials. Although there are many variations to the number of tiers within RTI models, students who do not respond eventually undergo formal identification and provision of special education services and appropriate accommodation. Before we discuss issues for future research and development, we address four relevant questions: First, what do we know about effective code-focused classroom instruction? Second, what do we know about Tier 1 instructional strategies that maximize reading outcomes? Third, what do we know about training code-focused skills through supplemental interventions that are powerful enough to improve reading in children with the most severe reading problems? Finally, what do we know about poor responders?

What Do We Know About Effective Code-Focused Classroom Instruction?

It is possible to combine what is known about reading growth with knowledge of the instructional factors that support reading growth and that can prevent RD for most children. In general, instruction to stimulate phonological awareness should begin by providing exposure to rhyming songs, books, and activities for children in preschool and the early part of kindergarten. Once children begin to understand the concept of rhyme (as shown by their ability to decided whether words rhyme or to generate rhyming words), they can begin to do a variety of sound comparison activities involving the first, last, and middle sounds of words. Tasks that require children to manipulate, segment, or blend individual phonemes would come next and are most appropriate for use immediately prior to or in conjunction with instruction in sound–letter correspondences and phonemic reading and writing. Table 5.3 provides some examples of phonological awareness activities along a continuum of difficulty.

TABLE 5.3	Phonological Awareness Activities along a Continuum of Difficulty	

Activity	Objective	
I Spy	Students will learn to identify rhyming words	Place some familiar objects or pictures that rhyme near the small group of children (e.g., "snake," "rake," "lake") *Model*: "I spy with my little eye, something that rhymes with snake. It's a lake." *Guided practice*: "Your turn. See if you can guess what I see. I spy with my little eye something else that rhymes with snake." *Extra support*: If child struggles, provide a forced choice such as, "Is it a pen or a rake?" *Enrichment/extension*: "Can you think of something else that rhymes with snake?" Read a book that has lots of rhyming words and have children identify the rhymes.
What starts with my sound?	Students will learn to isolate initial sounds	Place some common objects or pictures that begin with two easily distinguishable letters near the small group of children (e.g., "mom," "mat," "monster," "car," "can," "coat"). *Model*: "I can match these pictures with their starting sound. This letter says /m/ like moon. So I am going to put all the pictures that start with the /mmm/ sound with the letter." *Guided practice*: "Your turn to match the pictures with their starting sound. Say /mmm/ with me. Can you find something that starts with /mmm/?" *Extra support*: Give a forced choice, emphasizing the first sound: "Is it 'mmmmom' or 'car'?" This may be easier using continuous sounds like /mmm/ rather than stop sounds. *Enrichment/extension:* "Can you think of something else that starts with /mmm/?" Read a book that emphasizes alliteration such as *Fox in Socks* by Dr. Seuss (1965).
Guess my word/ I'm thinking of	Blending and segmenting	Place some objects or pictures that begin with two easily distinguishable sounds near the small group of children (e.g., "map," "mouse," "sock"). *Model*: "I am going to say these words in a funny slow way. See if you can guess my picture, 'mmaap.' " *Guided practice*: "Your turn to match the pictures with their starting sound. Say /mmm/ with me. Can you find something that starts with /mmm/?" *Extra support*: "Is it mouse or sock?" *Enrichment/extension:* "Can you think of something else that starts with /mmm/?"

(continued)

TABLE 5.3   *(continued)*

Activity	Objective	
Sound boxes/ Word building	Blending and segmenting	Place some objects or pictures that have two or three phonemes and that begin with two easily distinguishable letters near the small group of children (e.g., "bee," "bus," "rat," "rock").
		Model: "Today we are going to build some words with these blocks. First, I'll make 'bee.' " Move a marker as you say both sounds in /b/ /e/. "There are two sounds in 'bee.' "
		Guided practice: "Your turn to build 'be' with the blocks. Now let's try to build 'bus.' "
		Extra support: "Let's build it together."
		Enrichment/extension: "Can you build 'rock' all by yourself? What word has more sounds, bee or rock?"
		Include some decodable words.
Stand up when you hear your silly-sound-name	Manipulation	A good transition activity.
		Model: "Today I am going to call you to line up in a silly way. I am going to pretend everyone's name starts with a /mmm/ like Mary's. Mary, you come up and be the leader, because we are using your letter today!"
		Guided practice: Looking directly at her, ask Alexis, "Malexis, will you line up?"
		Extra support: And take his hand, and say, "Monathon, will you line up?"
		Enrichment/extension: "If your silly-sound-name is Marlos, line up."
Read-aloud books		Choose a predictable story with rhyming text (see Yopp, 1995, for an annotated bibliography of read-aloud books for developing phonemic awareness)

Similarly, instruction in word recognition should explicitly follow a scope and sequence that parallels phonological awareness instruction, beginning by teaching high utility, consonant letter–sound correspondences. Table 5.4 describes some examples of instructional activities that are useful for teaching word-reading skills systematically. Early on, preschool and kindergarten teachers may help children become aware of the spelling of their own names (Ehri, 2002). Further, to maximize children's attention to print and to letter–sound associations, research has shown teachers should make use of certain genres of books—alphabet books and print-rich storybooks (i.e., storybooks featuring interesting print features, like speech bubbles and font changes; see Smolkin, Conlon, & Yaden, 1988)—because these types of books allow more authentic and explicit opportunities to highlight print. For instance, Justice and her colleagues (2005) reported more than twice as many visual fixations on print for 3- to 5-year-olds in print-rich than typical picture-rich story books. Nevertheless, Justice's research highlights the need for teachers to reference the print because only about 5 to 7 percent of the time do children pay attention to print rather than pictures (Justice, Pullen, & Pence, 2008).

TABLE 5.4	Instructional Activities Useful for Teaching Word-Reading Skills
Phase	**Activity**
Letter–Sound Correspondence	T-**Each letter stands for a sound. When people read, they use letter sounds to help them figure out words. Let's learn the sound for the letter _m_.** (Hold up a card with the letter _m_ written on it. Point to the letter _m_.) **This letter's sound is /mmm/. What sound?**
	S-/mmm/
	T-(Point to the letter _m_ again). **What sound?**
	S-/mmm/
	T-**Let's practice the letter sounds we have learned so far.** (Teacher holds letter cards that contain letters in which the students have already been taught their sounds. She points to each letter and asks, "What sound?" Immediate corrective feedback is offered.)
Decoding	Once students have learned a few useful letter–sound correspondences (e.g., /m/, /t/, /s/, /a/) the decoding process is taught explicitly:
	T-(Writes the letter _m_ on the board) **What's the sound**?
	S-/m/
	T-(Writes the letter _a_ next to the _m_) **What's the sound?**
	S-/a/
	T-(Writes the letter _t_ next to the _a_) **What's the sound?**
	S-/t/
	T- **Blend it.** (Sweeping hand under the word)
	S-mat
	T- **Sound out the word.** (Sweeping hand under each letter)
	S-/m//a//t/
	T- **Blend it**. (Sweeping hand under the word)
	S-mat
	This instructional routine is implemented daily so students receive ample practice with the decoding process. Words are made up of previously learned letter sounds. After students have had practice with this process, the same words are organized in a list and students practice reading them fluently. These same words are incorporated in sentences and stories so students can practice and experience success at reading connected text.
Spelling	Once students know letter sounds (/m/, /t/, /s/, /a/), spelling activities can be implemented.
	T-**Spell the word _mat_. Write each letter's sound as you say the sound to yourself.**
	S-(Students write the word _mat_)
	T-(Models spelling the word _mat_ on the board as she says each sound. Students check their spelling. Teacher asks a student to use _mat_ in a sentence.)

(continued)

TABLE 5.4	(continued)

Phase	Activity
Advanced Decoding	When students use advanced decoding, they recognize chunks of words, also referred to as phonograms (e.g., *-an*, *-at*). It is important to note that beginning reading instruction should not begin with advanced decoding instruction. This is due to the fact that beginning readers who rely mostly on recognizing chunks of words to determine pronunciation are less skilled at word identification than beginning readers who analyze words fully, phoneme by phoneme. Relying on recognizing chunks of words, or phonograms, is less efficient and less generalizable than phonemic decoding. Therefore, it is important to begin reading instruction with decoding sound by sound (as described earlier).
	Once students are successful at decoding words by individual phonemes, advanced decoding can be introduced. When advanced decoding is taught, it is important to teach phonograms made up the letter sounds already learned by the students. For example, if the /a/ and /n/ are already known letter sounds, then the phonogram /an/ would be a good choice to teach.
	The instructional routine for advanced decoding is similar to the instructional routine for decoding:
	T-(Writes the letters *an* on the board and points to one at a time asking for each sound)
	S-/a/ /n/
	T-**Blend it.** (sweeping hand under the chunk).
	S-an
	T-Tell students this is a word family, and it will help us read other words.
	T-(Writes the letter *f* in front of *an* and points to the *f*) **What's the sound**?
	S-/f/
	T-(Sweeps hand under word) **Blend it.**
	S - fan
	T-(Writes the letter *m* in front of *an* and points to the *m*) **What's the sound**?
	S-/m/
	T-(Sweeps hand under word) **Blend it.**
	S – man
	T-(Writes the letter c in front of *an* and points to the c) **What's the sound**?
	S-/k/
	T-(Sweeps hand under word) **Blend it.**
	S - can

TABLE 5.4	(continued)

Phase	Activity
Sight Words—Fluency	*Teaching sight words:* There are two important ways to explicitly teach sight words.
	The first method involves selecting words from lists of high-frequency words or from selections that will soon be read and providing directed practice for children in reading these words. For high-frequency words, teachers typically put the words on cards, and then drill students until they are able to pronounce the words in less than one second. Sometimes, children are encouraged to "sound out" the words the first time they see them on the cards, and then, for irregular words, the teacher explains the parts of the words that "don't play fair." This procedure encourages the students to notice all the letters in a word's spelling.
	The second way to directly build fluency is to provide practice with the repeated reading of phrases or short paragraphs containing a few (not too many) words the student needs to learn. Typically, the teacher asks the student to reread about three times, and sometimes a stopwatch is used to record the improved reading time on each subsequent reading of the text. Material that is used to practice fluency using repeated reading should be read initially with at least 95 percent accuracy.
Analogy	Word walls are frequently used in classrooms. This technique can help most children learn to read and write the words posted on the walls when certain conditions are in place: the words are used often in reading and writing, words are organized or grouped according to a common letter pattern, meanings of words are discussed, and students have daily practice finding, writing, and chanting the words.
	To help students learn to read by analogy, teachers could group words by common spelling patterns and provide students ample practice reading and writing these words (e.g., *sack, lack, back, tack, slack, crack; night, bright, light, flight*). An activity could include students sorting word cards under the proper rime. For example, *sack, lack, tack, crack* would be sorted under the rime *–ack. Night, bright, flight* would be categorized under the rime *–ight*.
Context	When teaching students to use context, the preferred strategy is to encourage students to first analyze unknown words phonemically, and then guess a word that makes sense in the context of the passage and that matches the sounds identified in the unknown word. So, for example, if a child encountered the sentence, *The boy _____ his dog in the woods,* with the blank representing an unknown word, it is difficult to guess from context alone the right word to fill in the blank. However, if the child was able to do even a little phonemic analysis first, such as sounding out the first sound (ch) in the word, the range of words that fit the context is dramatically narrowed. As children become able to identify more of the phonemes in words, their choices become even more constrained by their knowledge of the sounds that must be present in whatever word they guess, and they become more accurate readers.

As children learn about letter–sound correspondences and can recognize their own name, teachers introduce frequent initial and ending sounds (e.g., m, s, t, n), followed by short vowels (e.g., a), followed by a blending routine (/m/ /a/ /t/ is "mat"). This careful instructional sequence provides children opportunities to begin to read words and simple sentences right away. Next, consonant digraphs and long vowels should be taught, followed by vowel digraphs and variant vowel digraphs and diphthongs. It is important to note that even when letter sounds are taught in isolation, it is essential to quickly offer opportunities for students to practice reading words using those letter sounds. Instruction in how to read irregular words is also important. Oftentimes, teachers use the terms *sight words, high-frequency words*, and *irregular words* interchangeably. However, this is not accurate. A *sight word* is any word that a student can read from memory. That is, a student has had sufficient practice and exposure to a word such that he or she has committed it to memorize and can read it automatically (Ehri, 2002). *Regular words* are those words that follow the most common letter–sound patterns and are easily decoded. *Irregular words* contain spelling patterns that "do not follow the rules" or that do not follow the most common letter–sound patterns. It is important to note that most letters in irregular words conform to common letter–sound conventions (e.g., all but the *s* in *island*, the *w* in *sword*, the *t* in *listen*). *High-frequency* words include a small number of words that appear frequently in print. High-frequency words can be regular (e.g., *that, with, and*) or irregular (e.g., *some, was, said*; Honig, Diamond, & Gutlohn, 2000).

Next, teachers can instruct children about syllable types and how to use morphemic analysis to help students to read multisyllabic words and become aware of the chunks of meaning within larger words. Other, more sophisticated, strategies include reading words by analogy and using context. When students are taught to read words by analogy, for example, it is imperative that the analogous word is stored in memory as a sight word. That is, when using the familiar word *moon* to read the unfamiliar word *spoon*, it is important that the students have had sufficient practice reading the word *moon* such that it is a sight word for them. Students need to be taught the strategy of looking for familiar words when they encounter new words (Gaskins, Ehri, Cress, O'Hara, & Donnelly, 1997).

Furthermore, children can be explicitly taught to use context as a clue in identifying unknown words. However, we should never encourage students to use context alone to guess at the identity of unknown words because normal text is not sufficiently redundant to make context by itself a reliable clue to the identity of specific words. Some books for beginning readers are written using highly predictable text, but if a child learns to rely solely on context to identify new words, he or she will not be well prepared when asked to read more natural text in which context does not constrain word choice to the same extent. Finally, opportunities for students to read aloud with feedback from a highly qualified teacher or well-trained tutor help students to become proficient readers.

What Do We Know About Tier 1 Instructional Strategies That Maximize Reading Outcomes?

First, we know that the effects of preventative early literacy overall, and of phonological awareness and word recognition training more specifically, appear strong in preschool and kindergarten before children have begun to read (Bus & Van Ijzendoorn, 1999; Lonigan et al., 2008; NRP, 2000). It also makes intuitive sense that it would be easier to prevent than to remediate reading difficulties. Within preschool and kindergarten, most children benefit from small-group instruction that is relatively brief (i.e., 15 minutes daily) and that includes engaging gamelike activities.

Second, we know that methods that integrate instruction in alphabetic knowledge or phonics to directly link newly acquired phonemic awareness to reading and spelling are more effective than those that do not (Bus & Van Ijzendoorn, 1999; Ehri et al., 2001; Lonigan et al., 2008; NRP, 2000). Thus, although most instructional programs in phonemic awareness begin with oral language activities, the most effective programs conclude by leading children to apply their newly developed ability to think about the phonemic segments in words to reading and spelling activities. The importance of the progression from oral to written language activities was illustrated in the first major demonstration of the effectiveness of training in phonemic awareness reported by Bradley and Bryant (1985). In this study, phonemic awareness was stimulated by using activities that required children to categorize words on the basis of similarities in their beginning, middle, and ending sounds (sound comparison tasks). However, in one of the conditions, this training was supplemented by work with individual plastic letters to illustrate the way new words could be made by changing only one letter (or sound) in a word. Children in this latter condition showed the largest benefit from the phonemic awareness training program. Although training in phonemic awareness, by itself, can produce significant improvement in subsequent reading growth (Lundberg, Frost, & Peterson, 1988), programs that directly illustrate the relevance of the training to reading and spelling activities consistently produce the largest gains in reading (Blachman, Ball, Black, & Tangel, 1994; Byrne & Fielding-Barnsley, 1995; Cunningham, 1990; Fuchs, Fuchs, Thompson, et al., 2001; Hatcher & Hulme, 1999).

It is recommended, therefore, that practitioners combine training in phonological awareness with instruction in how the alphabet works. This integration of orally based instruction in phonological awareness with activities involving print does not mean that training in phonological awareness is useful only if it precedes systematic and complete "phonics" oriented reading instruction. These activities should be included simply to help children learn to apply their newly acquired phonological awareness to reading and spelling tasks. The print-based activities that should accompany instruction in phonological awareness are necessarily very simple. For example, children who have been taught a few letter sounds and achieved a beginning level of phonemic awareness should be able to identify the first letter of a word when they hear it pronounced. They might also be led to substitute different letters at the beginning or end of a word like *cat* to make different words. They could also be asked to pronounce the "sounds" of the letters *c - a - t* and then blend them together to form a word. If children have learned to blend orally presented sounds together, they can be led to perform the same process when letters represent phonemes.

Third, researchers have shown that classroom teachers who use an explicit core reading instructional program with a strong and systematic emphasis on code-focused skills are more likely to maximize reading outcomes for most children than those teachers who use less explicit and less systematic programs. Foorman, Francis, Fletcher, Schatschneider, and Mehta (1998) evaluated the effectiveness of three types of core reading programs in nearly 70 classrooms. On average, the first and second graders taught with core reading programs that emphasized direct instruction and that included controlled vocabulary text showed more improvement in reading than children taught with a core program that was less direct (i.e., phonics was taught through trade books less explicitly and systematically) or children who were taught with a core program that was implicit. Although children's initial level of phonemic awareness moderated their rate of reading development, a majority of children responded well who were taught with the direct instruction core reading program.

Subsequent to the NRP report in 2000, most currently available core reading programs that claim to be research based also contain materials and procedures to provide explicit and systematic instruction in phonemic awareness and word recognition in kindergarten and first grade

(Al Otaiba, Kosanovich-Grek, Torgesen, Hassler, & Wahl, 2005). More evidence that this type of core reading program maximizes student outcomes comes from another large-scale kindergarten study, also conducted by Foorman and colleagues (Foorman et al., 2003). This multiyear study involved three cohorts and over 4,800 students who attended struggling schools whose teachers were provided professional development. Foorman and colleagues reported that children whose teachers used systematic and explicit reading curricula that explicitly linked phonemic awareness and the alphabetic principle in kindergarten achieved reading performance that was at the national average.

A fourth way to maximize the impact of Tier 1 instruction is to focus on a limited set of skills such as blending and segmenting and to teach these skills explicitly and systematically (Ehri et al., 2001). As we previously discussed, explicit instruction includes modeling, guided practice, and immediate corrective feedback, and systematic instruction is based on a scope and sequence that moves from easier to more difficult tasks. A number of factors influence the difficulty of blending and segmentation tasks, and there is not one particular sequence to which every teacher must adhere. Roughly, though, researchers (Chard & Dickson, 1999; Lonigan et al., 2008; Snider, 1995) have proposed that phonological instruction should begin with larger linguistic units and proceed to individual phonemes, as it is easier to blend and segment syllables and onset-rime units than individual phonemes. At the phonemic level, instruction should begin with simple, two- and three-phoneme words such as "no, sun, man," which are easier to blend or segment than words with initial blends such as "stop" or "flag." Similarly, Snider (1995) suggested that continuous sounds, which may be sung or stretched without distorting their sounds (e.g., m, s, and vowels) are easier to "stretch out" than stop sounds (e.g., b, t) and so should be used for initial instruction. Imagine how much easier it would be to teach a child to blend "mm-maaannn" than /b/ /a/ /t/, which a child might mispronounce as "buh" "a" "tuh."

The final way to maximize the effectiveness of code-focused classroom instruction is to ensure teachers have the requisite knowledge to use data to inform instruction. At least one study conducted by Piasta and colleagues (2009) showed that when classroom teachers had very little knowledge about how to teach code-focused skills, their students who received more code-focused instruction actually scored lower than children with less instruction. Thus, even with a good core reading program, teacher knowledge matters. Fortunately, we also know that professional development that helps teachers use child data to differentiate instruction is associated with stronger Tier 1 outcomes. In other words, if Joey does not know how to segment the initial sound of words and knows very few letter sounds, he would need different instructional activities and support than Suzy, who is able to blend individual phonemes to name a CVC word such as "cat." There is a growing body of evidence that teachers who learn how to group their students homogeneously for instruction and who individualize or differentiate what they do in small-group instruction have students with significantly greater reading outcomes (Al Otaiba et al., in press; Connor, Morrison, Fishman, Schatschneider, & Underwood, 2007).

What Do We Know About Training Code-Focused Skills Through Supplemental Interventions?

Experienced reading clinicians have favored phonemically based approaches to instruction for children with RD from very early in the history of the field (Clark & Uhry, 1995). However, research and case study information tended to emphasize how extremely difficult it is to teach these children generalized phonemic reading skills (Lovett, Warren-Chaplin, Ransby, & Borden, 1990; Lyon, 1985; Snowling & Hulme, 1989). In contrast to these earlier results, later work by

Lovett and her associates (Lovett et al., 2000) and by others (Foorman et al., 1998; Torgesen et al., 1999; Torgesen et al., 2001; Vellutino et al., 1996; Wise & Olsen, 1995) has reported significant success in building generalized phonemic reading skills in children with phonologically based RD. In fact, in a review of outcomes from intervention research with children identified because of difficulties acquiring accurate and fluent word-level reading skills, Torgesen (in press) concluded that intensive and skillfully delivered instructional interventions produced the largest gains in phonemic decoding ability, followed by gains in text reading accuracy, reading comprehension, and reading fluency.

Al Otaiba and her colleagues (Al Otaiba, Puranik, Zilkowksi, & Curran, 2009) synthesized the findings of phonological awareness intervention research studies delivered to young children with SI or LI to describe how effective various training approaches have been in improving their phonological and, when possible, early reading skills. Generally, students with SI were easier to remediate; the majority of these children made short-term improvements in phonological skills after receiving early intervention that combined speech articulation with phonological awareness training. However, there were few efforts to document their subsequent reading development. One study incorporated multiple treatment components (including rhyme, blending, and segmenting) and reported positive short- and longer-term effects (Warrick, Rubin, & Rowe-Walsh, 1993). By first grade, children who received intervention in kindergarten had caught up to same-age typically developing peers on all measures of phonological awareness, suggesting that explicit segmentation intervention in analyzing words to the level of the individual phonemes, as recommended by the NRP (2000) for typically developing children, may also support reading development for students with LI.

Both of the strongest research studies involving students with LI (Warrick et al., 1993) and SI (Moriarty & Gillon, 2006) included phonological awareness skills that are consistent with those taught in current core beginning reading programs and preschool curricula. However, for both students with LI and SI, there were large individual differences in response to interventions. It is important to note that the collaborative model in which children were seen only once a month was ineffective. An implication of Al Otaiba et al.'s review (2009) is that children with LI and SI likely will need ongoing intervention that combines speech production and phonological training provided by speech-language pathologists that is carefully aligned with the early phonological awareness, small-group instruction provided by the classroom teacher.

The most appropriate conclusion from instructional research with children with LI or RD is that it is clearly possible to have a substantial impact on the growth of their phonemic decoding skills if the proper instructional conditions are in place. These conditions appear to involve instruction that is more *explicit*, more *intensive*, and more *supportive* than what is usually offered in most public and private school settings (Torgesen, Rashotte, Alexander, Alexander, & MacPhee, 2003).

Instruction becomes more *explicit* when the teacher or clinician makes fewer assumptions about preexisting skills or children's abilities to make inferences about sound–letter regularities on their own. As Gaskins et al. (1997) have pointed out, "First graders who are at risk for failure in learning to read do not discover what teachers leave unsaid about the complexities of word learning. As a result, it is important to teach them procedures for learning words" (p. 325). Based on information already considered in this chapter, one way to make instruction in word-learning strategies more explicit is to provide direct instruction to increase children's level of phonemic awareness. Although some form of instruction in phonemic awareness characterizes all successful programs, there has been substantial variability in the way this instruction is provided. Another way to make instruction for children with RD more *explicit* is to provide direct instruction in sound–letter correspondences and in strategies for using these correspondences to decode words while reading text. Explicit instruction and practice in these skills is characteristic of *all* programs that have produced substantial growth in phonemic decoding skills in children with RD. In a direct test of the utility of this type of instruction, Iverson and Tunmer (1993) added explicit training in phonemic decoding to the popular *Reading Recovery* (Clay, 1979) program, which has traditionally placed less emphasis on instruction and practice in these skills. This carefully controlled study showed that a small amount of explicit instruction in phonics increased the efficiency of the *Reading Recovery* program by approximately 37 percent.

Yet another way in which the explicitness of instruction and practice for children with RD must be increased is a careful and systematic focus on building reading fluency. Many children with RD may require more opportunities to correctly pronounce new words before they can add them to their sight vocabulary (Reitsma, 1990). Research has demonstrated that practice repeatedly reading either individual words or text can lead to improvements in reading fluency for children with reading difficulties (Levy, Abello, & Lysynchuk, 1997; Meyer & Felton, 1999). The primary value of both of these types of interventions is that they provide children opportunities to repeatedly read new words within a short enough interval of time that the children can "remember" how they pronounced the words previously and learn to rely on their emerging orthographic representation of the word to identify it in print. An interesting new development to aid the provision of explicit practice to develop fluency is the use of texts that have been specifically engineered for this purpose (Hiebert & Fisher, 2002). These texts provide ample repetition of high-utility, high-frequency words within a thematic structure to ensure that students receive many opportunities, within a single reading of the text, to pronounce important words multiple times.

In addition to being more *explicit*, effective reading instruction for children with RD must be more *intensive* than regular classroom instruction. Increased intensity involves more teacher–student instructional interactions, or reinforced learning trials, per unit of time. Intensity of instruction can be increased either by lengthening total instructional time (thus increasing the number of instructional interactions per day or week), or by reducing teacher–pupil ratios (thus increasing the number of instructional interactions per hour). The most powerful method of increasing instructional efficiency for children with RD may be to substantially reduce the teacher–pupil ratio for part of the day (Elbaum, Vaughn, Hughes, & Moody, 1999).

There are actually a variety of ways to accomplish this reduction in teacher–pupil ratio for children who are struggling to learn to read. For example, Greenwood (1996) has obtained increased amounts of student engagement and increased reading achievement for at-risk students through the use of the ClassWide Peer Tutoring model. Others who have used peers effectively to increase the number of instructional interactions per hour for struggling readers are Doug and Lynn Fuchs and their colleagues (Fuchs, Fuchs, Mathes, & Simmons, 1997), and Patricia Mathes and her colleagues (Mathes, Torgesen, & Allor, 2001). Keep in mind that a small proportion of young children may not respond to peer tutoring (e.g., Al Otaiba & Fuchs, 2006), so it is important to monitor their progress and consider alternative interventions. Another method for increasing the intensity of instruction for struggling readers is small-group instruction provided by the regular classroom teacher during part of the reading block. In addition to the regular classroom teacher, this small-group instruction can also be provided by carefully trained paraprofessionals (Torgesen, 2002a) or by specialists such as a special education teachers, Title I reading intervention teachers, or speech/language pathologists. One interesting finding that has emerged from meta-analyses of intervention studies is that one-to-one interventions in reading have not consistently been shown to be more effective than small-group interventions (Elbaum et al., 1999; NRP, 2000; Wanzek & Vaughn, 2007).

A third way to make instruction more successful for children with RD involves the level of *support* provided within the instructional interactions. At least two kinds of special support are required. First, because acquiring word-level reading skills is more difficult for these children than others, they will require more *emotional* support in the form of encouragement, positive feedback, and enthusiasm from the teacher to maintain their motivation to learn. Second, instructional interactions must be more supportive in the sense that they involve carefully *scaffolded* interactions with the child. In her investigation of the characteristics of effective reading tutors, Juel (1996) identified the number of scaffolded interactions during each teaching session as one of the critical variables predicting differences in effectiveness across tutors. A scaffolded interaction is one in which the teacher enables the student to complete a task (e.g., read a word) by directing the student's attention to a key piece of information or breaking the task up into smaller, easier to manage ones. The goal of these interactions is to provide just enough support so the child can go through the processing steps necessary to find the right answer. In essence, the teacher leads the child to do all the thinking required to accomplish a task (decoding or spelling a word) that he or she could not do without teacher support. With enough practice, the child becomes able to go through the processing steps independently. Juel's finding about the importance of carefully scaffolded instructional interactions is consistent with the emphasis on these types of interactions in the teachers' manuals that accompany two instructional programs shown to be effective with children who have severe RD (Lindamood & Lindamood, 1998; Wilson, 1988).

Thanks to the hard work of researchers, a large array of programs and sets of materials have been developed specifically to help teachers provide effective instruction in phonemic awareness and word recognition for young children. Programs are available both to supplement the whole-class instruction provided by the teacher by providing more intensive small-group or individual intervention for students who are having difficulties learning to read (e.g., *Ladders to Literacy* by O'Connor, Notari-Syverson, & Vadasy, 2005; *Phonemic Awareness in Young Children: A Classroom Curriculum* by Adams, Foorman, Lundberg, & Beeler, 1997; *Earobics* by Cognitive Concepts, Inc., 1998; *Road to the Code* by Blachman, Ball, Black, & Tangel, 2000; *Phonological Awareness Training for Reading* by Torgesen & Bryant, 1993; *The Lindamood Phoneme Sequencing Program for Reading, Spelling, and Speech* by Lindamood & Lindamood, 1998; *Teacher-Directed Paths to Achieving Literacy Success* by Mathes, Allor, Torgesen, & Allen, 2001; and *Sound Partners,* by Vadasy et al., 2004).

Although a complete review of the efficacy of early code-focused interventions provided to students with RD is beyond the scope of this chapter; recently Wanzek and Vaughn (2007) completed a meta-analytic synthesis of this research published from 1995–2005. The extant research included 18 studies in which investigators had examined the impact of extensive interventions, operationalized as lasting over 100 hours and provided in small groups, on reading outcomes across the early grades (K–1). Specifically, Wanzek and Vaughn described some interesting findings with regard to intervention components that were associated with relatively higher effect sizes. Studies with the highest effects emphasized phonics instruction that incorporated either letter–sound identification with word blending or word patterns such as rimes. Some studies integrated encoding or spelling with phonics instruction. Wanzek and Vaughn found no clear relation between the effect size and duration of treatment, but as they suggested, the relationship may be confounded by the fact that children who continued to need more help were among those initially impaired. Similarly, due to the designs of the studies, it was not possible for Wanzek and Vaughn to directly compare the efficacy of small-group to one-on-one interventions. It was encouraging that in 14 of the 18 studies, school personnel implemented interventions, but in each case, personnel were trained and supported by research staff.

One example of these programs is *Sound Partners,* which is a well-researched explicit code-focused (K–2nd grade) supplemental tutoring intervention program designed to be implemented by volunteers or paraeducators for 30 minutes, four times each week (e.g., Jenkins, Vadasy, Firebaugh, & Profliet, 2000; Vadasy, Jenkins, Antil, Wayne, & O'Connor, 1997; Vadasy, Jenkins, & Pool, 2000; Vadasy, Sanders, & Abbott, 2008; Vadasy, Sanders, & Peyton, 2006). Vadasy and colleagues developed 100 scripted lessons that provide a systematic and structured routine to train letter–sound correspondences, decoding words with familiar sounds or from common word families, practicing sight words, demonstrating fluency on decodable text, and monitoring comprehension.

A second example is *Proactive Reading* (now published by SRA as *Early Interventions in Reading*, Mathes & Torgesen, 2005). As noted by Wanzek and Vaughn (2007), Mathes and coinvestigators conducted the only study that documented whether Tier 1 was effective (Mathes et al., 2005) and was one of three investigations including students who had not responded to previous Tier 1 instruction (one involved *Sound Partners,* Vadasy et al., 2002; another was conducted by Vaughn, Linan-Thompson, & Hickman, 2003). In their large-scale experiment, Mathes and colleagues (2005) gave first-grade teachers feedback about student progress in oral reading fluency and provided professional development regarding linking assessment data to instruction. They randomly assigned poor readers to continue enhanced classroom instruction or to participate in one of two supplemental small-group interventions: *EIR* or *Responsive Reading Instruction* (Denton & Hocker, 2006). *EIR* is a supplemental explicit training program designed for struggling readers (1st–2nd grades). There are 120 scripted lesson plans that include about 7 to 10 short, interrelated activities and that provide opportunities for children to apply skills in context. Both supplemental interventions taught code-focused skills, but *Responsive Reading Instruction* was less directive and required teachers to respond to individual students' strengths and weaknesses as they were observed during the lesson. Both interventions were delivered daily to small groups (of three children) by well-trained certified teachers and lasted 40 minutes a day for 30 weeks. (However, *EIR,* as published, is intended to be used for 4 to 5 days per week for about 45 minutes per lesson and can also be implemented by certified teachers or by well-trained paraeducators.) On average, these initially poor readers were able to achieve grade-level reading at the end of the year. Not surprisingly, the two intervention groups outperformed the enhanced classroom group on outcomes of phonological awareness, word reading, and oral reading fluency. By the end of the study only a small proportion of students read below the 30th percentile on a standardized test of word reading. If the study findings were extrapolated to the larger population, we would expect only about 3 percent of students in the enhanced classroom condition, 0.2 percent in the *EIR* intervention, and 1.5 percent in the *Responsive Reading Instruction* intervention would read below average. It is noteworthy that both interventions, teamed with enhanced classroom instruction, resulted in significant increases in children reading at grade level.

The What Works Clearinghouse (WWC) has published reviews of many currently available programs. The WWC is part of the Institute for Education Sciences, and it provides ongoing reviews of programs. A tutorial about how the WWC works is available at http://ies.ed.gov/ncee/wwc/help/tutorials/tour.asp.

What Do We Know About Poor Responders?

Research has consistently shown that there is always a small proportion of children whose improvement is very small, in contrast to peers who show stronger growth trajectories. In the research literature, these children are referred to alternately as either "nonresponders" or "treatment resistors" (see, for example, Al Otaiba & Fuchs, 2002; Al Otaiba & Torgesen, 2007; Torgesen, 2000). Two relevant reviews of the extent literature on nonresponders found a fairly consistent relationship between low initial phonological awareness and treatment nonresponsiveness (see Al Otaiba & Fuchs, 2002 or Nelson, Benner, & Gonzalez, 2003 for a discussion of characteristics of nonresponders). Of course, growth in word recognition ability requires knowledge and skills other than phonemic awareness. Additional characteristics that are correlated with treatment unresponsiveness include slow performance on rapid naming tasks, attention and behavior problems, poor phonological memory, poor orthographic processing, and low IQ or low verbal ability (Al Otaiba & Fuchs, 2002; Nelson et al., 2003). Thus, roughly 3 percent to 5 percent of the general population of students will likely be poor responders to supplemental interventions (Wanzek & Vaughn, 2009), and there is very little evidence about how to help children catch up to the performance of their peers without RD, particularly in terms of fluency and comprehension.

Thus special educators and speech language pathologists will likely need to develop expertise on using data to screen children, to monitor their progress to gauge the success of interventions, to tailor intervention, and also to collaborate on Individualized Education Planning for students with RD. It is likely that the influence of phonemic reading skill on the growth of fluent word recognition processes will be affected by a number of other factors such as size of oral vocabulary, amount of reading practice and breadth of print exposure, and effective use of context (Cunningham & Stanovich, 1998). Weaknesses in phonemic decoding ability may be compensated for by strengths in one of these latter factors, whereas extra strength in phonemic reading ability may enable growth in orthographic skills, even in the presence of weakness in one of these other variables. It is also possible that many children with phonologically based reading disabilities may have additional weaknesses that interfere specifically with the formation of orthographic representations for words (Wolf & Bowers, 1999).

Some researchers have expressed concern for limitations of using phonological awareness measures for universal screening at the beginning of kindergarten because many measures designed to be used at that time may be characterized by floor effects (Catts, Petcher, Schatschneider, Bridges, & Mendoza, 2009). This is problematic because floor effects will make it more difficult to accurately predict which children truly need extra help and to distinguish these children from those who simply lack literacy experience at the beginning of kindergarten. Even in first grade, poor responders may pass through multiple tiers before they are eligible to receive special education (Fuchs, Compton, Fuchs, & Bouton, in press; Fuchs, Fuchs, & Strecker, 2010). These researchers suggest that dynamic assessment, or DA, could be used to distinguish children who are unable to perform a task such as phonemic segmentation or phonemic decoding independently but who could learn the task after a brief teaching cycle of assistance or scaffolding by a well-trained examiner (for a more thorough discussion of DA, see Grigorenko & Sternberg, 1998). Thus, Fuchs et al. proposed DA as "an index of a child's readiness to change and as such it represents a unique means of differentiating performance among children at the low end of the achievement continuum" (in press).

Some preliminary work with kindergartners by Bridges and Catts (in press) shows that a DA phonological protocol could reduce the rate of false positives (children really did not need extra help to reach grade-level reading) associated with the DIBELS Initial Sound Fluency task by over a third. These authors were predicting outcomes on an end-of-year word-reading or word attack standardized assessment. At the same time they found that DA minimally increased false negatives (children who needed help but were not identified). Whereas these results suggest that the DA can improve the specificity as a secondary measure, Bridges and Catts (in press) cautioned that their DA measure alone showed relatively poor sensitivity among kindergarteners. Fuchs and colleagues (in press) examined whether DA could improve identification for first-grade poor responders beyond more traditional measures (IQ, vocabulary, phonological awareness, timed alphabetic skills) in predicting end-of-year decoding and comprehension. In a sample of over 300 first graders, they found that a DA decoding protocol did have construct validity relative to the traditional measures and that it predicted reading performance. However, the amount of unique variance was small (ranging from 1 percent on passage comprehension up to 2.3 percent on word attack). As researchers improve on these efforts to create more powerful DA methods, it is likely that the expertise of special educators and speech language pathologists may be needed if the DA protocols incorporate more intensive teaching trial and experimental teaching.

Finally, it seems clear that instructional methods must have a significant impact on the phonemic reading skills of these children if they are going to have a long-term effect on reading growth. This inference creates a dilemma of sorts for those who are interested in preventing or remediating reading disabilities. Instruction to build phonemic decoding skills, which are seen as essential in normal reading growth, is instruction directed toward the primary cognitive/linguistic *weakness* of most children with severe RD. There is a strong component of instructional theory in the area of learning disabilities (Hammill & Bartel, 1995) that emphasizes teaching to children's strengths rather than their weaknesses. Thus, we sometimes see recommendations to children with RD using "sight word," "visually based," or even other whole-language-like approaches that do not overly stress limited phonological abilities. Even though this may be an attractive instructional approach to many teachers, it is important to emphasize that we have converging evidence that teaching phonemic decoding skills is more effective than other methods of teaching students how to read (Lonigan et al., 2008; NRP, 2000).

ISSUES FOR FUTURE RESEARCH AND DEVELOPMENT

Although research over the past 40 years has made enormous progress in helping to develop appropriate diagnostic and instructional procedures for children who experience difficulties acquiring good word recognition skills, many important issues remain for further research and development. First, and foremost, is the need for stronger procedural guidelines for RTI, including improved screeners and a better understanding of how long students should stay in an intervention and how good versus poor response is best measured.

A second issue is the need for professional development for teachers, school psychologists, speech language pathologists, and special educators. All these individuals must understand how to use data to group children and to match their needs with interventions. Knowledge about how to link Tier 1 with supplemental interventions is also needed. Encouragingly, most of the instructional programs and materials currently available can be adapted for uses other than those for which they seem most clearly appropriate. That is, skillful teachers should be able to adapt "whole-class" materials to support instruction for small groups of at-risk children, and the more intensive material can also be adapted for whole-class instruction (Foorman & Torgesen, 2001).

A third issue is that special education is likely after RTI to have the most severe or most-resistant-to-treatment RD, but yet little is known about how effective interventions can be when delivered to students who have not been helped by Tier 1 and Tier 2. Only two studies to date shed light on this topic (Denton, Fletcher, Anthony, & Francis, 2006; O'Connor, 2000) and both suggest that we really don't have the answer of how to help all children achieve and stay on grade level. Findings from these two just-mentioned studies, and from another conducted by Linan-Thompson and colleagues (2003), suggest to us an analogy to the medical field. When doctors prescribe an antibiotic, if you don't take the whole dose, not only may you get sicker, but also the germs themselves become more difficult to fight on a local and global level. This is important because we still do not understand fully the amount and type of instruction and practice that will be required for *all* RD children to attain normal word-level reading ability. Even in studies that produce very large gains in phonetic reading ability (i.e., Torgesen et al., 2001), some children remain significantly impaired in this area at the conclusion of the study. Furthermore, even in a remedial effort that produced very large improvements in the accuracy of children's word recognition skills, the children, as a group, still remained very dysfluent readers when compared to average readers of their own age. Part of this problem with fluency may result from the nature of reading fluency itself (Torgesen et al., 2001), but part of it may also be amenable to better instructional practices in this area.

A fourth issue is that we need a better understanding of the range of individual differences in the level of word recognition ability and fluency required for good reading comprehension. We know that, in general, better phonemic reading ability and more fluent word recognition skills are associated with better reading comprehension (Share & Stanovich, 1995). We also know that better phonemic reading skills are reliably associated with more accurate and fluent word recognition ability (NRP, 2000). However, cases have been reported in which students seem able to develop good word recognition ability in the absence of strongly developed phonemic skills. In one particular case (Campbell & Butterworth, 1985), the student was highly motivated to learn to read, had substantially above-average general intellectual ability, and was particularly strong on measures of visual memory. If there prove to be certain limits on fluency of phonological processes in reading for many children, it will be very helpful to understand more fully what other routes to effective reading may be available.

A final issue arises from the movement toward school-based accountability for the reading achievement of all children in the United States. The provisions of the No Child Left Behind Act of 2002 required states to set reading standards by third grade to evaluate whether or not a child has attained adequate reading skills. Within each state, the effectiveness of both preventive and remedial programs in reading will ultimately be evaluated by determining the percentage of children who fail to meet standards for adequate reading ability by the end of third grade. Typically, the tests that states use to assess reading outcomes are measures of reading comprehension that are administered to classroom-sized groups. These tests usually include lengthy passages, and require both multiple choice and written answers to questions.

The new accountability standards require all students to be tested by the same measures. Thus, the effectiveness of instructional procedures for students with RD will ultimately be evaluated in terms of their ability to help these children respond adequately on complex, group-administered measures of silent reading comprehension. To date, none of the studies of intensive interventions for older students with word-level RD has included information about the success of students on these "high-stakes," state-administered reading achievement tests. Measures typically used in intervention research are administered one-to-one, involve shorter reading passages, and provide a number of supports not available during group-administered tests.

References

Adams, M. J. (1990). *Beginning to read: Thinking and learning about print*. Cambridge, MA: MIT Press.

Adams, M. J., Foorman, B., Lundberg, I., & Beeler, C. (1997). *Phonemic awareness in young children: A classroom curriculum*. Baltimore: Brookes.

Al Otaiba, S., Connor, C. M., Folsom, J., Greulich, L., Meadows, J., & Li, Z. (in press). Assessment data-informed guidance to individualize kindergarten reading instruction: Findings from a cluster-randomized control field trial. *Elementary School Journal*.

Al Otaiba, S., & Fuchs, D. (2002). Characteristics of children who are unresponsive to early literacy intervention: A review of the literature. *Remedial and Special Education, 23*, 300–316.

Al Otaiba, S., & Fuchs, D. (2006). Who are the young children for whom best practices in reading are ineffective? An experimental and longitudinal study. *Journal of Learning Disabilities, 39*, 414–431.

Al Otaiba, S., Kosanovich-Grek, M. L., Torgesen, J. K., Hassler, L., & Wahl, M. (2005). Reviewing core kindergarten and first grade reading programs in light of No Child Left Behind: An exploratory study. *Reading and Writing Quarterly, 21*, 377–400.

Al Otaiba, S., Puranik, C., Zilkowksi, R., & Curran, T. (2009). Effectiveness of early phonological awareness interventions for students with speech or language impairments. *Journal of Special Education, 43*, 107–128.

Al Otaiba, S. & Torgesen, J. K. (2007). Effects from intensive standardized kindergarten and first grade interventions for the prevention of reading difficulties. In S. R. Jimerson, M. K. Burns, & A. M. Van der Heyden (Eds.), *The handbook of response to intervention: The science and practice of assessment and intervention* (pp. 212–222). New York: Springer.

American Speech-Language-Hearing Association. (2001). *Roles and responsibilities of speech-language pathologists with respect to reading and writing in children and adolescents*. Rockville, MD: Author.

Apel, K., Wilson-Fowler, E. B., & Masterson, J. J. (2011). Developing word-level literacy skills in children with and without typical communication skills. In S. Ellis & E. McCartney (Eds.), *Applied linguistics in the primary school: Developing a language curriculum* (pp. 229–241). Cambridge, UK: Cambridge University Press.

Aram, D. M., & Hall, N. E. (1989). Longitudinal follow-up of children with preschool communication disorders: Treatment implications. *School Psychology Review, 18*, 487–501.

Biemiller, A. (1970). The development of the use of graphic and contextual information as children learn to read. *Reading Research Quarterly, 6*, 75–96.

Bird, J., Bishop, D. V., & Freeman, N. H. (1995). Phonological awareness and literacy development in children with expressive phonological impairments. *Journal of Speech and Hearing Research, 38*, 446–462.

Bishop, D. V., & Adams, C. (1990). A prospective study of the relationship between specific language impairment, phonological disorders, and reading retardation. *Journal of Child Psychology and Psychiatry, 31*, 1027–1050.

Blachman, B. (1989). Phonologic awareness and word recognition: Assessment and intervention. In A. G. Kamhi & H. W. Catts (Eds.), *Reading disabilities: A developmental language perspective* (pp. 133–158). Boston: College Hill Press.

Blachman, B. (2000). Phonological awareness. In M. Kamil, P. Mosenthal, P. Pearson, & R. Barr (Eds.), *Handbook of reading research* (Vol. 3, pp. 483–502). Mahwah, NJ: Erlbaum.

Blachman, B. A., Ball, E. W., Black, R. S., & Tangel, D. M. (1994). Kindergarten teachers develop phoneme awareness in low-income, inner-city classrooms: Does it make a difference? *Reading and Writing: An Inter disciplinary Journal, 6*, 1–17.

Blachman, B. A., Ball, E. W., Black, R. S., & Tangel, D. M. (2000). *Road to the code: A phonological awareness program for young children*. Baltimore: Brookes.

Boudreau, D. M., & Hedberg, N. L. (1999). A comparison of early literacy skills in children with specific language impairment and their typically developing peers. *American Journal of Speech-Language Pathology, 8*, 249–260.

Bowey, J., & Hansen, J. (1994). The development of orthographic rimes as units of word recognition. *Journal of Experimental Child Psychology, 58*, 465–488.

Bradley, L., & Bryant, P. (1985). *Rhyme and reason in reading and spelling*. Ann Arbor: University of Michigan Press.

Bridges, M. S., & Catts, H. W. (in press). The use of a dynamic screening of phonological awareness to predict risk for reading disabilities in kindergarten children. *Journal of Learning Disabilities*.

Bus, A., & Van Ijzendoorn, M. (1999). Phonological awareness and early reading: A meta-analysis of experimental training studies. *Journal of Educational Psychology, 91*, 403–411.

Byrne, B., & Fielding-Barnsley, R. (1995). Evaluation of a program to teach phonemic awareness to young children: A 2- and 3-year follow-up and a new preschool trial. *Journal of Educational Psychology, 87,* 488–503.

Campbell, R., & Butterworth, B. (1985). Phonological dyslexia and dysgraphia in a highly literate subject: A developmental case with associated deficits of phonemic processing and awareness. *The Quarterly Journal of Experimental Psychology, 37,* 435–475.

Carlisle, J. (2004). Morphological processes that influence learning to read. In A. Stone, E. Silliman, B. Ehren, & K. Apel (Eds.), *Handbook of language and literacy* (pp. 318–339). New York: Guilford Press.

Catts, H. W. (1991). Early identification of dyslexia: Evidence from a follow-up study of speech-language impaired children. *Annals of Dyslexia, 41,* 163–177.

Catts, H. W. (1993). The relationship between speech-language impairments and reading disabilities. *Journal of Speech & Hearing Research, 36,* 948–958.

Catts, H. W., Fey, M. E., Tomblin, J. B., & Zhang, X. (2002). A longitudinal investigation of reading outcomes in children with language impairments. *Journal of Speech, Language, and Hearing Research, 45,* 1142–1157.

Catts, H. W., & Hogan, T. P. (2002, November). *At what grades should we assess phonological awareness?* Paper presented at annual meetings of the American Speech, Hearing, and Language Association, San Francisco, CA.

Catts, H. W., Petscher, Y., Schatschneider, C., Bridges, M. S., & Mendoza, K. (2009). Floor effects associated with universal screening and their impact on the early identification of reading disabilities. *Journal of Learning Disabilities, 42,* 163–176.

Catts, H. W., Wilcox, K. A., Wood-Jackson, C., Larrivee, L. S., & Scott, V. G. (1997). Toward an understanding of phonological awareness. In C. K. Leong & R. M. Joshi (Eds.), *Cross-language studies of learning to read and spell: Phonologic and orthographic processing* (pp. 31–52). Dordecht: Kluwer Academic Press.

Chard, D. J., & Dickson, S. (1999). Phonological awareness: Instructional and assessment guidelines. *Interventions in School and Clinic, 34,* 261–170.

Clark, D. B., & Uhry, J. K. (1995). *Dyslexia: Theory and practice of remedial instruction* (2nd ed.). Baltimore: York Press.

Clay, M. M. (1979). *Reading: The patterning of complex behavior.* Auckland, New Zealand: Heinemann.

Cognitive Concepts, Inc. (1998). *Earobics auditory development and phonics program.* Evanston, IL: Author.

Connor, C. M., Morrison, F. J., Fishman, B. J., Schatschneider, C., & Underwood, P. (2007). The early years: Algorithm-guided individualized reading instruction. *Science, 315,* 464–465.

Cunningham, A. E. (1990). Explicit versus implicit instruction in phonemic awareness. *Journal of Experimental Child Psychology, 50,* 429–444.

Cunningham, A. E., & Stanovich, K. E. (1998). The impact of print exposure on word recognition. In J. L. Metsala & L. C. Ehri (Eds.), *Word recognition in beginning literacy* (pp. 235–262). Mahwah, NJ: Erlbaum.

Denton, C. A., Fletcher, J. M., Anthony, J. L., & Francis, D. J. (2006). An evaluation of intensive intervention for students with persistent reading difficulties. *Journal of Learning Disabilities, 39,* 447–466.

Denton, C. A., & Hocker, J. L. (2006). *Responsive reading instruction: Flexible intervention for struggling readers in the early grades.* Longmont, CO: Sopris West.

Ehri, L. C. (1998). Grapheme-phoneme knowledge is essential for learning to read words in English. In J. Metsala & L. Ehri (Eds.), *Word recognition in beginning reading* (pp. 3–40). Hillsdale, NJ: Erlbaum.

Ehri, L. C. (2002). Phases of acquisition in learning to read words and implications for teaching. In R. Stainthorp & P. Tomlinson (Eds.), *Learning and teaching reading* (pp. 7–28). London: British Journal of Educational Psychology Monograph Series II.

Ehri, L. C., Nunes, S. R., Willows, D. M., Schuster, B. V., Yaghoub-Zadeh, Z., & Shanahan, T. (2001). Phonemic awareness instruction helps children learn to read: Evidence from the national reading panel's meta-analysis. *Reading Research Quarterly, 36,* 250–287.

Ehri, L. C., & Robbins, C. (1992). Beginners need some decoding skill to read words by analogy. *Reading Research Quarterly, 27,* 12–26.

Elbaum, B., Vaughn, S., Hughes, M. T., & Moody, S. W. (1999). Grouping practices and reading outcomes for students with disabilities. *Exceptional Children, 65,* 399–415.

Fletcher, J. M., Shaywitz, S. E., Shankweiler, D. P., Katz, L., Liberman, I. Y., Stuebing, K. K., et al. (1994). Cognitive profiles of reading disability: Comparisons of discrepancy and low achievement definitions. *Journal of Educational Psychology, 86,* 6–23.

Foorman, B. R., Chen, D., Carlson, C., Moats, L., Francis, K. D., & Fletcher, J. M. (2003). The necessity of the alphabetic principle to phonemic awareness instruction. *Reading and Writing, 16,* 289–324.

Foorman, B. R., Francis, D. J., Fletcher, J. M., Schatschneider, C., & Mehta, P. (1998). The role of instruction in learning to read: Preventing reading failure in at-risk children. *Journal of Educational Psychology, 90,* 37–55.

Foorman, B. R., & Torgesen, J. (2001). Critical elements of classroom and small-group instruction promote reading success in all children. *Learning Disabilities Research & Practice, 16,* 203–212.

Fuchs, D., Compton, D. L., Fuchs, L. S., & Bouton, B. (in press). The construct and predictive validity of a dynamic assessment of young children learning to read: Implications for RTI frameworks. *Journal of Learning Disabilities.*

Fuchs, D., Fuchs, L. S., Mathes, P. G., & Simmons, D. C. (1997). Peer-assisted learning strategies: Making classrooms more responsive to academic diversity. *American Educational Research Journal, 34,* 174–206.

Fuchs, D., Fuchs, L. S., McMaster, K., & Al Otaiba, S. (2003). Identifying children at risk for reading failure: Curriculum-based measurement and the dual discrepancy approach. In L. Swanson, K. R. Harris, & S. Graham (Eds.), *Handbook of Learning Disabilities* (pp. 431–449). New York: Guilford.

Fuchs, D., Fuchs, L. S., & Strecker, P. M. (2010). The "blurring" of special education in a new continuum of general education placements and services. *Exceptional Children, 76,* 301–323.

Fuchs, D., Fuchs, L. S., Thompson, A., Al Otaiba, S., Yen, L., Yang, N., et al. (2001). Is reading important in reading-readiness programs? A randomized field trial with teachers as program implementers. *Journal of Educational Psychology, 93,* 251–267.

Fuchs, L. S., & Fuchs, D. (1998). Treatment validity: A unifying concept for reconceptualizing the identification of learning disabilities. *Learning Disabilities Research and Practice, 13,* 204–219.

Gaskins, I., Ehri, L. C., Cress, C., O'Hara, C., & Donnelly, K. (1997). Procedures for word learning: Making discoveries about words. *The Reading Teacher, 50,* 312–327.

Glushko, R. J. (1981). Principles for pronouncing print: The psychology of phonography. In A. M. Lesgold & C. A. Perfetti (Eds.), *Interactive processing in reading* (pp. 61–84). Hillsdale, NJ: Erlbaum.

Good, R. H., Simmons, D. C., & Kame'enui, E. J. (2001). The importance and decision-making utility of a continuum of fluency-based indicators of foundational reading skills for third grade high-stakes outcomes. *Scientific Studies of Reading, 5,* 257–288.

Good, R. H., Simmons, D. C., Kame'enui, E. J., Kaminski, R. A., & Wallin, J. (2002). *Summary of decision rules for intensive, strategic, and benchmark instructional recommendations in kindergarten through third grade* (Technical Report No. 11). Eugene: University of Oregon.

Good, R. H., Wallin, J., Simmons, D. C., Kame'enui, E. J., & Kaminski, R. A. (2002). *System-wide percentile ranks for DIBELS benchmark assessment* (Technical Report No. 9). Eugene: University of Oregon.

Gough, P., & Walsh, S. (1991). Chinese, Phoenicians, and the orthographic cipher of English. In S. Brady & D. Shankweiler (Eds.), *Phonological processes in literacy: A tribute to Isabelle Y. Liberman* (pp. 199–234). Hillsdale, NJ: Erlbaum.

Greenwood, C. R. (1996). Research on the practices and behavior of effective teachers at the Juniper Gardens Children's Project: Implications for the education of diverse learners. In D. L. Speece & B. K. Keogh (Eds.), *Research on classroom ecologies* (pp. 39–67). Mahwah, NJ: Erlbaum.

Grigorenko, E. L., & Sternberg, R. J. (1998). Dynamic testing. *Psychological Bulletin, 124,* 75–111.

Hammill, D. D., & Bartel, M. R. (1995). *Teaching children with learning and behavior Problems.* Boston: Allyn & Bacon.

Hatcher, P. J., & Hulme, C. (1999). Phonemes, rhymes, and intelligence as predictors of children's responsiveness to remedial reading instruction: Evidence from a longitudinal study. *Journal of Experimental Child Psychology, 72,* 130–153.

Hiebert, E. H., & Fisher, C. W. (2002, April). *Text matters in developing reading fluency.* Paper presented at the International Reading Association, San Francisco, CA.

Høien, T., Lundberg, I., Stanovich, K. E., & Bjaalid, I. (1995). Components of phonological awareness. *Reading and Writing, 7,* 171–188.

Honig, B., Diamond, L., & Gutlohn, L. (2000). *Teaching reading sourcebook.* Novato, CA: Arena Press.

Iversen, S., & Tunmer, W. E. (1993). Phonological processing skills and the reading recovery program. *Journal of Educational Psychology, 85,* 112–126.

Jenkins, J. R., Vadasy, P. F., Firebaugh, M., & Profilet, C. (2000). Tutoring first-grade struggling readers in phonological reading skills. *Learning Disabilities Research & Practice Special Issue: Research to Practice: Views from Researchers and Practitioners, 15,* 75–84.

Juel, C. (1996). What makes literacy tutoring effective? *Reading Research Quarterly, 31,* 268–289.

Justice, L. M., Meier, J., & Walpole, S. (2005). Learning new words from storybooks. *Language, Speech, and Hearing Services in Schools, 36,* 17–32.

Justice, L. M., Pullen, P. C., & Pence, K. (2008). Influence of verbal and nonverbal references to print on preschoolers' visual attention to print during storybook reading. *Developmental Psychology, 44,* 855–866.

LaBerge, D., & Samuels, S. J. (1974). Toward a theory of automatic information processing in reading. *Cognitive Psychology, 6*, 293–323.

Laxon, V., Coltheart, V., & Keating, C. (1988). Children find friendly words friendly too: Words with many orthographic neighbours are easier to read and spell. *British Journal of Educational Psychology*, 58, 103–119.

Levy, B. A., Abello, B., & Lysynchuk, L. (1997). Transfer from word training to reading in context: Gains in reading fluency and comprehension. *Learning Disability Quarterly, 20*, 173–88.

Linan-Thompson, S., Vaughn, S., Hickman-Davis, P., & Kouzekanani, K. (2003). Effectiveness of supplemental reading instruction for second-grade English language learners with reading difficulties. *The Elementary School Journal, 103*, 221–238.

Lindamood, P., & Lindamood, P. (1998). *The Lindamood phoneme sequencing program for reading, spelling, and speech.* Austin, TX: PRO-ED, Inc.

Lonigan, C., Schatschneider, C., & Westberg, L. (2008). Results of the national early literacy panel research synthesis: Identification of children's skills and abilities linked to later outcomes in reading, writing, and spelling. In *Developing early literacy: Report of the National Early Literacy Panel* (pp. 55–106). Washington, DC: National Institute for Literacy.

Lovett, M. W., Lacerenza, L., Borden, S. L., Frijters, J. C., Seteinbach, K. A., & DePalma, M. (2000). Components of effective remediation for developmental reading disabilities: Combining phonological and strategy-based instruction to improve outcomes. *Journal of Educational Psychology, 92*, 263–283.

Lovett, M. W., Warren-Chaplin, P. M., Ransby, M. J., & Borden, S. L. (1990). Training the word recognition skills of reading disabled children: Treatment and transfer effects. *Journal of Educational Psychology, 82*, 769–780.

Lundberg, I., Frost, J., & Petersen, O. (1988). Effects of an extensive program for stimulating phonological awareness in preschool children. *Reading Research Quarterly, 23*, 263–284.

Lyon, G. R. (1985). Identification and remediation of learning disability subtypes: Preliminary findings. *Learning Disabilities Focus, 1*, 21–35.

Mathes, P. G., Allor, J. H., Torgesen, J. K., & Allen, S. H. (2001). *Path to achieving literacy success: Teacher-directed small-group early reading lessons (Teacher-directed PALS).* Longmont, CO: Sopris West.

Mathes, P. G., Denton, C. A., Fletcher, J. M., Anthony, J. L., Francis, D. J., & Schatschneider, C. (2005). The effects of theoretically different instruction and student characteristics on the skills of struggling readers. *Reading Research Quarterly*, 40, 148–182.

Mathes, P. G., & Torgesen, J. K. (2005). *SRA early interventions in reading.* Columbus, OH: SRA/McGraw-Hill.

Mathes, P. G., Torgesen, J. K., & Allor, J. H. (2001). The effects of peer-assisted literacy strategies for first-grade readers with and without additional computer assisted instruction in phonological awareness. *American Educational Research Journal, 38*, 371–410.

Meyer, M. S., & Felton, R. H. (1999). Repeated reading to enhance fluency: Old approaches and new directions. *Annals of Dyslexia, 49*, 283–306.

Moriarty, B. C., & Gillon, G. T. (2006). Phonological awareness intervention for children with childhood apraxia of speech. *International Journal of Language and Communication Disorders, 41*, 713–34.

National Reading Panel (NRP). (2000). *Teaching children to read: An evidence-based assessment of the scientific research literature on reading and its implications for reading instruction.* Rockville, MD: NICHD Clearinghouse.

Nelson, J. R., Benner, G. J., & Gonzalez, J. (2003). Learner characteristics that influence the treatment effectiveness of early literacy interventions: A meta-analytic review. *Learning Disabilities Research & Practice, 18*, 255–267.

O'Connor, R. E. (2000). Increasing the intensity of intervention in kindergarten and first grade. *Learning Disabilities Research & Practice, 15*, 43–54.

O'Connor, R. E., Notari-Syverson, A., & Vadasy, P. F. (2005). *Ladders to literacy: A kindergarten activity book* (2nd ed.). Baltimore: Brookes.

Perfetti, C. A. (1985). *Reading ability.* New York: Oxford University Press.

Piasta, S. B., Connor, C. M., Fishman, B., & Morrison, F. J. (2009). Teachers' knowledge of literacy concepts, classroom practices, and student reading growth. *Scientific Studies of Reading, 13*, 224–248.

President's Commission on Special Education. (2002). *A new era: Revitalizing special education for children and their families.* Retrieved January 3, 2011, from http://www2.ed.gov/inits/commissionsboards/whspecialeducation/index.html

Puranik, C., Petscher, Y., Al Otaiba, S., Catts, H. W., & Lonigan, C. (2008). Development of oral reading fluency in children with speech or language impairments: A growth curve analysis. *Journal of Learning Disabilities, 41*, 545–560.

Raynor, K., Foorman, B. R., Perfetti, C. A., Pesetsky, D., & Seidenberg, M. S. (2001). How psychological science informs the teaching of reading. *Psychological Science in the Public Interest, 2,* 31–73.

Reitsma, P. (1990). Development of orthographic knowledge. In P. Reitsma & L. Verhoeven (Eds.), *Acquisition of reading in Dutch* (pp. 43–64). Dordrecht: Foris.

Scarborough, H. S., & Dobrich, W. (1990). Development of children with early language delay. *Journal of Speech & Hearing Research, 33,* 70–83.

Share, D. L., & Stanovich, K. E. (1995). Cognitive processes in early reading development: A model of acquisition and individual differences. *Issues in Education: Contributions from Educational Psychology, 1,* 1–57.

Smolkin, L. B., Conlon, A., & Yaden, D. B. (1988). Print salient illustrations in children's picture books: The emergence of written language awareness. *National Reading Conference Yearbook, 37,* 59–68.

Snider, V. E. (1995). A primer on phonemic awareness: What it is, why it's important, and how to teach it. *School Psychology Review, 24,* 443–455.

Snow, C. E., Burns, M. S., & Griffin, P. (Eds.). (1998). *Preventing reading difficulties in young children.* Washington, DC: National Academy Press.

Snowling, M., & Hulme, C. (1989). A longitudinal case study of developmental phonological dyslexia. *Cognitive Neuropsychology, 6,* 379–401.

Stanovich, K. E., Cunningham, A. E., & Cramer, B. B. (1984). Assessing phonological awareness in kindergarten children: Issues of task comparability. *Journal of Experimental Child Psychology, 38,* 175–190.

Torgesen, J. K. (2005). Recent discoveries from research on remedial interventions for children with dyslexia. In M. Snowling & C. Hulme (Eds.), *Presentations and publications* (pp. 521–537). Oxford, UK: Blackwell Publishers.

Torgesen, J. K. (2000). Individual differences in response to early interventions in reading: The lingering problem of treatment resisters. *Learning Disabilities Research & Practice, 15,* 55–64.

Torgesen, J. K. (2002a, February). *The effects of group size and teacher training and experience on reading growth in first grade children at-risk for reading difficulties.* Paper presented at meetings of the Pacific Coast Research Conference, San Diego, CA.

Torgesen, J. K. (2002b). The prevention of reading difficulties. *Journal of School Psychology, 40,* 7–26.

Torgesen, J. K., & Bryant, B. (1993). *Phonological awareness training for reading.* Austin, TX: Pro-Ed.

Torgesen, J. K., Burgess, S., & Rashotte, C. A. (1996, April). *Predicting phonologically based reading dis-*

abilities: What is gained by waiting a year? Paper presented at the annual meetings of the Society for the Scientific Study of Reading, New York.

Torgesen, J. K., & Morgan, S. (1990). Phonological synthesis tasks: A developmental, functional, and componential analysis. In H. L. Swanson & B. K. Keogh (Eds.), *Learning disabilities: Theoretical and research issues* (pp. 263–276). Hillsdale, NJ: Erlbaum.

Torgesen, J. K., Rashotte, C. A., & Alexander, A. (2001). Principles of fluency instruction in reading: Relationships with established empirical outcomes. In M. Wolf (Ed.), *Dyslexia, fluency, and the brain* (pp. 333–355). Parkton, MD: York Press.

Torgesen, J. K., Rashotte, C. A., Alexander, A., Alexander, J., & MacPhee, K. (2003). Progress towards understanding the instructional conditions necessary for remediating reading difficulties in older children. In B. Foorman (Ed.), *Preventing and remediating reading difficulties: Bringing science to scale* (pp. 275–298). Parkton, MD: York Press.

Torgesen, J. K., Wagner, R. K., Rashotte, C. A., Burgess, S. R., & Hecht, S. A. (1997). The contributions of phonological awareness and rapid automatic naming ability to the growth of word reading skills in second to fifth grade children. *Scientific Studies of Reading, 1,* 161–185.

Torgesen, J. K., Wagner, R. K., Rashotte, C. A., Lindamood, P., Rose, E., Conway, T., et al. (1999). Preventing reading failure in young children with phonological processing disabilities: Group and individual responses to instruction. *Journal of Educational Psychology, 91,* 579–593.

Trieman, R., Goswami, U., & Bruck, M. (1990). Not all nonwords are alike: Implications for reading development and theory. *Memory and Cognition, 18,* 559–567.

Vadasy, P. F., Jenkins, J. R., Antil, L. R., Wayne, S. K., & O'Conner, R. E. (1997). Community-based early reading intervention for at-risk first graders. *Learning Disabilities Research & Practice, 12,* 29–39.

Vadasy, P. F., Jenkins, J. R., & Pool, K. (2000). Effects of tutoring in phonological and early reading skills on students at risk for reading disabilities. *Journal of Learning Disabilities, 33,* 579–590.

Vadasy, P. F., Sanders, E. A., & Abbott, R. D. (2008). Effects of supplemental early reading intervention at 2-year follow-up: Reading skill growth patterns and predictors. *Scientific Studies of Reading, 12,* 51–89.

Vadasy, P. F., Sanders, E. A., & Peyton, J. A. (2006). Paraeducator-supplemented instruction in structural analysis with text reading practice for second and third graders at risk for reading problems. *Remedial and Special Education, 27,* 365–378.

Vadasy, P. F., Sanders, E. A., Peyton, J. A., & Jenkins, J. R. (2002). Timing and intensity of tutoring: A closer look at the conditions for effective early literacy tutoring. *Learning Disabilities Research & Practice, 17*, 227–241.

Vadasy, P. F., Wayne, S. K., O'Connor, R. E., Jenkins, J. R., Pool, K., Firebaugh, M., et al. (2004). *Sound partners: A supplementary, one-to-one tutoring program in phonics-based early reading skills.* Longmont, CO: Sopris West.

Vaughn S., & Linan-Thompson, S. (2003). Group size and time allotted to intervention: Effects for students with reading difficulties. In B. Foorman (Ed.), *Interventions for children at-risk for reading difficulties or identified with reading difficulties* (pp. 299–324). Parkton, MD: York Press.

Vaughn, S., Linan-Thompson, S., & Hickman, P. (2003). Response to instruction as a means of identifying students with Reading/Learning disabilities. *Exceptional Children, 69*, 391–409.

Vellutino, F. R., Scanlon, D. M., Sipay, E. R., Small S. G., Pratt, A., Chen R., et al. (1996). Cognitive profiles of difficult-to-remediate and readily remediated poor readers: Early intervention as a vehicle for distinguishing between cognitive and experiential deficits as basic causes of specific reading disability. *Journal of Educational Psychology, 88*, 601–638.

Wagner, R. K., Torgesen, J. K., & Rashotte, C. A. (1994). The development of reading-related phonological processing abilities: New evidence of bidirectional causality from a latent variable longitudinal study. *Developmental Psychology, 30*, 73–87.

Wanzek, J., & Vaughn, S. (2007). Research-based implications from extensive early reading interventions. *School Psychology Review, 36*, 541–561.

Wanzek, J., & Vaughn, S. (2009). Students demonstrating persistent low response to reading intervention: Three case studies. *Learning Disabilities Research & Practice, 24*, 151–163.

Warrick, N., Rubin, H., & Rowe-Walsh, S. (1993). Phoneme awareness in language-delayed children: Comparative studies and intervention. *Annals of Dyslexia, 43*, 153–173.

Wilson, B. A. (1988). *Wilson Reading System, Instructor manual.* Millbury, MA: Wilson Language Training.

Wise, B. W., & Olsen, R. K. (1995). Computer-based phonological awareness and reading instruction. *Annals of Dyslexia, 45,* 99–122.

Wolf, M. A., & Bowers, P. G. (1999). The double-deficit hypothesis for the developmental dyslexias. *Journal of Educational Psychology, 91*, 415–438.

Yopp, H. K. (1988). The validity and reliability of phonemic awareness tests. *Reading Research Quarterly, 23*, 159–177.

Chapter 6

Perspectives on Assessing and Improving Reading Comprehension

Alan G. Kamhi

This chapter and the one that follows by Carol Westby focus on reading comprehension. The reading and literacy skills necessary for academic, economic, and social success involve not just the ability to accurately and fluently recognize words but also the ability to construct and extract meaning from texts. Although the contribution of comprehension skills for successful reading has always been recognized by cognitive psychologists, in the last 10 years a number of federal initiatives have called for more thorough and systematic investigations of comprehension processes and the development of interventions that target them (Pressley, Graham, & Harris, 2006; RAND Reading Study Group [RRSG], 2002). These initiatives often mention the gap that exists between research on the mechanisms that underlie comprehension and the intervention strategies used to improve reading comprehension difficulties (McNamara, 2007; RRSG, 2002).

The gap is best seen in how the processes and products of comprehension are viewed by researchers and practitioners. The products of comprehension are the indicators and measures of what the reader knows and understands after reading a text. The processes of comprehension are the cognitive activities and knowledge sources the reader uses to arrive at the products (Rapp, van den Broek, McMaster, Kendeou, & Espin, 2007). These processes and knowledge sources were discussed in Chapter 1 in the section on discourse and text-level processes. Interventions are often designed to improve the cognitive processes that occur *during* reading, yet comprehension assessments and determinations of intervention effectiveness, such as recall or question-based tasks, are product-based measures that occur *after* reading (Rapp et al., 2007). Thus, unlike decoding, where instruction and assessment target the same skill (letter recognition, phoneme awareness, alphabetic knowledge, word-level reading), comprehension instruction and assessment often do not coincide.

The difference between the products and processes of comprehension is one of the many challenges that confront educators faced with helping struggling readers. Many others will be considered in this chapter. My principal aim in discussing these challenges is not to discourage educators from tackling comprehension problems, but to provide teachers and practitioners (i.e., special educators and speech-language pathologists [SLPs]) with an understanding of the factors that need to be considered in designing instruction and intervention to improve comprehension performance.

DEFINING COMPREHENSION

Defining comprehension would seem to be a straightforward task. It is not. Not only are there different levels of understanding (e.g., basic/literal, elaborated/analytic, and highly elaborated/creative), but comprehension, especially deep understanding, also depends on thinking and reasoning processes that are specific to a discipline or subject area (Kintsch, 1998; RRSG, 2002; Snow, 2010). A definition of comprehension must reflect the processes as well as the products of comprehension. Most definitions focus only on the processes of comprehension. The Research and Development (RAND) Reading Study Group (RRSG, 2002), for example, succinctly defined comprehension as "the process of simultaneously constructing and extracting meaning through interaction and engagement with print." According to Snow (2010), the definition was intended to emphasize the importance of three key elements: accurate word-level decoding, a process that integrates inferences and information not in the text (world knowledge) with text information to construct meaning, and the importance of an active, engaged reader.

The cognitive and linguistic processing that occur during comprehension events have been studied extensively by researchers (e.g., Rapp et al., 2007; RRSG, 2002). This research has made it clear that successful comprehension is determined by three factors: reader abilities, text factors, and the comprehension task that measures the products of comprehension (Snow, 2010). In clear cases of comprehension, the three dimensions of comprehension are aligned. Mismatches in any pair of these dimensions results in comprehension failure. Variations in the age and developmental level of the reader, the nature and complexity of the text being read, and the particular comprehension task means that there may be as much variability in comprehension performance within students as across students. Variability is also caused by differences in contextual factors such as the setting or the reading event (home, school, park), how noisy or distracting the setting is, whether there are time constraints to produce responses, and the purpose and expectation of the reading event (pleasure, school, work, standardized test). Reader abilities, text, and task factors are discussed in more detail in the next few sections.

Reader Abilities

As discussed in previous chapters, the two most important factors for reading comprehension are the ability to accurately and fluently decode words and the ability to understand spoken language. It is not coincidental that the Simple View of Reading (Gough & Tunmer, 1986) defines reading comprehension as the product of these two components. The importance of decoding and language knowledge (e.g., vocabulary and grammar) for comprehension is indisputable, but focusing on these two components can often lead to less emphasis and attention directed toward other factors that significantly affect listening and reading comprehension, such as background knowledge, level of engagement (attention, interest, and motivation), and inferencing abilities.

As discussed in Chapter 1, background knowledge is a crucial element in constructing meaning. Indeed, the best predictor of comprehension is often familiarity with content knowledge domains (Hirsch, 2006; RRSG, 2002; Willingham, 2006). Familiarity with the content of a passage is, in fact, so important that poor decoders do better than good decoders when they have more knowledge of a topic than good readers (Moravcsik & Kintsch, 1993; Recht & Leslie,

1988; Yekovich, Walker, Ogle, & Thompson, 1990). Based on findings such as these, Hirsch (1996, 2006) has argued that a knowledge deficit is the primary cause of the education gap in American schools.

The role of motivation in comprehension has been emphasized in the work of Guthrie (2003), who has noted that background knowledge is likely to be richer in areas of personal interest and readers are more likely to try to understand texts when they are interested in the topic. A recent study by Oakhill and Petrides (2007) found evidence supporting the role of interest for comprehension, but the findings revealed a provocative sex difference. Boys' comprehension was more affected by interest than girls' comprehension. Fifth-grade boys answered 60 percent of comprehension questions correctly on the high-interest passage compared with 38 percent for the low-interest one. Their performance on the high-interest passages was comparable to girls, who performed at the same 60 percent for high- and low-interest passages.

Clark and Kamhi (2008, 2009) attempted to replicate these findings using different measures of interest (ranking vs. forced choice) on passages from the *Qualitative Reading Inventory* and passages that we created. Unlike Oakhill and Petrides (2007), we did not find that interest influenced comprehension performance. Both boys and girls performed similarly for high- and low-interest passages. Every educator can cite examples of how students are influenced by interest and motivation, but these factors are strongly influenced by reader ability and the comprehension task. Perhaps our students were a more homogeneous group of readers than those in the British study by Oakhill and Petrides (2007).

There is a rich literature demonstrating the influence of inferencing abilities on comprehension (Graesser, Singer, & Trabasso, 1994; Laing & Kamhi, 2002; Magliono, Trabasso, & Graesser, 1999; Trabasso & Magliono, 1996). Inferencing abilities are important for comprehension because critical information is often not explicitly mentioned in texts. Poor readers have particular difficulty constructing explanatory inferences, which provide causal connections between actions and events in a story, as opposed to simpler predictive and associative inference. Westby devotes considerable attention in her chapter to inferencing abilities.

Text Factors

Text factors include readability and clarity of writing, text structure/genre, and display characteristics such as font size and type, layout, and use of graphics. For example, well-written textbooks have good topic sentences and good concluding sentences, which make it possible for readers to skim long, detailed chapters. As people get older, font size becomes a critical factor in reading. Children who may not like to read books will often enjoy reading comic books or magazines and surfing the Web. There is no doubt that text factors significantly affect reading, but they are rarely the cause of specific reading difficulties.

Task Factors

What does it mean to understand a simple sentence? Is the task to understand individual word meanings, phrases, clauses, or the entire sentence or use previous knowledge to interpret the sentence? Snow (2010) suggests that the challenge of reading comprehension is caused in large part by the difficulty of defining its borders—where reading comprehension begins and ends. The problem does not just occur with longer narrative and expository texts. As Snow shows, it also occurs with a simple sentence that may be found in a first-grade reader:

Alex and Ali ran to the swings and jumped on.

Snow asks us to consider: What would be considered adequate comprehension of this sentence? At minimum, one should create a mental representation of two people moving quickly to use some playground equipment, but is the inference that Alex and Ali are probably children part of the comprehension process or does this go beyond basic comprehension? What about assigning gender to Alex and Ali because Alex could be short for either Alexandra or Alexander, and Ali could be a boy's name or a nickname for Alison? If one assumes that Ali is a boy, is it part of the comprehension process to infer that he is Arabic, or is this an inference that goes well beyond basic comprehension? Is it necessary to infer that Alex and Ali actually started swinging, or does this go beyond comprehension into the realm of prediction? In short, what type of response would be considered sufficient to indicate comprehension of this simple sentence?

The challenge for researchers and educators interested in comprehension is not only to answer the previous question, but also to answer the much more difficult question of how to determine comprehension of longer and more complex texts like newspaper reports, scientific articles, or what constitutes comprehension of an array of texts like conflicting scientific articles or the entire works of a novelist. There are several different levels of comprehension, ranging from literal interpretations to analytic and creative interpretations (Adler & Van Doren, 1972) or a simple representation of an event to a deep understanding of a worldview (Snow, 2010).

A Model of Comprehension

A model of comprehension must capture the differences between literal understanding of words and sentences and the specialized language and conceptual knowledge required to understand complex disciplinary texts. Snow (2010) suggests that reading comprehension might be thought of as a set of four concentric circles, with the center circle being basic word-level reading processes that produce an accurate representation of the word and fluent access to word meaning. The second circle contains the core comprehension processes that lead to the construction of a text-based meaning (Kintsch, 1998). Core comprehension requires text memory, making text-based inferences, and linking text information to world knowledge. Some researchers (e.g., Shanahan & Shanahan, 2008) prefer a pyramid model with three levels rather than four. The base of the pyramid represents the highly generalizable basic literacy skills that are reflected in the first two concentric circles. Instruction that focuses on these basic, core comprehension skills will help students activate relevant background knowledge before reading and encourage self-monitoring to ensure that the focus is on constructing meanings and not just on reading words.

In the concentric circle model, the third circle contains somewhat elaborated comprehension processes that go beyond text-based representations, eventually leading to deeper understandings (Snow, 2010). In this intermediate literacy phase, which begins in the upper elementary grades, students show more varied comprehension responses to texts (Shanahan & Shanahan, 2008). Students develop the ability to maintain attention to extended discourse, monitor their comprehension, and use various fix-up procedures when they don't understand something (e.g., rereading, requesting help, using the dictionary). They also begin to use author intention as a general strategy for critical response. The majority of American students are able to demonstrate these intermediate literacy skills by the end of middle school, but many struggling high school students have not mastered these skills (Shanahan & Shanahan, 2008).

Much of the strategy-based instruction that is common in the reading literature, such as visualization, generating questions while reading, and making text-to-text connections is focused on these intermediate elaborated comprehension skills. For example, Palinscar and Brown's (1984) reciprocal teaching approach teaches students to predict, question, clarify, and summarize texts. As students read, they ask themselves if they understand what they have read so far, clear up ambiguities by asking teachers or checking the dictionary, and eventually summarize the main idea of the passage. Other approaches that focus on elaborated comprehension processes include reader response (Karolides, 1997) and Questioning the Author (Beck & McKeown, 2002).

The outermost circle and the highest level of the pyramid consist of highly elaborated comprehension processes required for disciplinary studies and deep learning from texts (Shanahan & Shanahan, 2008; Snow, 2010). The only readers who reach this level are those with extensive background knowledge and disciplinary training. Whereas ordinary readers will be able to use moderately elaborated comprehension processes to understand the texts they read (e.g., novels, political commentaries, health and science articles), only those with disciplinary training can read for purposes of literary criticism, critical reviews (e.g., journal article critiques), or writing articles, chapters, or academic texts. For Shanahan and Shanahan (2008), after these authors the pyramid narrows at this level because disciplinary reading abilities are the most specialized and least generalizable. For example, a high school student who does exceptionally well in the sciences and math, might do poorly in English or social studies and vice versa. The majority of students in our schools will be able to demonstrate basic and intermediate comprehension skills, but many will never reach the level of proficiency necessary to understand challenging texts in science, history, literature, math, or technology (Grigg, Donahue, & Dion, 2007; Shanahan & Shanahan, 2008).

The representation of four kinds of reading as concentric circles with clear boundaries should be viewed cautiously because some comprehension events may not fall clearly on one side of a boundary (Snow, 2010). The model should also not be viewed as endorsing an approach to reading instruction that starts in the middle and moves slowly outward. The construction of meaning, new learning, and interpretation should be part of the earliest reading instruction before children have mastered the code.

Shanahan and Shanahan's (2008) model, in contrast, is presented as a view of how literacy progresses. They take issue with the prevailing assumption prevalent in education that basic literacy skills automatically evolve into more advanced reading skills (i.e., deep understanding). They point out that "we have spent a half century of education beholden to the generalist notion of literacy learning—the idea that if we just provide adequate basic skills, kids with adequate background knowledge will be able to read anything successfully" (p. 41). This view was feasible 30–40 years ago because schools were able to produce a sufficiently educated population for the nation's economic needs. In the last generation, however, the expansion of information-based technologies and changes in workplace demands have increased the importance of advanced literacy skills. Despite the growing need for higher-level literacy skills, high school students are reading at lower levels than they did in 1992 (Grigg et al., 2007). Shanahan and Shanahan (2008) are obviously very interested in improving disciplinary literacy skills in high school students. I will discuss their multiyear project that has been implemented in some Chicago high schools in the section on instruction.

ASSESSING READING COMPREHENSION[1]

It is generally agreed by reading specialists (e.g., Barr, Blachowicz, Katz, & Kaufman, 2002; Richek, Caldwell, Jennings, & Lerner, 2002; Ruddell, 2002) that a comprehensive assessment

[1]Portions of this section on assessment were adapted, with permission, from a previous chapter I wrote on reading comprehension entitled, "Finding Beauty in the Ugly Facts about Reading Comprehension." The chapter appeared in H. Catts and A. Kamhi (Eds.), *The Connections between Language and Reading Disabilities* (pp. 201–213), Mahwah, NJ: Erlbaum, 2005.

of reading needs to provide information about how well students can (1) read accurately and fluently; (2) relate text information to previously stored knowledge of the world and other texts; (3) recall, paraphrase, and provide the gist of texts; (4) use inferences to build cohesion and interpret texts; (5) construct literal, critical, and creative interpretations; (6) determine when comprehension is occurring or not occurring; and (7) select and use appropriate fix-up strategies. To obtain information about all these skills, several descriptive, criterion-oriented assessments are required. These assessments include informal reading inventories (IRIs), using a running record, portfolio assessment, dynamic assessment, curriculum-based assessment, and think-aloud procedures. Detailed descriptions of these procedures can be found in any of the resources cited earlier. For example, with the think-aloud procedure, students are asked to comment about what they read after each sentence or paragraph.

An important purpose of assessment is to plan instruction to help students read and learn better. Much has been written about the kinds of questions teachers should ask to assess and facilitate understanding and learning. For example, it is often suggested that teachers should ask questions that require high-level thinking as well as questions that require memory for directly stated information (Barr et al., 2002). Although this advice seems to have merit, it is not easy to implement. Sanders (1966), for example, has noted that if the text is trivial or simplistic, it is difficult to come up with a "thinking" question. Another more serious problem is that it is hard to align questions with levels of thinking. It may be more important to differentiate between questions that address important text information and questions that target incidental details. Studies have shown that most of the questions teachers ask involve "retrieval of the trivial factual makeup of stories" rather than important information about story plots, events, and sequences (Guszak, 1967, p. 233).

Instead of focusing on levels of thinking, one can differentiate questions according to their relationship to the text as a whole. For example, questions can be categorized as either text-related or beyond-the-text (Barr et al., 2002). Text-related questions are designed to follow the author's train of thought and assess the students' comprehension of the passage as a whole. These questions require factual as well as inferential knowledge. Beyond-text questions may question the author's intent or attempt to relate the text to personal experiences or other books, ideas, and issues. Barr et al. (2002, pp. 177–178) provided examples of these questions for *Charlotte's Web*. Text-related questions include, "What is a runt pig?" "Why was Fern's father going to do away with the pig?" and "How did Fern feel when she found out her father was going to kill the pig?" Examples of beyond-text questions are, "Why would Fern's father believe it was okay to kill the pig?" "If you were Fern, would you be willing to take care of the pig?"

Beyond-text questions are somewhat similar to the types of questions recommended by educators interesting in probing children's response to texts (Kamhi, 1997; Ruddell, 2002). Questions such as, "What made the book interesting?" and "Why did you like/not like the book?" focus attention on affective reactions to texts. A related approach called Questioning the Author (QtA), developed by Beck and her colleagues (Beck, McKeown, Sandora, Kucan, & Worthy, 1996), also encourages reader response questions by responding to questions like, "What is the author trying to say here?" and "Did the author explain this clearly?"

QtA, as well as other approaches that encourage personal responses to texts, not only uncover areas of learning strengths and weaknesses, but they also function as a way to teach and improve reading and learning in students with diverse abilities and needs. Beck et al. (1996) used QtA in a year-long study of 23 inner-city fourth-grade children and found that it had a significant impact on the way teachers and students viewed reading. One teacher commented, "Thanks to Questioning the Author, I now expect my students to think and learn and explain rather than memorize, dictate, and forget" (p. 410). The changes were particularly dramatic for the low-ability students. One teacher could not believe how involved all her students had become with the story. "They read ahead and even the slower, less motivated students are joining in the discussion with enthusiasm and vigor" (p. 410). One of the other important outcomes of QtA was an improvement in students' ability to construct meaning and monitor their understanding of texts.

Determining the best questions to ask to assess understanding and learning has challenged educational experts for a very long time. There is no simple prescription for the kinds of questions that will provide accurate measures of understanding and learning, but some combination of text-related and beyond-text questions is clearly necessary. Asking beyond-text questions should encourage students and teachers to broaden their view of reading and recognize the opportunities for learning that reading provides.

In the best of all possible worlds, the kind of assessment described in the previous pages would occur in classrooms and schools throughout the country. The reality, however, is that it is much more common for educators to assume that a student's comprehension abilities can be captured by one test and test score. In many cases, a student's reading abilities (decoding and comprehension) are reduced to one score. The National Assessment of Educational Progress (NAEP) is an example of a reading measure that reduces reading to one standard score. There are many others. But if comprehension is influenced by variability in reader abilities, texts, and the comprehension task, it cannot ever be captured or reduced to one number or score. The variability in comprehension is reflected in recent studies (Cutting & Scarborough, 2006; Francis, Fletcher, Catts, & Tomblin, 2005; Keenan, Betjemann, & Olson, 2008) showing that commonly used measures of reading comprehension do not measure the same thing. Some measures of reading comprehension (e.g., *The Peabody Individual Achievement Test* and *Woodcock-Johnson Passage Comprehension*) are heavily influence by decoding skill, whereas others (e.g., *Qualitative Reading Inventory-QRI*) are more influenced by general language and cognitive processes (e.g., inferencing and metacognitive abilities).

Measures of comprehension are also heavily influenced by specific subject or content knowledge (e.g., Hirsch, 2006; Willingham, 2006). Indeed, Geiser (2008) has found that a student's specific subject knowledge is a better indication of curriculum learning and a better predictor of college performance than general measures of reasoning or reading comprehension. Summarizing a decade of research at the University of California, Geiser found that admissions criteria that reflected student mastery of curriculum content, such as high school grades and performance on subject-area SAT tests, were stronger predictors of success in college and less biased toward poor and minority applicants than tests of general reasoning and comprehension such as the SAT. Another benefit of subject-specific tests is that they can be used to show that students can meet subject-specific learning goals despite performing poorly on general measures of reading comprehension.

An appreciation of the difficulty in measuring reading comprehension will hopefully lead educators to recognize that comprehension and reading ability should not be reduced to one number or score. Assessments of reading should differentiate word recognition skills from basic comprehension abilities. Subject-specific knowledge should be measured separately by discipline-specific assessments. Distinct measures of word-level reading, basic comprehension abilities, and discipline-specific knowledge will allow educators to tailor instruction and intervention to improve specific areas of deficiency.

COMPREHENSION INSTRUCTION

There are many challenges in providing effective comprehension instruction. Unlike word recognition with its well-defined scope of knowledge (e.g., letters, sounds, words) and processes (decoding), comprehension is influenced by knowledge and skills (language, background knowledge, inferencing abilities) that do not lend themselves to systematic instructional programs. Comprehension is also influenced by text and engagement factors such as attention, interest, and motivation. Because comprehension is influenced by so many factors, it is actually relatively easy to devise instructions that show measurable gains in some aspect of understanding. The problem is that measurable gains may be limited to certain subject areas and reflect literal, relatively shallow interpretations of simple texts. As discussed previously, there is a big difference between a simple representation or literal interpretation of a series of words and a response that requires a deep understanding of a novel, scientific article, or opinion essay. Instruction that targets simpler comprehension responses is obviously going to show measurable gains much quicker than those that target deeper understandings. Deciding what to target is thus one of the major issues confronting teachers and practitioners trying to improve comprehension abilities in struggling readers.

The goals that teachers and practitioners choose to target will be strongly influenced by their professional background (educator, reading specialist, SLP), instructional experiences (e.g., strategy- vs. content-oriented approaches), and the age and ability level of students. SLPs, for example, should be comfortable targeting the language aspects of comprehension that Westby discusses in the following chapter. Reading and special education teachers often have training in strategy instruction, so they are likely to target the use of strategies to facilitate comprehension. Those who teach adolescents are most likely to target subject and disciplinary literacy. The remainder of this chapter will review some of the key components of strategy instruction and content-focused disciplinary literacy.

Strategy Instruction

The most frequent comprehension instruction involves the teaching of comprehension strategies because for many educators, comprehension is viewed as strategic (e.g., Duffy, 2003; Pressley, 2002; Swanson, 1999), and strategy instruction has proven to be effective (National Institute of Child Health and Human Development [NICHD], 2000; Vaughn, Gersten, & Chard, 2000). As discussed previously, Palinscar and Brown's (1984) reciprocal teaching approach was one of the first to emphasize strategy instruction. Many educators use the seven strategies identified by the National Reading Panel (NRP; NICHD, 2000) to improve comprehension: (1) comprehension monitoring, (2) cooperative learning, (3) graphic and semantic organizers, (4) self-questioning, (5) story structure analysis, (6) summarizing, and (7) answering questions. A brief synopsis of each of these strategies is provided in the sections to follow. More detailed information about these and other strategies can be found in textbooks on reading or learning disabilities (e.g., Bursuck & Damer, 2007; Richek et al., 2002; Ruddell, 2002).

COMPREHENSION MONITORING.   Comprehension monitoring requires students to determine when they are having difficulty understanding something and know which "fix-up" strategy to use to address the problem. Bursuck and Damer (2007) describe several comprehension monitoring and fix-up strategies based on the work of Armbruster and colleagues (2001). Students learn to identify where the difficulty occurs, know what the difficulty is, restate the difficult sentence or passage in their own words, look back through the text, and look forward in the text for information that might help resolve the difficulty.

COOPERATIVE LEARNING.   The teacher divides the class into small groups comprised of students with different reading levels and perspectives. The group works on a well-structured, clearly defined learning activity. Literature circles are often used for these activities. Four or five students who have read the same book are assigned roles by the teacher. The roles can include discussion director, summarizer, literacy reporter (finds memorable passages), illustrator, vocabulary enricher (finds meanings of difficult words), connector (finds links between the book and other books and sources of information on the topic), and investigator (uncovers background information related to the book). Cooperative learning is often difficult to implement in the classroom because of behavioral management issues (Dunston, 2002). Careful planning, close monitoring, and well-structured tasks are crucial for providing effective instruction in cooperative learning groups (Bursuck & Damer, 2007).

GRAPHIC AND SEMANTIC ORGANIZERS.   Graphic and semantic organizers help students identify the critical elements in a text and provide them with a visual representation of these elements. The first step for constructing graphic organizers is to determine the critical elements or content of a text. Teachers begin by helping students identify the critical information in a text. The purpose of a graphic organizer is to clarify interrelationships among ideas and information (Bursuck & Damer, 2007). Friend and Bursuck (2006) give an example of a story about Native Americans and colonists who had different ideas about the land. Native Americans shared the land, whereas colonists owned individual pieces. The graphic organizer/concept map they created looked like this:

Attribute	Native American	Colonists
land	shared	owned
	lived close to it without changing it	cleared it
	respected it	used it

Once a graphic organizer is created, teachers can distribute partially completed concept maps to students and then introduce the various concepts as the text is being read.

SELF-QUESTIONING.   Self-questioning has proven to be an effective way for readers to become actively engaged with text. There are many different questions students can ask themselves. They can ask self-monitoring questions (e.g., "Does this make sense?" "What does this word mean?" "Is this what I thought the passage was about?"), factual questions (who, what, where, when), inferential questions (why, how), and beyond-text questions about the author's intent or how the text relates to personal experiences or other books, ideas, and issues. Teachers play an important role in determining the kinds of questions children will ask. As discussed in the previous section, beyond-text questions such as those used by Beck and her colleagues (Beck et al., 1996) taught students to think and learn and explain rather than memorize, dictate, and forget.

STORY STRUCTURE ANALYSIS.   Students learn to identify the framework or schema of a story, including the story elements of setting, characters, motivation, problems, plot, and theme. Story maps are a useful way to represent these story elements (Friend & Bursuck, 2006). Westby (Chapter 7) goes into considerable detail about this topic.

SUMMARIZING.   Summaries provide a synthesis of important ideas in text by helping students identify the main idea in expository texts and recognizing the key story elements in narrative texts. Summarizing can be done periodically after each paragraph or at the end of a text (Bursuck & Damer, 2007).

ANSWERING QUESTIONS.   Students are taught to ask text-explicit and text-implicit questions to guide their understanding. The Question-Answer Relationship (Raphael, 1986) approach divides questions into two broad categories: *In the Book* questions and answers use words that are in the text, whereas *In My Head* questions and answers are not in the text. There are two types of *In the Book* questions: (a) *Right There* questions, where the answers are easy to find because the words used in the question are the same as the words in the answer, and (b) *Think and Search* questions, where the answer is in the story, but you have to find it, and the words in the question and the answer are not the same. There are also two types of *In My Head* questions: (a) *Author and You* questions, where the reader uses previous knowledge with text information to create an answer, and (b) *On my Own* questions, where the reader uses previous experience to respond. The teacher models the use of each question type with various texts.

MULTIPLE STRATEGY INSTRUCTION.   Not surprisingly, The NRP report (NICHD, 2000) found that readers benefit more when multiple strategies are taught together, as they are in approaches like Palinscar and Brown's (1984) reciprocal teaching. Multiple strategy instruction should include teaching students when specific strategies are most effective—before, during, or after reading (Bursuck & Damer, 2007; Duffy, 2003; NICHD, 2000). *Before-reading* strategies include activating background knowledge, previewing the text, and asking questions about it. *During-reading* strategies are monitoring comprehension, using fix-up strategies, generating questions about the reading, periodic summarizing, visualizing what is happening, taking notes, and constructing responses to the text. *After-reading* strategies include generating questions about the text, recalling and summarizing key elements from the text, and extending the knowledge gained from the text to other activities (Bursuck & Damer, 2007).

EVALUATION OF STRATEGY INSTRUCTION.   Despite the hundreds of studies that have found strategy instruction is effective in improving comprehension (NICHD, 2000), there are still questions about how comprehension strategies work and what they do for comprehension (Catts, 2009; Willingham, 2006). Catts questions, for example, how two common strategies, finding the main idea and summarization, could directly cause better comprehension. The ability to find the main idea and summarize are more likely to be the product or result of comprehension rather than the cause. To know what the main idea of a passage is, one must understand the passage. Comprehension strategies often function as activities that focus attention on what is important for understanding texts, such as understanding the purpose of reading, using prior knowledge to predict what might happen in the text, and generating questions that help the reader create meanings and interpret texts (Catts, 2009; Willingham, 2006).

Although comprehension strategies may be helpful in facilitating comprehension, they do not address deficiencies in background and language knowledge or motivational factors that research has shown are the most significant causes of comprehension problems (Guthrie, Wigfield, & Perencevich, 2004; Hirsch, 2006; Snow, 2010). In addition, strategies are often taught as ends in themselves rather than as a means to construct meaning (Torgesen, 2007). Students may spend too much time and effort focusing on how they should process a text rather than on the text itself. Focusing on processing a text might not affect good students who have enough cognitive resources to focus on meaning construction, but students with language and learning disabilities may not benefit much from strategy instruction if their attention is focused primarily on the reading process rather than the text.

Content Goals and Disciplinary Literacy

Many researchers now believe that a focus on content goals and disciplinary literacy, rather than strategies per se, is the most effective way to create engaged readers who read for meaning

(Bulgren, Deshler, & Lenz, 2007; Guthrie et al., 2004; Moje, 2008; Shanahan & Shanahan, 2008; Snow, 2010). When content goals are prominent in reading, students focus on gaining meaning, building knowledge, and understanding deeply, rather than on simply answering a series of comprehension questions. The importance of motivation and content knowledge for deep comprehension led Guthrie and his colleagues (Guthrie et al., 2004; Guthrie, 2008) to develop Concept Oriented Reading Instruction (CORI). The premise of CORI is that motivated students usually want to understand texts fully and process information deeply. One of the key components of CORI is choice. Students are given choices of texts to read, choices of responses to texts (presentations, papers, projects), and choices of partners to collaborate with during instruction and responses (assignments). Choice leads to ownership and increased motivation. Students are given the opportunity to work collaboratively, with lots of opportunities for discussion, questioning, and sharing.

An excellent description of the CORI program can be found at the following Web site: http://www.cori.umd.edu. This Web site describes two 6-week phases of CORI that focus on hidden worlds of the woodlands and wetlands. Each phase has four stages: (1) observe and personalize (2 weeks), (2) search and retrieve (1 week), (3) comprehend and integrate (2 weeks), and (4) communicate to others (1 week). In the first stage, students begin by activating background knowledge. They are asked to relate personal experiences to stories and texts about the theme of hidden worlds. Then the class takes a field trip to local woods and observes the habitats of hidden worlds for animals and plants. Back in class, they are asked to relate the texts about hidden worlds to their field observations. Engagement and motivation are fostered by allowing children to focus on animals and plants of interest.

In the Search and Retrieve stage, students gather information from different texts and media to answer personal questions about survival of classes of animals. They then conduct an experiment on preferences for darkness among beetles. After demonstrating knowledge related to their personal questions, students are asked about similarities and differences in the animals in the field or experiment and the animals in the texts.

In the Comprehend and Integrate stage, students consolidate their knowledge by summarizing the gist of the information from their field experiences and the texts they have read. The final stage involves teaching an audience what they learned about woodland animals from their experiences and texts and writing a report about the content they learned from their experiences and texts.

CORI has been implemented at the elementary school level as well as with adolescents in middle and high schools (Guthrie et al., 2004; Guthrie, 2008). The approach is unique in the way it combines strategy instruction with practices of literacy engagement and emphasizes content of particular disciplines. Importantly, Guthrie and his colleagues have conducted a number of studies demonstrating the effectiveness of the program with readers of varying abilities and ethnic-racial groups (e.g., Guthrie et al., 2009).

Despite the promise of CORI, many barriers make it difficult to integrate disciplinary literacy instruction with more familiar strategy-based instructions. Two major obstacles are knowledge of the literacy skills that characterize different disciplines and the preparation of teachers capable of delivering needed instruction (Duncan, 2009; Shanahan & Shanahan, 2008). A third obstacle is that reading specialists may take issue with the view that disciplinary literacy should be a part of literacy instruction because it goes beyond basic reading skills (cf. Moje, 2008). I think it is difficult to talk meaningfully about improving adolescent literacy skills without recognizing the differences that exist in reading and understanding texts in history, science, literature, and math. These differences are briefly discussed in the following section.

DIFFERENTIATING DISCIPLINARY LITERACIES.   History educators believe that deep subject learning in historical studies requires students to think analytically and critically about the contexts in which texts or ideas were produced (Wineburg, 1991). Historians examine texts for attribution, asking questions like, "Who wrote the text" and "What was the writer's background and biases?" Their goal is to figure out what story a particular author wanted to tell; they are keenly aware that they are reading an interpretation of historical events and not "Truth" (Shanahan & Shanahan, 2008). Not surprisingly, high school students accept history textbooks without much critique, whereas historians rated them as less trustworthy than historical fiction (Wineburg, 1991).

Scientific literacy, in contrast to history, requires that students be able to predict, observe, analyze, and summarize (Lemke, 1990). Shanahan and Shanahan (2008) found that for chemists, the most important aspect of reading was relating text information to formulas, graphs, charts, or diagrams. Alternative representations of an idea were essential for full understanding of a concept.

The study of English literature requires interpreting figurative language and recognizing symbols, irony, and satire, as well as knowledge of social and historical contexts of the author (Lee, 2001). Deep reading of literature also involves the identification of literary devices that signal emotions, motives, and goals as well as how an author constructs a world that the reader simultaneously enters and stands apart from (Lee & Spratley, 2006).

In contrast to these other disciplines, writing and reading mathematical texts depend heavily on accuracy and precision (Bass, 2006). Even function words must be read carefully because "the" might have a very different meaning than "a." Math texts thus cannot be read for gist; math reading requires a precision of meaning because each word has a particular meaning (Shanahan & Shanahan, 2008).

To further differentiate disciplinary literacy, Shanahan and Shanahan (2008) asked experts about the specific literacy challenges in vocabulary, comprehension, fluency, and writing they felt that students experience when they read their disciplinary texts. For vocabulary, the mathematicians and chemists noted the challenge of words that had both general and specific meanings, with mathematicians feeling strongly that the precise mathematical definition needed to be learned to understand the mathematical meaning. For example, "prime" has a specific mathematical meaning and a general meaning, but the general meaning (i.e., perfect, chief, highest grade) aids in the understanding of the mathematical meaning. In contrast, historians made no mention of words with general and specific meanings. History does not have much of a technical vocabulary; technical terms were often borrowed from other fields. The level of difficulty of the general vocabulary could be quite high, however.

DISCIPLINARY LITERACY INSTRUCTION.   The differences Shanahan and Shanahan (2008) discovered in the texts of these different disciplines offer unique challenges for students and teachers who are unaware of these differences. Discipline-specific strategies were created by the experts and teachers during the second year of their study. Shanahan and Shanahan (2008) found, however, that the experts and high school teachers were less than enthusiastic in embracing strategy instruction because the instruction "seemed a little contrived" (p. 54). They may have been more successful if they had attempted to implement a version of CORI, which as discussed earlier, emphasizes engagement and content more than strategy instruction.

In her review of the literature on disciplinary teaching, Moje (2007) discussed the work of other content-area literacy researchers and the programs they have developed (e.g., Borasi & Siegel, 2000; Bulgren et al., 2007; Conley, 2008; Lee & Spratley, 2006). These researchers are less interested in generic comprehension strategies than in (1) specifying the reasoning and thinking skills members of a discipline use to comprehend or produce oral and written texts, and (2) determining the best way to teach these skills to students (Moje, 2007). Much of the work in this area has focused on history learning, beginning with Wineburg's (1991) study discussed in the previous section.

Moje (2007) also discussed a branch of disciplinary literacy that identifies the specific linguistic differences, not just in vocabulary as mentioned previously, but in grammatical and structural properties of texts. Schleppegrell and colleagues (Schleppegrell & Achugar, 2003; Schleppegrell, Achugar, & Oteiza, 2004), for example, have analyzed the grammar of history textbooks to help history teachers improve content learning. Teachers who helped students make sense of the specific grammatical abstractions in history texts reported increased critical reading and comprehension, but specific effects were not described. (Moje, 2007). Moje suggested that this functional linguistics approach should be used to analyze academic as well as everyday texts.

It should be clear that basic-level reading skills are not sufficient for the information-based technology and workplace demands of the 21st century. Students need to be able to access, interpret, critique, and produce oral and written texts on paper as well as electronic media. They also need to exhibit these skills in specific subject areas and disciplines. Programs like CORI will clearly help improve specific subject and content knowledge. Knowledge of disciplinary literacy practices also has the potential to have a significant impact on subject area instruction. Instruction will improve as researchers and teachers become more knowledgeable of the specific disciplinary literacy practices that have the most impact on learning and understanding.

Summary and Conclusions

This chapter began by noting the many challenges that confront educators and practitioners faced with helping struggling readers improve their understanding of texts. These challenges stem directly from the multifaceted nature of comprehension. As discussed in the first part of the chapter, comprehension is often quite variable because it is influenced by reader abilities, engagement, text and task factors, and the context in which the reading event is occurring. This means that comprehension abilities cannot be assessed with one measure. Assessments that reduce comprehension performance to one number or grade level are particularly problematic because they promote the view that comprehension is a stable and consistent ability. It is not. Even good students will show differences in comprehension performance, depending on subject content and the nature of texts. Poor readers will perform less well overall, but will still show relative strengths with certain subject areas and texts.

The multifaceted nature of comprehension means that every measure of comprehension will have its strengths and limitations. Some measures may provide good indications of vocabulary and sentence-level language abilities, but provide little information about text-level processing. Others may provide useful information about inferencing abilities and constructing beyond text meanings, but provide no information about language abilities. Some measures may indicate how well students can construct literal meanings, but no information about students' ability to construct deeper meanings. Other measures may assess how well students can relate text information to previously stored knowledge. Knowledgeable teachers and practitioners will know the strengths and limitations of different comprehension assessments and use these assessments to provide information about a student's strengths and weaknesses as well as the specific factors that contribute to these comprehension strengths and weaknesses.

The many factors that affect comprehension (i.e., reader abilities, engagement, and text and task factors) make it difficult to decide what to target in instruction or intervention. For young children, the emphasis needs to be on building vocabulary and background knowledge while they are developing their decoding skills. As children get older, they will still need instruction on vocabulary and background knowledge, but will also need more explicit instruction in how texts are constructed and how language cues signal meaning at sentential and discourse levels (Snow, 2010). Middle and high school students will benefit from explicit instruction in the literacy skills required by different disciplines.

The focus of instruction should always be on meaning construction. Too much focus on strategy use sometimes takes the focus away from meaning construction. Strategy use should always be taught as a way to facilitate meaning construction. For example, when reading texts, students should be taught to ask beyond-text questions that address author's intent (QtA) and help them relate the text to personal experiences and background knowledge (Barr et al., 2002; Beck & McKeown, 2002). By en-

couraging personal responses to texts, teachers and practitioners will be providing the skills students need to construct literal, critical, and creative interpretations of subject and disciplinary texts.

In conclusion, reading comprehension is clearly a complex topic. The importance of high-quality teachers and a good classroom environment cannot be overemphasized. A recent study found that increasing class quality by one standard deviation for one year raised earnings by $1,520 (9.6%) at age 27 (Chetty et al., 2010). This translates into a lifetime earnings gain of approximately $39,100 for the average individual. For a classroom of 20 students, this is a benefit of $782,000. The two factors that contributed most to class quality were good teachers and class size. Improved classroom environments also lead to other gains such as better health, better peers, and less crime. A good reading specialist and classroom environment will presumably lead to even greater financial, social, and health gains for struggling readers. Excellent teachers and practitioners know that there is no simple prescription for improving understanding and interpretations of subject and disciplinary texts. They also know that their knowledge about what they are teaching is one of the most important factors for successful instruction and intervention. This is why you are reading this chapter and this book. So take a little break, stretch your legs, have a cup of coffee, and get back to it. There are four chapters left.

References

Adler, M., & Van Doren, C. (1972). *How to read a book.* New York: Simon & Schuster.

Armbruster, B., Lehr, F., & Osborn, J. (2001). *Put reading first: The research building blocks for teaching children to read.* Washington, DC: Partnership for Reading.

Barr, R., Blachowicz, C., Katz, C., & Kaufman, B. (2002). *Reading diagnosis for teachers: An instructional approach* (4th ed.). Boston: Allyn & Bacon.

Bass, H. (2006). *What is the role of oral and written language in knowledge generation in mathematics? Toward the improvement of secondary school teaching and learning. Integrating language, literacy, and subject matter.* Ann Arbor: University of Michigan Press.

Beck, I. L., & McKeown, M. G. (2002). Questioning the author: Making sense of social studies. *Educational Leadership, 60,* 44–47.

Beck, I. L., McKeown, M. G., Sandora, C., Kucan, L., & Worthy, J. (1996). Questioning the author: A yearlong classroom implementation to engage students with text. *Elementary School Journal, 96,* 385–414.

Borasi, R., & Siegel, M. (2000). *Reading counts: Expanding the role of reading in mathematics classrooms.* New York: Teachers College Press.

Bulgren, J., Deshler, D. D., & Lenz, B. K. (2007). Engaging adolescents with LD in higher order thinking about history concepts using integrated content enhancement routines. *Journal of Learning Disabilities,* *40,* 121–133.

Bursuck, W., & Damer, M. (2007). *Reading instruction for students who are at risk or have disabilities.* Boston: Allyn & Bacon.

Catts, H. W. (2009). The narrow view of reading promotes a broad view of comprehension. *Language, Speech, and Hearing Services in the Schools, 40,* 178–183.

Chetty, R., Friedman, J., Hilger, N., Saez, E., Schanzenbach, D., & Yagan, D. (2010). *How does your kindergarten experience affect your earnings? Evidence from project Star.* Cambridge, MA: Harvard Working Paper.

Clark, M. K., & Kamhi, A. (2008, November). *The validity of prior knowledge assessment in the QRI-4: Influence of gender, interest, and prior knowledge on reading comprehension.* Poster session presented at the American Speech-Language-Hearing Association Annual Convention, Chicago, IL.

Clark, M. K., & Kamhi, A. (2009, June). *The influence of prior knowledge on reading comprehension.* Poster session presented at the 16th Annual Meeting of the Society for the Scientific Study of Reading, Boston, MA.

Conley, M. (2008). *Content area literacy: Learners in context.* Boston: Allyn & Bacon.

Cutting, L. E., & Scarborough, H. S. (2006). Prediction of reading comprehension: Relative contributions of word recognition, language proficiency, and other cognitive skills can depend on how comprehension is measured. *Scientific Studies of Reading, 10,* 277–299.

Duffy, G. (2003). *Explaining reading: A resource for teaching concepts, skills, and strategies.* New York: Guilford.

Dunston, P. (2002). Instructional components for promoting thoughtful literacy learning. In C. Block & M. Pressley (Eds.), *Comprehension instruction research-based best practice* (pp. 135–151). New York: Guilford.

Duncan, A. (2009, October). *Teacher preparation: Reforming the uncertain profession.* Presentation at Teacher's College, Columbia University.

Francis, D., Fletcher, J., Catts, H., & Tomblin, B. (2005). Dimensions affecting the assessment of reading comprehension. In S. Paris & S. Stahl (Eds.), *Children's reading comprehension and assessment* (pp. 369–394). Mahwah, NJ: Erlbaum.

Friend, M., & Bursuck, W. (2006). *Including students with special needs: A practical guide for classroom teachers.* Boston: Allyn & Bacon.

Geiser, S. (2008). *Back to the basics: In defense of achievement (and achievement tests) in college admissions.* Berkeley, CA: University of California Center for Studies in Higher Education.

Gough, P. B., & Tunmer, W. E., (1986). Decoding, reading, and reading disability. *Remedial and Special Education, 7,* 6–10.

Graesser, A. C., Singer, M., & Trabasso, T. (1994). Constructing inferences during narrative text comprehension. *Psychological Review, 101,* 371–395.

Grigg, W., Donahue, P., & Dion, G. (2007). *The nation's report card: 12th-grade reading and mathematics 2005* (NCES 2007–468). Washington, DC: U.S. Department of Education, National Center for Education Statistics.

Guszak, F. J. (1967). Teacher questioning and reading. *The Reading Teacher, 21,* 227–234.

Guthrie, J. T. (2003). Concept-oriented reading instruction: Practices of teaching reading for understanding. In A. P. Sweet & C. E. Snow (Eds.), *Rethinking reading comprehension* (pp. 115–140). New York: Guilford.

Guthrie, J. T. (Ed.). (2008). *Engaging adolescents in reading.* Thousand Oaks, CA: Corwin.

Guthrie, J. T., McRae, A., Coddington, C. S., Klauda, S. L., Wigfield, A., & Barbosa, P. (2009). Impacts of comprehensive reading instruction on diverse outcomes of low-achieving and high-achieving readers. *Journal of Learning Disabilities, 42,* 195–214.

Guthrie, J. T., Wigfield, A., & Perencevich, K. C. (Eds.). (2004). *Motivating reading comprehension: Concept-oriented reading instruction.* Mahwah, NJ: Erlbaum.

Hirsch, E. D., Jr. (1996). *The schools we need & why we don't have them.* New York: Doubleday.

Hirsch, E. D., Jr. (2006). *The knowledge deficit: Closing the shocking education gap for American children.* New York: Houghton Mifflin.

Kamhi, A. (1997). Three perspectives on comprehension: Implications for assessing and treating comprehension problems. *Topics in Language Disorders, 17,* 62–75.

Karolides, N. J. (Ed.). (1997). *Reader response in the elementary classroom: Quest and discovery.* Mahwah, NJ: Erlbaum.

Keenan, J. M., Betjemann, R. S., & Olson, R. K. (2008). Reading comprehension tests vary in the skills they assess: Differential dependence on decoding and oral comprehension. *Scientific Studies of Reading, 12,* 281–300.

Kintsch, W. (1998). *Comprehension: A paradigm for cognition.* New York: Cambridge University Press.

Laing, S., & Kamhi, A. (2002). The use of think-aloud protocols to compare inferencing abilities in average and below-average readers. *Journal of Learning Disabilities, 35,* 436–438.

Lee, C. D. (2001). Is October Brown Chinese? A cultural modeling activity system for underachieving students. *American Educational Research Journal, 38,* 97–141.

Lee, C. D., & Spratley, A. (2006). *Reading in the disciplines and the challenges of adolescent literacy.* New York: Carnegie Corporation.

Lemke, J. L. (1990). *Talking science: Language, learning, and values.* Norwood, NJ: Ablex.

Magliano, J. P., Trabasso, T., & Graesser, A. C. (1999). Strategic processing during comprehension. *Journal of Educational Psychology, 91,* 615–629.

McNamara, D. S. (Ed.). (2007). *Reading comprehension strategies: Theory, interventions, and technologies.* Mahwah, NJ: Erlbaum.

Moje, E. B. (2007). Developing socially just subject-matter instruction: A review of the literature on disciplinary literacy teaching. *Review of Research in Education, 31,* 1–44.

Moje, E. B. (2008). Foregrounding the disciplines in secondary literacy teaching and learning: A call for change. *Journal of Adolescent & Adult Literacy, 52,* 96–107.

Moravcsik, J. E., & Kintsch, W. (1993). Writing quality, reading skills, and domain knowledge as factors in text comprehension. *Canadian Journal of Experimental Psychology, 47,* 360–374.

National Institute of Child Health and Human Development (NICHD). (2000). *Report of the National Reading Panel. Teaching children to read: An evidence-based assessment of the scientific research literature on reading and its implications for reading instruction: Reports of the subgroups* (NIH Publication No. 00-4754). Washington, DC: U.S. Government Printing Office.

Oakhill, J. V., & Petrides, A. (2007). Sex differences in the effects of interest on boys' and girls' reading comprehension. *British Journal of Psychology, 98,* 223–235.

Palinscar, A. S., & Brown, A. L. (1984). Reciprocal teaching of comprehension fostering and comprehension-monitoring activities. *Cognition & Instruction, 1,* 117–175.

Pressley, M. (2002). Metacognition and self-regulated comprehension. In A. Farstrup & S. Samuels (Eds.), *What research has to say about reading instruction* (pp. 291–309). Newark, DE: International Reading Association.

Pressley, M., Graham, S., & Harris, K. (2006). The state of educational intervention research as viewed through the lens of literacy intervention. *British Journal of Educational Psychology, 76,* 1–19.

RAND Reading Study Group (RRSG). (2002). *Reading for understanding: Toward a research and development program in reading comprehension.* Santa Monica, CA: RAND. Retrieved July 2010, from http://www.rand.org/pubs/monograph_reports/MR1465/index.html

Raphael, T. (1986). Teaching question-answer relationships. *The Reading Teacher, 39,* 516–520.

Rapp, D. N., van den Broek, P., McMaster, K. L., Kendeou, P., & Espin, C. A. (2007). Higher-order comprehension processes in struggling readers: A perspective for research and intervention. *Scientific Studies of Reading, 11,* 289–312.

Recht, D. R., & Leslie, L. (1988). Effect of prior knowledge on good and poor readers' memory of text. *Journal of Educational Psychology, 80,* 16–20.

Richek, M., Caldwell, J., Jennings, J., & Lerner, J. (2002). *Reading problems: Assessment and teaching strategies* (4th ed.). Boston: Allyn & Bacon.

Ruddell, R. (2002). *Teaching children to read and write: Becoming an effective teacher* (3rd ed). Boston: Allyn & Bacon.

Sanders, N. M. (1966). *Classroom questions: What kinds?* New York: Harper & Row.

Schleppegrell, M. J., & Achugar, M. (2003). Learning language and learning history: A functional linguistics approach. *TESOL Journal, 12,* 21–27.

Schleppegrell, M. J., Achugar, M., & Oteíza, T. (2004). The grammar of history: Enhancing content-based instruction through a functional focus on language. *TESOL Quarterly, 38,* 67–93.

Shanahan, T., & Shanahan, C. (2008). Teaching disciplinary literacy to adolescents: Rethinking content-area literacy. *Harvard Educational Review, 78,* 40–59.

Snow, C. E. (2010). Reading comprehension: Reading for learning. In P. Peterson, E. Baker, & B. McGraw (Eds.). *International encyclopedia of education* (3rd ed., pp. 413–418). Oxford, UK: Elsevier.

Swanson, H. L. (1999). Reading research for students with LD: A meta-analysis of intervention outcomes. *Journal of Learning Disabilities, 32,* 504–532.

Torgesen, J. K. (2007). *Research related to strengthening instruction in reading comprehension.* Presented at Reading First Comprehension Conference. Retrieved from http://www.fcrr.org/science/sciencePresentations Torgesen.shtm

Trabasso, T., & Magliano, J. P. (1996). Conscious understanding during comprehension. *Discourse Processes, 22,* 255–287.

Vaughn, S., Gersten, R., & Chard, D. (2000). The underlying message in LD intervention research: Findings from research syntheses. *Exceptional Children, 67,* 99–114.

Willingham, D. T. (2006). How knowledge helps: It speeds and strengthens reading comprehension, learning—and thinking. *American Educator, 30,* 1–12.

Wineburg, S. S. (1991). On the reading of historical texts: Notes on the breach between school and the academy. *American Educational Research Journal, 28,* 495–519.

Yekovich, F. R., Walker, C. H., Ogle, L. T., & Thompson, M. A. (1990). The influence of domain knowledge on inferencing in low-aptitude individuals. *Psychology of Learning and Motivation, 25,* 259–278.

Chapter 7

Assessing and Remediating Text Comprehension Problems

Carol E. Westby

In a culture where written language is prominent and readily available, basic literacy is a natural extension of an individual's linguistic development.

—FILLION & BRAUSE, 1987, P. 216

The United Nations proclaimed 2003–2012 the Literacy Decade, with the subtheme "Literacy as Freedom," because in the 21st century, people cannot be truly free if they are not literate. In many parts of the world, large numbers of persons have not had opportunities to learn to read and write. In the United States, we anticipate that everyone, particularly children, have had opportunities to become literate. Although 99 percent of persons in the United States are considered literate, many are functionally illiterate. People who are functionally illiterate can decode print. They have some ability to read and write, but not enough to fully function in everyday life. They have difficulty with crucial tasks such as filling out job applications, reading maps, understanding bus schedules, or reading newspaper articles, and of course, they have difficulty with the literacy demands of middle school and beyond. Nationally, the functional illiteracy rate is 21 percent, but in some areas of the country as many as one-third of adults are functionally illiterate. Functionally illiterate adults comprise not only those who have language/learning impairments but also students who have inadequate teaching or who because of social/emotional, motivational, or family issues dropped out of school. Lack of functional literacy severely limits the job opportunities of adolescents and adults and results in many living in poverty.

In the last century, the definition of what it means to be literate has changed (Morris & Tchudi, 1996; Obanya, 2003). When the United States was colonized in the 17th through the 19th centuries, being literate for the majority of the population meant knowing one's letters—the ability to decode and encode, to say the words on a printed page, and to say what the words meant. This *basic literacy,* which involves *reading along the lines,* is what has been associated with the 3 Rs (reading, writing, and 'rithmatic). Such literacy has functioned as a memory support for list making, remembering religious texts, or transmitting simple directions on familiar topics. By the latter third of the 20th century, basic literacy was no longer sufficient in a technological, global economy. Persons needed to be able to *read between the lines* of what was written. They had to be able to move beyond literal meanings, to interpret texts, and to use writing not simply to record, but also to interpret, analyze, synthesize, and explain. This reading between the lines has been termed *critical literacy.* Even in early elementary school, students must be able to do more that retell the events of a story or the steps in an experiment. In literature, they must be able to determine story theme, interpret characters' motivations, and perceive interrelationships among themes, and in social studies and science, they must be able to predict and explain events. Even critical literacy, however, is not sufficient to meet the literacy demands of society in the 21st century. Not only must persons possess critical literacy, which involves reading between the lines, but they must also have *dynamic literacy*, which involves *reading across the lines*—that is, reading multiple texts, comparing and contrasting their content, and integrating their ideas—and *reading beyond the lines* by acting on the content gained from texts and interrelating the content for problem-raising and problem-solving matters.

Literacy has traditionally been defined as the ability to comprehend and produce printed texts. In the 21st century, literacy is not limited to printed texts; now it encompasses comprehension and production of a wide variety of communication modalities. Knowledge is encountered in multiple forms—in print, in images, in video, in combinations of forms in digital contexts— and persons must also be able to represent their knowledge in an equally complex manner. A group of scholars meeting in New London, New Hampshire, in 1994, coined the term *multiliteracies* (New London Group, 1996) to highlight the proliferation of multimodal ways of making meaning where the written word is part and parcel of visual, audio, and spatial patterns.

Today's students are surrounded by multimodal literacy. Even traditional print materials are incorporating multimedia. For example, *The Invention of Hugo Cabret* (Selznick, 2007), the winner of the 2008 Caldecott Award for picture books, is a 24-chapter, 526-page book, nearly 300 of which are pictures. The story is carried as much by the pictures as by the printed text. To interpret the pictures adequately, readers/viewers need to be able to interpret facial expressions to make inferences about characters' intentions and behavior, and they also need to be alert to how the artist uses perspectives, close-ups, and distant views to convey information. A Web site devoted to the book is found at www.theinventionofhugocabret.com. Links from the Web site take students to videos and old movie clips related to the story and to sites that sell model automatons (robots) to build. Students must be able to interpret the significance of the movements, visual effects, sound effects, and music in the videos. If they decide to purchase an automaton, they must evaluate the pictures and text descriptions provided to make their choice, and once they receive the automaton kit, they must be able to integrate the information in the printed text with the graphics to put it together. Many textbooks also now come with CDs/DVDs and referenced links to Web sites.

A great deal of attention has been devoted to literacy instruction during the first decade of the 21st century. Federal mandates under the No Child Left Behind Act (NCLB) required changes to the ways reading was taught. The *Report of the National Reading Panel* (National Institute of Child Health and Human Development, 2000) listed components that are essential for reading proficiency (phonemic awareness, phonics, fluency, vocabulary, and comprehension). To meet the literacy goals of NCLB, educators increased the frequency and intensity of teacher-directed activities, focusing particularly on phonological/phonemic awareness and fluency. Despite the emphasis placed on skill development in response to NCLB, a study reviewing the effects of Reading First (which funded literacy programs for children in kinder-garten through third grade in high-poverty schools), *Reading First Impact Study: Interim Report* (2008), indicated that the program did not increase the percentages of students in grades 1, 2, or 3 whose reading comprehension scores were at or above grade level. Grover Whitehurst, director of the Institute of Education Sciences, the Education Department's research arm, suggested that it was possible that "in implementing Reading First, there was a greater emphasis on decoding skills and not enough emphasis, or maybe not correctly structured emphasis, on reading comprehension" (Glod, 2008). Whitehurst further suggested that the program's approach might be effective in helping students learn building-block skills but that it did not take children far enough along to have a significant impact on comprehension. Although fluent decoding is a foundation for literacy, it is not sufficient to ensure comprehension. This chapter focuses on the cognitive and linguistic underpinnings for proficiency in multiliteracies and strategies for developing the language and schema knowledge essential for promoting comprehension and production of multiliteracies.

COGNITIVE AND LINGUISTIC UNDERPINNINGS FOR LITERACY

The relations between oral language and written language are fundamental and reciprocal; reading and writing are initially dependent on oral language and eventually extend oral language abilities (Flood & Lapp, 1987). Young children use their oral language skills to learn to read, whereas older children use their reading ability to further their language learning—they read to learn (Westby, 1985). Once children are able to decode and read words and simple sentences, their focus should shift from decoding, or learning to read, to comprehension, or reading to learn. To read to learn, students must learn how to learn from reading; they must learn how to use their language, cognitive abilities, and background knowledge to comprehend text so they can acquire new knowledge (Brown, 1982; Pearson & Fielding, 1991).

Reading to learn, or comprehending texts, requires understanding a literate language style, which involves comprehension of novel words and increasingly complex sentences; yet, more than comprehension of novel words and complex sentences is required for reading to learn. Readers must also possess and acquire ever-increasing knowledge of their physical and social world, and they must combine their linguistic knowledge with their world knowledge to create mental models or mental representations for the information encountered in the texts (Perfetti, 1997; Yuill & Oakhill, 1991). Readers must be able to recognize individual words, understand grammatical and semantic relations between words, and integrate ideas in the text and with past knowledge to make inferences to aid integration and fill in implicit information. The linguistic components of a text, the words and sentences, are the microstructures of a text, and the content information or content schemata and the overall organization of this content are the macrostructures of a text (the content schema macrostructure—the gist and theme of the text; and the text grammar macrostructure).

Linguistic Skills for Literacy

The academic language of schooling is not the conversational language of everyday communication. Academic language involves specialized sets of words, complex grammar, and organizational strategies that are used for higher-order thinking processes and to describe complex concepts and abstract relationships (Zwiers, 2008). Conversational language is used primarily to meet needs (requesting and commanding), to accomplish daily tasks, and to share personal information. In contrast, academic language is used to analyze, evaluate, synthesize, persuade, and explain. Students must discuss complex concepts such as relationships among characters in literature, causes and effects of major events in social studies, and geological forces that change the planet in science, and they must describe abstract relationships that cannot be pointed to or illustrated, such as, "Electromagnetic waves are waves that are capable of traveling through a vacuum, unlike mechanical waves, which require a medium to transport their energy."

Academic discourse is more lexicalized, that is, in each clause, it has more vocabulary words that carry the meaning of the text than oral, conversational language (Unsworth, 1999). Contrast the following two texts. The first is from a middle school student giving an oral book report; the second is from a high school science text. The first has a lexical density of 1.4 (number of words carrying meaning per clause). In the second, nearly all the words carry meaning.

> Like I *reckon //* he would have been really *nice //* but now that he's been to all the *towns* and *seen* like there's no *life* or anything *//* and he *comes* into the *valley* and *sees Ann* and *sees life //* and he just *wanted power* over her *//* because he's never had *power* or anything before.

> *Plant cells* are *shaped* like a *box* and *contain chlorophyll.//* The *chlorophyll* is a *green material.//* When the *chlorophyll* is *struck* by *sunlight*, it *makes food* for the *plant.//* The *plant cell consists* of a *cell wall, mitochondrion, and chloroplast.//* Animal cells are *rounded* and have a *fluid shape.//* An *animal cell consists* of a *nucleus, chromosomes, vacuole, cell membrane,* and *cytoplasm.*

> (http://www.macmillanmh.com/science/2005/student/summary.php?isbn=0022812148&id=702&level1=A&level2=1&level3=1)

Written texts also make use of nominalization, which is substitution of one grammatical class or one grammatical structure for another (frequently substituting nouns for verbs; Halliday & Martin, 1993). For example, "his documentation of the treachery" versus "he documented the treachery." Here the words (lexical items) are the same. What has changed is their place in the grammar. Nominalization is used extensively in social studies and science texts, particularly in defining technical terms, for example, "The process in green plants and certain other organisms by which carbohydrates are synthesized from carbon dioxide and water using light as an energy source is called photosynthesis." Here the technical term *photosynthesis* is a nominalized form referring to a series of events. Although the language used in social studies is usually not technical, it can be very abstract, such as "The *condemnation* of dissenting *perspectives* led to American *revolution.*" Nominalized concepts required an understanding of the events that underly the nominalized form. Science and social studies bundle together many events into abstract concepts such as convection currents, electromagnetic force, the American Revolution, and the civil rights movement. Each of these concepts requires understanding of a sequence of other events.

Academic discourse also makes use of more complex syntactic patterns than conversational discourse. It employs more passive voice, particularly in math and science, for example, "The radius *is* then *plugged* into the formula for the area of the circle." It makes greater use of all types of dependent clauses. The variety of adverbial clauses increases as students develop understanding of more complex connectives. Adverbial clauses with *when, while, so,* and *because* develop early; clauses with *if–then, although,* and *unless* develop later (Owens, 2007). Adjectival and noun clauses increase throughout the school years (Nippold, Hesketh, Duthie, & Mansfield,

2005). Dependent clauses are used increasingly in academic texts from the middle elementary school years such as,

- Adverbial: *Although several precautions were taken*, the key was lost.
- Adjectival (relative): The colonists, *who felt they did not have representation*, dumped the tea into Boston Harbor.
- Noun: *Where the rebels were going* was unknown.

And as students advance in school, they encounter texts with multiple dependent clauses, even in literature, for example,

> Gravel crackled beneath their feet as Snape and Yaxley sped toward the front door, which swung inward at their approach, though nobody had visibly opened it. (Rowling, 2007, p. 2)

This sentence has one independent clause, two dependent adverbial clauses, and one dependent adjective clause.

Cognitive Understanding for Text Comprehension

If students recognize the vocabulary words and understand the syntax used to present the facts in a text, they can comprehend the individual pieces of information. To gain meaning from the overall text, however, a student must have a content schema (a mental model for the facts presented in the text) and a text schema (superordinate organization for the presentation of the content information). One can have a content schema for the social structure of ant or bee colonies, the metamorphosis process of caterpillars and tadpoles, or the activities at a birthday party. This content information may be organized into various text structures, such as descriptions, stories, or explanations. The speed of reading and comprehension of a text becomes easier when the reader possesses intuitive knowledge of the text content schema and grammar structure of a text (Kieras, 1985).

The role of schemata in text comprehension has been extensively studied (Anderson, 1994; Bartlett, 1932; Bransford, 1994; Kintsch, 1998; Rumelhart, 1980; Stein & Glenn, 1979; Van Dijk & Kintsch, 1983). Schemata are hierarchically organized sets of facts or information describing generalized knowledge about a text, an event, a scene, an object, or classes of objects (Mandler, 1984). (Note: Some authors use the term *script* to refer to an event schema—the stereotypical knowledge structures that people have for common routines such as going to a restaurant, taking a subway, or going to a party [Beaugrande, 1980; Bower, Black, & Turner, 1979; Nelson, 1985; Schank & Abelson, 1977]. A script can be viewed as a specific type of schema.) Our schema knowledge enables us to behave appropriately in familiar situations, and when our schema information is applied to discourse (oral or written), it enables us to make the *inferences* necessary to comprehend the text—it enables us to read between the lines. If you have an elaborated schema or script for restaurants and you read the sentence, "John was hungry. He looked in the Yellow Pages," you know that John may be intending to call a restaurant for reservations or to order a pizza—you also know that he is not intending to eat the Yellow Pages. The ability to draw inferences is essential for critical and dynamic literacy. Although children who are poor comprehenders (despite adequate decoding skills) are less able than good readers to answer all types of questions about texts, they exhibit particular difficulty answering questions that require them to draw inferences (Oakhill & Yuill, 1996). In fact, when both good and poor comprehenders were able to refer to the text to answer questions, there was no difference between the good and poor comprehenders on literal questions. The availability of the text made little difference in the poor comprehenders' ability to answer the inferential questions. This deficit in inferencing may be related to lack of relevant schema knowledge, to difficulty in accessing relevant schema knowledge and integrating it with the text because of processing limitations, or because they may be unaware that inferences are necessary.

Activation of background schema knowledge is a fundamental aspect of comprehension. Comprehension and production of the discourse or texts require the ability to make a variety of inferences (Snow, 2002) that involve an understanding of the physical and psychological temporal and cause–effect relations between people, objects, and events (Cain & Oakhill, 2007; Tapiero, 2007). Readers rely on their schema knowledge when making inferences from texts. The ability to make inferences is essential for critical and dynamic literacy. Following is one classification for the types of inferences that are required for comprehension:

- *Anaphoric reference:* A pronoun or noun phrase that refers to a previous text entity, such as, "The wolf stopped Little Red Riding Hood in the forest. *He* asked *her* where *she* was going."
- *Bridging/relational inference:* Requires readers to integrate semantically or conceptually related information across sentences, for example, "Morgan sat at the kitchen table doing addition problems. She could hear the TV. It was her favorite show. Morgan sighed and got to work." Readers must deduce here that Morgan was doing her homework, the TV was not in the kitchen, and Morgan wanted to watch her favorite TV show.
- *Explanation-based/causal inference:* Requires readers to infer the antecedent or consequences of an action, for example, inferring that Martin Luther King held his march in Washington, DC, because he wanted to have laws changed, and Washington was where the laws of the country were written.
- *Predictive:* Forecasts what events will unfold, for example, predicting that pigs in stories will get away from wolves or predicting what people will do when they hear a violent storm is coming.
- *Goal inference:* Infers intentions of an agent, for example, wolves and foxes in stories generally want to eat pigs, ducks, and geese; in *The Wolf's Chicken Stew* (Kasza, 1987), the wolf is bringing food to the baby chickens because he wants to fatten them up to eat them.
- *Elaborative inference:* Considers properties and associations that cannot be explained by causal relationships, for example, a straw house will not be very strong—it would not survive a windstorm; a brick house would be sturdier and could not be destroyed easily.

The types of inferences necessary for comprehending academic texts are not unique to academic texts; similar inferences are needed in many social interactions. Students must be able to recognize emotional cues of persons in their environments. They must be able to interpret these cues correctly-understanding what triggered the emotions, and predicting what might result from the emotions (Ford & Milosky, 2003). In fact, much of the knowledge required for text inferencing likely develops first in social interactions. When making inferences in both social and academic contexts, persons make connections between something that is observable and something that is not. In doing so, they must make a distinction between what occurs in the real world (the observation) and what occurs in one's mind. To make appropriate inferences, persons must have a theory of mind (ToM), which is defined as being able to infer the full range of mental states (beliefs, desires, intentions, imagination, emotions, etc.) that cause action. A theory of mind involves an interpersonal component, which is the ability to reflect on the contents of the minds of others, and an intrapersonal component, which is the ability to reflect on one's own mind (Lucariello, 2004). Employing the interpersonal component of ToM enables readers to make inferences about characters in stories or persons in history. When employing intrapersonal ToM, readers note what they know and do not know, and they make decisions and plans regarding their learning and goals.

Narrative content can be described in terms of *landscape of action* and *landscape of consciousness* (Bruner, 1986). In narratives with primarily a landscape of action, temporally patterned sequences of actions are reported in the third person with minimal information about the psychological states of characters. In narratives with primarily a landscape of consciousness, the story is told from the perspectives of the various characters. A landscape of consciousness represents a linguistic coding of ToM. Most stories have aspects of both a landscape of action and a landscape of consciousness; however, some focus on one landscape more than another. Folktales and stories told by young children generally are primarily landscapes of actions. As children mature, they include more aspects of the landscape of consciousness in their stories, and comprehension of stories beyond the third-grade level becomes increasingly dependent on an understanding of a landscape of consciousness. The following excerpt from *The Bunyans* (Wood, 1996) is an example of writing characteristic of the landscape of action:

> One summer, Little Jean and Teeny wanted to go to the beach. Ma Bunyan told them to follow a river to the ocean. But all the rivers flowed west back then, so they missed the Atlantic Ocean and ended up on the other side of the country instead.
>
> Ma Bunyan tracked them out to the Pacific Ocean, where she found Teeny riding on the backs of two blue whales and Little Jean carving out fifty zigzag miles of the California coast.
>
> When Ma Bunyan saw what her son had done, she exclaimed, "What's the big idea, sir?" From that time on, the scenic area was known as Big Sur.

In contrast, a great deal of the story Too Many Tamales (Soto, 1993) has a landscape of consciousness. Maria fears that she has lost her mother's ring:

> Maria didn't dare look into Teresa's mouth. She wanted to throw herself on the floor and cry. The ring was now in her cousin's throat, or worse, his belly. How in the world could she tell her mother?
>
> But I have to, she thought. She could feel tears pressing to get out as she walked into the living room where the grownups were chatting.

Interpretation of a landscape of action requires only the use of familiar cognitive processes to explain the physical world (e.g., balls break windows, hurricane winds generate high tides, dogs chase cats). Interpretation of landscape of consciousness requires understanding of human intentionality and how humans (or animals with human characteristics) deal with the vicissitudes of life (Feldman, Bruner, Renderer, & Spitzer, 1990). This requires that readers have a ToM, that is, an awareness that mind exists apart from the physical world and what the mind does. In addition, interpretation of the landscape of consciousness aspects of narratives requires interpretation of two types of linguistic phenomena: (1) mental state terms such as *remember, forget, hypothesize, think, believe*, and (2) tropes, which are figures of speech such as metaphor, irony, metonym (a word used to evoke an idea through association, e.g., "He gave up the **sword**." is used to convey the idea that he left the military).

Texts are not created equal. Bruner (1985) suggested that there are two general types of cognitive functioning—narrative and paradigmatic, or logical-scientific. These modes of thought are reflected in narrative and a variety of expository texts. These texts represent different ways of knowing. Consequently, they differ in their content and overall organization or text grammar structures. Table 7.1 summarizes the differences between narrative and expository texts. Narrative texts are generally described in terms of causal event chains or story grammars.

TABLE 7.1	Comparison of Narrative and Expository Texts

Text Differences	
Narrative	**Expository**
Purpose to entertain	Purpose to inform
Familiar schema content	Unfamiliar schema content
Consistent text structure; all narratives have same basic organization	Variable text structures; different genres have different structures
Focus on character motivations, intentions, goals	Focus on factual information and abstract ideas
Often require multiple perspective taking—understanding points of view of different characters	Expected to take the perspective of the writer of the text
Can use pragmatic inferences (i.e., inference from similar experiences)	Must use logical-deductive inferences based on information in texts
Connective words not critical—primarily *and, then, so*	Connective words critical—wide variety of connectives, e.g., *because, before, after, when, if-then, therefore*
Each text can stand alone	Expected to integrate information across texts
Comprehension is generally assessed informally in discussion	Comprehension often assessed in formal, structured tests
Can use top-down processing	Relies on bottom-up processing

Expository texts are generally described in terms of text functions/organization, such as description, procedural, comparison/contrast, description, problem/solution, and argumentation. Because of the differences that exist between narrative and expository texts, readers must use different strategies to comprehend the texts.

The structure and content of most stories in Western culture conform to a stereotypical pattern. They begin with a setting, followed by an event or perception (initiating event) to which a character reacts (emotionally, cognitively, and/or behaviorally). The initiating event motivates a character to establish a goal to cope with the event or perception. To achieve the goal, the character must implement a series of attempts that yield consequences or outcomes to which characters respond emotionally (e.g., relieved), cognitively (e.g., decided to forgive), and/or behaviorally (e.g., returned home). The reader uses knowledge of this pattern to make comprehension a very rapid and efficient process. It is not clear whether a story grammar is a macrostructure text grammar or a content schema (Mandler, 1982). Most stories follow content schemata that have to do with events and goal-directed activities of characters. The text grammars specify how to take these events and activities and generate stories. Although the order of characters' activities may be modified to produce different stories, there is a strong relationship between the order of the story events and the order in which the events appear in the story text. The story content schemata and story text grammars or macrostructures facilitate students' abilities to recognize the gists or themes of passages. The gist or theme of a text represents the overall coherent topic of the text and its essential points. The macrostructure also facilitates readers' abilities to keep the gist or theme in mind and to use this information to construct text coherence by relating each sentence to preceding and following sentences and to the overall theme or gist. Research has shown that readers make use of story grammar or schema knowledge in the comprehension of narrative texts (Pearson & Fielding, 1991). Research on narrative abilities has shown that students with reading disabilities are not as knowledgeable or efficient in using story content schemata and text grammars to tell, retell, or comprehend stories. Students with reading disabilities tell shorter, less complete, less organized stories; comprehend and remember less of stories; and make fewer inferences about stories (Feagans & Short, 1984; Graybeal, 1981; Hansen, 1978; Liles, 1985, 1987; Merritt & Liles, 1987; Roth & Spekman, 1986; Weaver & Dickinson, 1979; Williams, 1998).

Just as there are schemata for concepts that enable us to predict the specifics of content, there are also schemata for types of discourses or texts that enable us to predict the text genre and organization of information within the text. Each type of text has its own organization or macrostructure. When readers know the macrostructure of the text they are reading, they are better able to predict what will come next and comprehend the material (Chambliss, 1995; Horowitz, 1985a, b; Meyer, 1987; Scardamelia & Bereiter, 1984; Thorndyke, 1977). For narrative texts, the narrative content often determines the text structure. Although the structure of expository texts is not as predictable as narrative text grammars, expository texts still follow some text grammar rules that govern the placement and order of information within text. A number of expository text grammar structures have been proposed. Because the function and content of expository texts is so variable, unlike a story grammar, which can fit most content schemata, there must be different expository grammars for different types of texts. Common expository text grammars include structural organizations for comparison–contrast, problem–solution, cause–effect, temporal order, descriptive, and enumerative texts (Horowitz, 1985a, b; Meyer, 1987; Piccolo, 1987; Richgels, McGee, Lomax, & Sheard, 1987). The various expository text patterns are often signaled by headings, subheadings, and specific words (Finley & Seaton, 1987).

As students advance in school, they are exposed to more and more expository texts (Otto & White, 1982). In early grades, the focus is typically on narrative texts. Even the material presented in history and science lessons is often presented in a narrative mode. By junior high and high school levels, however, narrative material usually appears only in literature/language arts courses. The information in all other classes is presented in a variety of expository formats. Students experience more difficulty understanding expository passages than they do narrative passages (Dixon, 1979; Hall, Ribovich, & Ramig, 1979; Lapp & Flood, 1978; Saenz & Fuchs, 2002; Spiro & Taylor, 1987; Vacca, Vacca, & Grove, 1991). Compared to expository prose, narratives are read faster, are more absorbing, and are easier to comprehend and recall (Freedle & Hale, 1979; Graesser & Goodman, 1985). Minimal research has been done exploring learning disabled students' abilities with expository text. Considering the difficulties they experience with narrative text, however, one would expect similar and likely greater difficulties with comprehension of expository texts.

Expository text usually contains content that is novel to the reader; consequently, the reader cannot readily apply content schema knowledge to aid comprehension (Kieras, 1985; Spiro & Taylor, 1987). Therefore, unlike comprehending narrative text, comprehending expository text is not primarily a matter of matching the content to a previously known pattern, but rather involves dealing with the passage content at the level of individual facts. Once readers have processed the individual facts, they may organize them into schemata. Even if a content schema is available to the reader, this schema provides no strong expectations about the text grammar form of the material. For example, no textual rules state in what order one must describe the facts about ant and bee colonies. This relative independence of content facts, content schemata, and text grammars marks a major difference between expository prose and stories. Because the content schema and text grammar are generally not available to the student prior to the first reading of an expository text, processing of expository texts is much more a bottom-up process than the top-down processing used in comprehending narrative texts, where the content schema and text grammar guide the reader's comprehension (Meyer & Rice, 1984). Bottom-up processing puts more of a load on the memory and integrative processes of readers because they must hold facts in memory, organize the facts into content schema, and attempt to search for a text structure that may facilitate their processing of the content schema (Beaugrande, 1984; Britton, Glynn, & Smith, 1985). Comprehending expository texts requires that readers use the individual facts of the text to construct a content schema, a text grammar or macrostructure, and the coherence relations among the sentences of the text.

Narrative and expository prose differ in the types of ideas and connections represented, and consequently, these two types of texts require different kinds of knowledge on the part of readers. Narrative texts unfold primarily in terms of goals and the reasons for these goals, whereas expository texts have more physical state ideas linked by consequences, property, and support relationships (Black, 1985; Graesser & Goodman, 1985). To understand texts, one must understand the content ideas and relationships among the content ideas that underlie the text. For narrative texts, one must understand human motivations and goal-seeking behavior. For expository texts, one must comprehend a variety of logical relationships (Black, 1985; Bruce & Newman, 1978; Voss & Bisanz, 1985).

ASSESSING LANGUAGE AND COGNITIVE SKILLS FOR TEXT COMPREHENSION

The discussion in the first section of this chapter has summarized the language and cognitive skills that are essential for reading to learn—for comprehending text. They include a literate style of language and schema knowledge (including content schemata and text grammar schemata). This section will address assessment of each of those aspects of language and cognition essential for text comprehension.

Assessing Literate Language Style (Text Microstructures)

Literate language style involves more explicit language and more complex syntactic sentence structures than oral conversational speech (Horowitz & Samuels, 1987; Nippold et al., 2005; Scott, 1994). Although no specific linguistic analysis system is designed to identify a literate language style as opposed to an oral style, some systems capture components of a literate style. In addition, some specific aspects of language are associated with literate style that can be noted in a language sample.

Hunt's terminal-unit (T-unit) analysis has been a popular linguistic analysis system to code increasing syntactic development during the school years (Hunt, 1965). A *T-unit* is defined as a main clause plus any subordinate clauses or nonclausal structures that are attached to it. Subordinate clause structure is associated with a literate language style and has been shown to increase with a culture's exposure to literacy (Kalmar, 1985). One way that T-unit length increases through adolescence is through the use of subordinate clauses. Some data on mean length of T-unit for orally produced narrative and expository texts are available. Several narrative databases are available when using the Systematic Analysis of Language Transcripts (SALT) software to analyze language samples (Miller, 2010). The samples for the databases were collected in a variety of ways: telling stories from picture books or single pictures, retelling, or telling personal stories. Depending on the database, normative information is available on children from ages 4 to 13 years.

Nippold and colleagues (Nippold et al., 2005) have reported mean T-unit lengths for children ages 8, 11, 13, and 17 and adults 25 and 44 based on oral expository texts collected by asking persons to explain how to play their favorite game using the following protocol:

- What is your favorite game or sport?
- Why is that your favorite game?
- I'm not too familiar with that game, so I would like you to tell me all about it. For example, tell me what the goals are, and how many people may play a game. Also, tell me about the rules that players need to follow. Tell me everything you can think of about the game so that someone who has never played before will know how to play.
- Now I would like you to tell me what a player should do to win the game. In other words, what are some key strategies that every good player should know?

(Note: The SALT system is adding the expository data based on students explaining how to play a game. At this point the data includes only students in the age range of 12 years, 7 months to 15 years, 9 months.)

A T-unit analysis accompanied by noting the following aspects of language occurring in each T-unit provides some sense of the degree to which a student is using a literate language style. The following sentences were written as parts of stories generated by students in response to a wordless video, *Baby Bird*, a video in the Max the Mouse series (available from www.store.discoveryeducation.com):

1. Types of subordinate clauses, for example,
   Dependent clauses that work as adverbs:
   While Max went to the store, the bird ate all the food in the house.
   Max fed the bird *until he had no food left.*
   After the bird was full grown, it took off with Max's house.
   Although Max fed the bird a lot of food, the bird was still crying.
   Max kept feeding the bird *because he wanted it to be quiet.*
   The bird took off into the sky *as Max stepped onto his porch.*
      Dependent clauses that work as adjectives:
   The yellow bird *that had eaten all of Max's food* flew off with the house.
   Once there as a mouse named Max *who found a little yellow bird.*
   The bird flew to Mexico *where Max got a job making sombreros.*
      Dependent clauses that work as nouns:
   Max explained to his girlfriend Maxine *how the bird had eaten all his food.*
   Max's friends didn't know *what happened to him.*
      In addition to noting the types of dependent clauses, one should also consider clausal density, which is the average number of clauses per T-unit. Increases in clausal density reflect gains in the use of all types of subordinate clauses.
2. Connectives: *And, then,* and *and then* are not included in the tally because it cannot be determined if they are being used in their logical sense or only to keep the conversation going. Literate connectives coded include, but are not limited to, *when, since, before, after, while, because, so, as a result, if, until, but, therefore, however, although, unless.*

3. Elaboration of noun phrases:
   Modifiers: Note the words in the noun phrase immediately preceding the head noun (e.g., The *two, expensive, big, white* cockatoos).
   Qualifiers: Note the words that follow the noun (e.g., The big white cockatoos *in the pet store window*).

   Eisenberg and colleagues (Eisenberg et al., 2008) reported that in a study of noun phrase use in oral narratives, by age 5 all children produced simple designating noun phrases (*this boy, his shoe*). By age 8 all children produced simple noun phrases with adjectives (*the little boy, the kitchen counter*). And by age 11 all children produced complex noun phrases with noun postmodification such as prepositional phrases (*face like aliens*) or clauses (*a dog that had fur*).

4. Mental/linguistic verbs: These are verbs that denote cognitive processes (e.g., *think, know, forget, remember, consider, hypothesize*) and linguistic processes (e.g., *say, report, promise*). Verb tenses other than present and present progressive.

5. Adverbs: Adverbs often code aspects of tone, attitude, and manner that in oral language would be coded through stress and intonation. Cook-Gumperz and Gumperz (1981) noted that adverbs provide information about the necessary tone of voice to use when reading (*angrily, hotly, ominously*), and that children will recycle passages in which their previous reading intonation did not agree with the adverb.

6. Emotional words: Although not specifically associated with a literate language style, it is useful to note the use of emotional words because they reflect an awareness of landscape of consciousness.

Assessing Knowledge of Narrative Content Schemata and Text Grammar Schemata (Text Macrostructures)

Two general questions need to be asked with respect to students' schema knowledge in relation to reading. First, do the students have the necessary schemata, and can they retrieve the relevant schema information in response to visual and language cues so they can recognize or interpret the situation or comprehend the text or discourse? Second, can the students retrieve and organize schema information to initiate and carry out a task when little or no contextualized information is provided? In a sense, these two questions represent aspects of receptive and expressive schema knowledge and use.

One can evaluate students' schema knowledge for a particular situation or concept and for a particular text genre. Evaluation of students' schemata crosses both knowledge of world events and situations and knowledge of the structure of stories and other texts. As children develop, they acquire increasing understanding of their physical and social world. This knowledge is first coded in narrative texts and later in exposition and other genres. As their knowledge and understanding of the world increase and change, the structure of their narrative texts changes to reflect the changing construct of their thought. Children first read to learn through narrative, and research suggests that children learn more readily through narrative than through expository text (Freedle & Hale, 1979).

Traditionally, two approaches have been used to assess children's schema knowledge: (1) comprehension-based measures (e.g., asking questions about settings, characters, events) and (2) productive measures that require students to generate a story. Comprehension-based measures tend to tap students' schema understanding, whereas productive measures tend to tap students' ability to use schema knowledge to produce a text. In the literature, all productive measures have tended to be grouped together, whether the student is retelling a story, developing an original story with no stimulus provided, or describing the story in a wordless picture book. These do not, however, place the same demands on the storyteller. Telling a story from a wordless picture book requires only that a student recognize the story content schema. It does not require that the student generate story content schema and organize it into a text grammar structure. The pictures in the book lay out the story, and if students do little more than describe the pictures, their "story" contains the story grammar elements. For this reason, stories students tell when they are provided with highly structured stimuli (wordless picture books or films) are more similar to the comprehension-based measures because they focus on students' understanding or comprehension of content schema, but not on students' abilities to use story grammars. In this chapter, the schemata assessment section has been divided into (1) assessment of recognition/comprehension of content schemata and (2) assessment of ability to organize content schema and text grammar in stories and expository texts.

What conceptual knowledge is needed for a student's understanding and production of narratives? A narrative relates a time-ordered sequence of events that are interrelated in some way. The speaker/listener must, therefore, have an understanding of temporal relationships and two types of cause–effect relationships: physical and psychological. Physical cause–effect relationships obey the laws of the physical world (e.g., heavy rains cause floods or a dropped glass breaks). Psychological cause–effect relationships are the result of motivations or intentions of characters within the narrative. Behavior that is motivated or intentional is planned behavior. Understanding of planning or intentional behavior is essential for understanding story narratives because stories relate characters' plans to reach goals (Bruce, 1980; Wilensky, 1978). Recognition of the plans of characters in narratives requires (1) knowledge that people plan, (2) perspective taking (knowing what others are seeing), (3) person perception (knowing traits or attributes of others), and (4) role taking (knowing intentions, thoughts, and feelings of others).

Narratives also require that the story producer and receiver deal conjunctively with what happened in the action of the story and what the protagonists were thinking or saying. Preschool children begin to deal conjunctively with action and thought in play scripts when they alternate between describing the ongoing action and attitudes of characters in the play, taking on the roles of characters in the actual play activity, and acting as a stage manager (Wolf & Hicks, 1989). The distinction between what is intended and what is actually done is a difficult one for young children, particularly when there is a disjunction between what is said and what is done (Bruner, 1985). Trickery tales—that is, tales of deceit—involve a disjunction between action and intention. Abrams and Sutton-Smith (1977) reported that children become fully able to comprehend trickster tales between 8 and 10 years of age. In addition to knowledge of temporal and cause–effect relationships, planning, and role taking, comprehension of trickster tales requires that the child (1) realize that deception can exist, (2) recognize that messages can be intentionally false and that the intention is more important than the content or consequence of the message, and (3) be able to detect deceit by noting visual and vocal cues that suggest the speaker's words are not truthful and that the speaker is attempting to mask his or her true intentions (DePaulo & Jordan, 1982).

Table 7.2 presents aspects of the development of narrative structure in the first column, the development of physical and social schema knowledge about the world that underlies the narrative structure in the second column, and a narrative example in the third column.

TABLE 7.2	Narrative Development	
Narrative Structure	**Narrative Content**	**Example Stories**
Preschool		
Description: Unconnected sentences; order not important	Labels/simple descriptions of objects, characters, surroundings, ongoing actions; no interrelationships among the elements mentioned	The coyote was hungry for sheep. He had his tongue out. He has sharp teeth. The sun was going down. The sheep was happy. The coyote was sitting on the hill. The sheep was talk till he say a coyote.
Action sequence: Series of actions, generally with a temporal sequence; centering may be present—story may have a central character or a central theme (actions that each character takes)	Characters engage in a series of actions that may be chronologically, but not causally, related; characters act independent of one another	There was a kid traveling and he went away and came to a river. And he started following the river. And there were two seals. And the seals were jumping up and down the water. And the seals went up the shore. And the boy got on the seals.
Reactive sequence: Cause–effect sequences of events; chaining of actions	Awareness of cause–effect relationships; set of actions that automatically cause other changes, but with no planning involved (e.g., a rock rolled down the mountain and people ran)	The coyote was chasing the sheep. And the sheep was scared. And the sheep was climbing up the hills. And the coyote was running after the sheep. He was getting hungry and hungry. And the sheep was running and running cause the coyote keeps running after the sheep.
Early Elementary		
Abbreviated episode: Centering and chaining present; stories have at least an initiating event (problem), response (character's reaction to problem), and consequence	Stories with goals or intentions of characters, but planning must be inferred; awareness of psychological causality for primary emotions (happy, mad, sad, surprised, disgusted, afraid); awareness of what causes emotions and what might be done in response to them; developing theory of mind (awareness that people think and feel, which allows for some perspective taking; scriptal knowledge of common characters (e.g., wolves are bad and eat pigs; princes are good and save princesses from dragons)	A UFO came from outer space. Then the UFO came upon a big house. There were some scientists working in a building next to the big house. The UFO wanted to study earth people. One of the scientists was taken by the UFO and put in a big locker. Then the UFO went back into the back hole and was never seen again.

TABLE 7.2 (Continued)		
Narrative Structure	**Narrative Content**	**Example Stories**
Complete episode: Centering and chaining present; story has an initiating event, internal response, plan, attempt (carrying out plan), and consequence	Stories with goals, intentions, and plans for reaching the goals; further development of psychological causality (secondary or cognitive emotions, e.g., jealousy, guilt, shame, embarrassment); further perspective taking—awareness of character attributes with story elements of setting and events that enable child to comprehend/predict novel behaviors of characters; understanding of longer time frames (days, weeks); meta-awareness of the need to plan; understanding of need to justify plans	For a whole month there has been a real big giant that has been throwing things in the houses, and smashing homes and getting people, and throwing them. But one day there was one man that wanted to solve the problem. So he got all the men. And they started up the mountain with torches to see what they can do about it. So they were about 10 feet from him. One of the men threw a torch at him and lit the giant on fire. And the giant fell down the mountain. And they never see him again.
Later Elementary		
Complex episodes: Like complete episode, but with obstacle(s) to goal and multiple attempts to reach goal	Increases in working memory permit more complex stories, including overcoming obstacles through more elaborated plans and multiple attempts to reach goals and ability to take perspective of more than one character; developing ability to perceive character growth (understanding that attributes change over course of story as result of events); ability to detect deception/trickery and to deceive and trick; awareness of time cycles (seasons, years); developing awareness of multiple meanings for words and literal versus figurative meanings	Once upon a time there was a village in the mountains. And there was a gorilla that escaped from the zoo. And they went hunting for it. And it was on top of a ledge. And they started chasing it with guns and with swords. It ran up the hill. And then it fell over the edge. And then the men tried to get it, but it jumped and it wrecked their house. And then they started chasing it up the mountain again. And he started to ski down cause he found a pair of skis at the top. And then the people got skis too. So they chased him on skis. And they chase him right to the zoo. And he got back. He got caught in the zoo again. And he was there again.
Multiple sequential episodes: More than one "chapter" chapters are arranged in chronological order; at least one episode should be at least complete	Sequence of episodes: ability to deal with extended periods of time and more complex planning	(Not included because of length)

(continued)

TABLE 7.2	(Continued)		
Narrative Structure	**Narrative Content**		**Example Stories**
Adolescent/Adult			
Interactive episodes: Two or more characters with interactive goals	Increase in working memory that permits holding of ideas from beginning of first episode while a second episode is introduced. Permits flashbacks and flash-forwards in stories that involve understanding of time and space and comprehension of allegory, which requires comprehension of multiple meanings.		An old man and an old lady lived on a ranch. There was nothing to do except watch the cows. The old man got bored. He decided to drive into town to find some excitement. The old man found some friends and he played cards with them. While he was gone, an oilman came to the ranch. The oilman asked the old lady if he could drill a well. His men worked real hard and dug a deep well. They hit oil and paid the old lady a lot of money. She used the money to build a new house. Late at night the old man came home. He had lost all his money in the card game. He wondered what his wife had done all day.
Embedded episodes: One narrative structure embedded within another. (An interactive episode may be embedded.)	Ability to engage in metanarrative discussion (i.e., discussion of narrative structure and interpretation of characterization, themes, and plots)		

Assessing Recognition/Comprehension of Content Schemata

Assessing schema recognition involves evaluation of students' understanding of the information listed in the middle column of Table 7.2. A relatively quick way to evaluate students' ability to recognize and comprehend schema knowledge is to have the children tell stories from wordless picture books or DVDs. Many of the wordless books by Mercer Mayer (such as *One Frog Too Many, Frog Goes to Dinner*, and *A Boy, a Dog, a Frog and a Friend*) are especially useful for this purpose. Each story has several characters. The characters encounter a number of situations that trigger feelings that in turn trigger planned actions of the characters. The artist vividly depicts the characters' emotional experiences. To understand the stories, students must recognize what the characters are doing on each page. They must realize the relationships between activities on any two adjacent pages, as well as the relationships among all the actions in the book. They must understand temporal sequence and physical and psychological cause–effect relationships and plans and reactions of characters.

The *Max the Mouse* wordless DVDs (available from www.store.discoveryeducation.com) are useful for obtaining oral and written stories. For students in third grade and above, one can obtain a written narrative from students using these short videos. Each of the Max stories is about 2 to 3 minutes long, and the majority of them have a complete single episode structure. Some of them include two characters with conflicting goals. These are several values in collecting written samples. It is easy to collect written samples from an entire class. The video can be shown in a language arts class, and all the students in the class can be asked to write the story about the video. Students who are frequently resistant to the idea of writing a story are often willing to write in response to a video. This provides the evaluator with a quick way of comparing a particular student's performance with the performance of the class in general. In addition, it provides a way to compare written and oral narrative schema recognition skills.

Evaluation of children's schema knowledge using wordless picture books and videos can be done in two ways: having children tell or write the story in the book or video or asking children comprehension questions about the book or video. When using a book, children are given the picture book and permitted to look through it and then tell the story that happened in the book as they go through the book page by page. The evaluator sits across from the child so that he or she cannot see the book and tells the child, "I can't see the book so make sure to tell the story so that I will understand it. Make it the kind of story we would read in a book." Because children suspect that the evaluator does know the story in the book, the use of a classroom peer as a listener is an even better strategy. To reduce memory load when telling the story from a video, the students watch the story through twice before telling or writing it. The following stories exemplify students' differing schema recognition/comprehension abilities. The first story was told by a fourth-grade boy with high-average reading ability:

> Jerry Bert smiled when he found out that he had a new present. He looked at the tag and then he said, "Look, my name's on this. I'll open it up. Oh my gosh, another frog." [The other] the other frog, named Sandy, frowned. [um,] Then what was his name, what was the boy's name? [Examiner: Jerry]. Jerry lifted the baby frog out of the box. His dog, his pet dog, Patty, looked at it. The other frog, Sandy, was very mad. He didn't want another frog in his life. Jerry Bert said, [um um,] "Sandy, meet my new frog. His name is Bert." Then all of a sudden, Sandy bit onto Bert's leg. Bert started crying and then, [um,] I keep forgetting, Jerry saved the little frog. He told Sandy not to ever do that again. And so they went for a little hike. They pretended they were all pirates and all part of a team. So they went down to a lake. Sandy frowned as she sat onto the turtle's back. [And] and Bert smiled. Sandy kicked Bert off. Bert started crying. Then Jerry said, "Sandy don't you dare do that again." Sandy was ashamed of herself. She didn't get to ride on the boat. They all got on the boat and went for a ride. Kerplunk. Sandy jumped onto the boat. Bert was a little scared when he saw this. Nobody else noticed. All of a sudden, Sandy kicked Bert off. Bert screamed as he flew off the boat. The turtle looked at Sandy as he was very mad. Suddenly, [um] suddenly the turtle told Jerry. Jerry was mad. And then Jerry was surprised. He looked at Sandy and he was very very sad. So they went off looking for him. They couldn't find him anywhere, so they decided to go home. Everybody was mad at Sandy. Sandy was ashamed of herself. Jerry went home and he was very sad. He lied down on his bed and started crying. All of a sudden he heard something going "whee" in the sky. He saw something coming. It was flying toward him out of the window. It came right in and landed right on Sandy's head. Then they became friends.

Even without seeing the book, this story provides sufficient information for the listener to determine the theme and major activities of the characters. The student infers that a box with a ribbon and a tag is a present, identifies the expression on the character' faces, gives reasons for feelings, and infers the consequences of feelings. In so doing, the student is exhibiting the ability to project into the roles of the characters.

Students with a less developed schema knowledge will tell the story as a series of actions. They may realize that the book is presenting a story about several characters, but they appear unaware of the interrelationships of activities from one page to the next, and they do not recognize goal-directed behavior of the characters. Their stories consist of descriptions of the drawings, but with minimal interpretation. The following is part of the story told by a second-grade boy with an attention deficit disorder and language delay:

> The boy has a present and he's opening it. And he's looking at the tag. And the dog's sitting down and the frog's sitting down. And now after he opens it, [he] he has something. [And the and the] and the frog has a frown because he thinks it doesn't look good, and the turtle is sad because he can't see it. And the dog is happy. And the frog is happy, and the boy is happy. And now the boy had a bad face. A bad face on his face cause the big frog is biting the little frog's leg. And the turtle's sad and the dog is sad. And the turtle is taking both frogs walking. And now the turtle is taking both frogs and the big frog kicks the little frog off. And now the big frog is all alone in the forest. And someone got buried. I wonder who it was. The big frog maybe. And now they're in the water and the big one is jumping on that. The turtle is sleeping and the dog is sleeping. . . .

In a second method for assessing narrative content understanding, the clinician asks questions that focus on a variety of schema relationships using guidelines for questions proposed by Tough (1981). This method is useful for younger children, for hesitant or shy children, and for children who have difficulty organizing extended verbal responses. The questions fall into four categories:

1. Reporting: What was the boy doing here? What happened here? Tell me about this picture.
2. Projecting: What is the boy saying to the big frog? What is the frog thinking? How does the boy feel?
3. Reasoning: Why is the frog thinking that? Why does the boy feel angry? Why did the big frog bite the little frog? Why did the tree fall down?
4. Predicting: What will happen next? What will the big frog do now?

Paris and Paris (2001) have used a similar procedure with several wordless picture books, including one of the Mercer Mayer frog books, with children in kindergarten through second grade. Children told the story in a book, then the evaluator returned to pages in the book and asked five explicit and five implicit questions. The following questions are generic and can be used with any wordless picture book. The explicit questions address primary story components; the implicit questions require inferencing. The following questions are based on *A Boy, A Dog, and A Frog* (Mayer, 2003), but are easily adapted for any wordless book.

Explicit Questions

1. (Book Closed, Characters): Who are the characters (people, animals) in this story?
2. (Book Closed, Setting): Where does this story happen (take place)?
3. (Initiating Event): Tell me what happens at this point in the story. Why is this an important part of the story?
4. (Problem): If you were telling someone this story, what would you say is going on now? Why did this happen?
5. (Outcome Resolution): What happened here? Why does this happen?

Implicit Questions

1. (Feelings): Tell me what the people/animals are feeling in this picture. Why do you think so?
2. (Causal inference): Why did the frog follow the footprints?
3. (Dialogue): What do you think the boy would be saying here? Why would he be saying that?

4. (Prediction): This is the last picture in the story. What do you think happens next? Why do you think so?

5. (Book Closed, Theme): In thinking about everything that you learned after looking at this story, if you had a friend who wanted to catch an animal for a pet (a frog, a wild kitty, a baby quail), what would you tell him/her so he/she wouldn't have the problems the boy in this story had?

Responses to each question are scored on a 0 to 2 point scale. For example, students are asked "How does the frog feel?" while looking at a picture from *A Boy, A Dog, and A Frog* of a frog sitting alone on a lily pad.

> 0 point: Fails to identify the point of the question or make an inference. "The frog's sitting in the water."

> 1 point: Picture level response. The answer is correct but is based on only a single page. "The frog's sad. See his face."

> 2 points: Narrative level responses. The answer takes into account the overall narrative; connects information across pages. "The frog's sad because the boy left, and now the frog's all alone."

The assessment is available online at http://www.ciera.org/library/reports/inquiry-3/3-012/3-012.pdf. Data is provided on kindergarten, first-, and second grade students on the explicit and implicit questions. The questions cannot be matched to the books Paris and Paris used, but you can develop your own assessment tool using the framework. In doing so, my colleagues and I have found that students we have used this with score similar to Paris and Paris's students.

For students in third grade and above, one should ask questions regarding how more than one character feels about a situation. Between ages 9 and 11 students are developing the ability to attend to what characters think, feel, and want, and they are developing the awareness that different characters have different viewpoints on the same situation (Emery, 1996). Understanding of characters' emotions, thoughts, and beliefs are the glue that ties the action of stories together; hence, understanding of these emotional and mental states is critical for the understanding of the landscape of consciousness aspects of stories. Students often exhibit difficulty comprehending the landscape of consciousness, particularly when the consciousness of more than one character must be tracked. Students tend to have difficulty making inferences about characters for the following reasons:

- They focus on what happened instead of why it happened.
- They misinterpret character feelings because they are considering only their own perspective—they think the characters are just like them.
- They focus on only one part of the story instead of the whole.
- They focus on the perspective of only one character.

For students with language and reading difficulties at third grade and above, it is important to explore students' abilities to interpret the landscape of consciousness that is essential for making character inferences. The evaluator can ask questions that require students to focus on the way of behavior, attending to more than one character. The evaluator can read a story, such as *The Talking Eggs* (San Souci, 1989), a southern (African-American or Cajun) version of the Cinderella tale, and ask questions as the story is being read. There are two sisters in the story— Rose, the older sister, who was cross, mean, and not very bright, and Blanche, the younger sister, who was sweet, kind, and sharp. Blanche is told to bring Rose a drink of water. When she gives it to Rose, Rose responds, "This water's so warm, it's near boilin'," shouted Rose, and she dumped the bucket out on the porch.

- Why did Rose act this way?
- What was Blanche thinking when this occurred?
- What did Blanche want at this point?
- How is Rose feeling now?

Blanche runs into the woods. An old woman finds her and takes Blanche to her cabin. "The old woman sat down near the fireplace and took off her head."

- How did Blanche feel?
- Is that the way you would have felt?
- In what way is Blanche different from you?
- Because Blanche is different from you in this way, how do you think she felt?

Blanche is given eggs that turn into treasures. She takes all the treasures home to her sister and mother. To understand what might happen next in the story, it is essential that students understand the evil nature of the mother and Rose. They must be aware that the mother and Rose are not totally happy with the events—they are jealous and greedy.

- How did the mother and Rose feel when Blanche brought all the treasures home? (If the student replies simply, "happy," pursue with additional questions.)
- What else might Rose and her mother want? Be thinking? Be feeling?

If the student doesn't provide further relevant information, say

- Think about what happened so far in the story that clues us in to other feelings the characters might be having.
- What about how they treated Blanche at the beginning of the story?
- What does that tell you about what they might be thinking now?

Informal reading inventories, such as the *Qualitative Reading Inventory-V* (QRI-V) (Leslie & Caldwell, 2011), provide another way to assess students' ability to make inferences. This instrument provides several narrative and expository passages at each grade level that a student can read or listen to. Students retell the passage and are asked both explicit (literal) and implicit (inferential) questions about the passages. The information students include in their retellings are checked off according to their role in the text macrostructure (e.g., setting, goal, events, and resolution for narratives and main ideas and details for expository texts). Dewitz and Dewitz (2003) suggested a strategy for analyzing the nature of students' error responses to the questions. The strategy is particularly useful in understanding how students attempt to interpret inferential questions. Errors can be coded as:

- Failure to link ideas across a passage, that is, failure to make relational inferences
- Failure to make causal inferences
- Failure to properly parse or interpret syntax
- Excessive elaboration or overreliance on prior knowledge
- Failure to know a key vocabulary word
- No response—did not answer

Table 7.3 shows an analysis of a fifth-grade boy's responses to questions about the fourth-grade Johnny Appleseed passage. Although the student easily decoded the text, he correctly answered only three of eight questions. He relied heavily on his prior knowledge, rather the information in the text, when answering the questions, and he made only one correct inference.

TABLE 7.3	Analysis of Responses to Questions

Question	Explicit/ Implicit	Correct/ Incorrect	Relational	Causal Prior	Causal Text	Faulty Elaboration	Syntax	Vocab	NR
What was John Chapman's main goal?	I	I	R*			X			
Why did John choose to apples to plant instead of some other fruit?	I	C	R*						
Where did John get most of his seeds?	E	I				X			
Why would John be able to get seeds from cider makers?	I	I		R*				X	
How do we know that John cared about planning apple trees?	I	I	R*			X			
How did John get to many places?	E	C							
Name one hardship John suffered?	E	I				X			
Why should we thank Johnny Appleseed?	E	C							

R* indicates the type of inference required for a correct answer

Assessing Ability to Organize Schema Content and Text Grammars

If students are unable to tell a story from a wordless picture book or respond appropriately to questions asked about story content schemata, they will not be able to produce a coherent story themselves when no stimuli or stimuli with limited structure are provided (e.g., a single picture). Many students, however, are able to recognize the schema information presented in wordless picture books and print, and they can comprehend questions asked about stories they have listened to or read, but are unable to retrieve and organize schema knowledge when there is minimal environmental support. Ability to generate organized schema knowledge can be assessed by having students tell stories when minimal contextual cues are available. Students can be asked to tell stories about poster pictures or book covers, or they can be given small figures and asked to make up a story about them. They can be asked to tell a story of a personal experience or to make up an imaginary story without any visual or toy supports. Producing stories of this type requires not only that the students have content schema knowledge of their physical and social world, but also that they also have text grammar schema knowledge for the structure of narratives.

Westby (1984) modified the Glenn and Stein system (1980) by including the information from Applebee (1978) and Botvin and Sutton-Smith (1977). This modified structural hierarchy is presented in the first column of Table 7.2. Analysis of narrative level can be done quickly by following the binary decision tree in Figure 7.1 (modified from Stein & Policastro, 1984). To use this binary decision tree, read through a child's story, then ask the following questions:

1. "Does the story have a temporally related sequence of events?" If it does not, then the story is an isolated description.
2. If the story does have a temporally related sequence of events, then ask, "Does the story have a causally related sequence of events?" If it has a temporally related sequence of events but does not have a causally related sequence of events, then the story is an action sequence.
3. If the story does have a causally related sequence of events, then ask, "Does the story imply goal-directed behavior?" If the story has a causally related sequence of events but does not imply goal-directed behavior, then the story is a reactive sequence.
4. If the story does imply goal-directed behavior, then ask, "Is planning or intentional behavior made explicit?" If the story implies goal-directed behavior but does not make the planning of this behavior explicit, then the story is an abbreviated episode.
5. If the story does make the planning or intentional behavior explicit, then ask, "Is the story elaborated by having multiple attempts or consequences, multiple sequential episodes, or embedded episodes, or is the story told from the point of view of more than one of the characters?" If the story does make intentional behavior explicit but is not elaborated, then the story is a complete episode.
6. If the story is elaborated, how is it elaborated? Is one aspect of the story elaborated? For example, is there an obstacle in the attempt path and multiple attempts? Does the story have multiple episodes—are they sequential or embedded? Is the story told from the perspective of more than one character?

One standardized test of narrative skills is available for children ages 6 to 11 years, the Test of Narrative Language (TNL; Gillam & Pearson, 2004). The test was designed to assess two types of difficulties exhibited by children with language disorders of (1) difficulties in narrative comprehension (reflected in remembering the critical elements of stories and understanding the gist of stories and in difficulty drawing inferences, and (2) difficulties in narrative production. At the macrostructure level, this is reflected in incomplete references to characters and story contexts; in

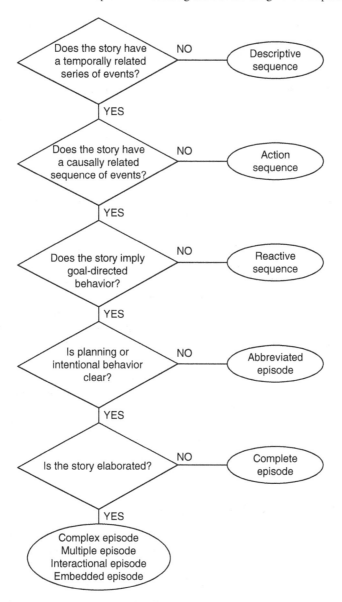

FIGURE 7.1 Story Grammar Decision Tree

fewer story grammar propositions related to character plans, actions, complications, and reactions; and in lower holistic scores. At the microstructure level, this is reflected in restricted vocabulary, fewer complex sentences, more grammatical errors, and fewer or problematic cohesive ties.

The TNL uses three formats for assessment of narrative comprehension and production: a no-picture format, a sequenced-picture format, and a single-picture format. In the no-picture format the examiner reads a story about a family going to McDonalds, then asks the child literal and inferential questions about the story. After answering the questions, the child is asked to retell the story. In the sequenced-picture format the child looks at a five-picture sequence of a boy building a boat and tripping and breaking it on the way to school while the examiner reads a story about the pictures. The child is then asked literal and inferential questions about the story. The child is shown a five-picture sequence of a boy who is late for school and asked to tell a story about the pictures. The child receives points for mentioning specific information about each of the pictures, for relating temporal relationships and causal relationships, for grammatical correctness, and for the degree to which the story is organized and makes sense.

For the single-picture format the child is shown a picture of two children who find a dragon guarding a treasure. The examiner reads a story about the picture and then asks the child literal and inferential questions. The child is then shown a picture of an alien spaceship landing in a park and is asked to tell a story about the picture. The child receives points for telling where and when the story occurs; identifying the aliens and humans; including dialogue; indicating a problem, conflict, or event that motivates the humans to act; referring to actions and events; indicating temporal and causal relationships among the events; providing consequences and an ending; describing objects in the picture; appropriately referencing characters; using correct grammar; and producing a coherent story that makes sense.

The TNL appears to provide a quick way to evaluate narrative skills of elementary school children. The range of formats (no picture, sequence pictures, single picture) allows SLPs to know how students do with varying levels of scaffolding. For most children, telling a story about a sequence of pictures is easier than telling a story about a single picture. A picture sequence stimulus provides children with a story they must recognize; they then generate language to code the story. A single-picture stimulus requires that children both generate the conceptual content of a story and linguistically code that content. The five-picture sequence stories are much shorter and less complex than wordless picture books and videos, and very few inferencing questions are asked, so the TNL may not capture the more complex narrative demands of upper elementary texts. All tasks in the TNL involve measures of both macrostructure and microstructure elements, but there are not separate macrostructure and microstructure scores. Children exhibit differing narrative skills, with some having difficulty primarily at the microstructure level and others having difficulty primarily at the macrostructure level. Narrative intervention must address these two levels and the interactions between them.

FACILITATING TEXT COMPREHENSION

The individualized education plans (IEPs) developed for students with language/learning disabilities are typically required to link to curriculum standards and benchmarks. Consequently, speech-language pathologists frequently use curricular content in their intervention activities. The concept of response to intervention (RTI) is being employed for students who are exhibiting difficulties with classroom content as well as those students who have been identified with disabilities. The purpose of RTI is to ensure that all children receive just the right instruction or intervention to be successful. RTI models typically identify three tiers of educational service/intervention (Fuchs, Fuchs, & Vaughn, 2008). Tier 1 refers to the core education programs for all students at each grade level. Tier 2 services typically represent supplemental research-based targeted services for those students who are not making adequate progress with Tier 1 services. Tier 3 services are typically reserved for students who, even with Tier 2 supports, fail to make adequate progress. In many instances, these students are referred for evaluation for special education services. Under the Individuals with Disabilities Education Act (IDEA), up to 15 percent of students served by special education personnel do not need to be qualified as special education students—they can be Tier 2 students. RTI and IDEA are resulting in increasing numbers of speech-language pathologists working closely with general education teachers, assisting them in differentiating instruction for diverse students in classrooms. Differentiating instruction means creating multiple paths so that students of different abilities, interests, or learning needs experience equally appropriate ways to absorb, use, develop, and present concepts as a part of the daily learning process (Tomblinson, 2001). SLPs can assist in differentiating instruction for students who experience difficulties comprehending the curriculum by:

- Identifying what is required in the learning task, such as vocabulary knowledge, syntactic understanding, the ability to make inferences, and the ability to work independently or in a group
- Determining students' strengths and weaknesses
- Developing differentiated lesson objectives (based on state standards and benchmarks) for what should be learned for all students, some students, or a few students
- Describing strategies for teachers and SLPs to use in differentiated instruction in science and social studies

Instruction can be differentiated in three ways:

- ***Content or topic.*** What information should the students learn? In any particular unit, what is the most important information for students to learn? What are the key points that the teacher would like everyone to understand (including those with language-learning disabilities); what additional content could most of the students in the class learn; and what content might only a few of the high-functioning or gifted students learn (Schumm, Vaughn, & Leavel, 1994; Watson & Houtz, 2002)? Figure 7.2 shows differentiated content for a unit on seasons.
- ***Process or activities.*** Differentiating processes means varying learning activities or strategies to provide appropriate methods for students to explore the concepts. Differentiation at this level is particularly important for students with language-learning impairments. How might the SLP need to work with the teacher to teach the vocabulary and syntactic patterns

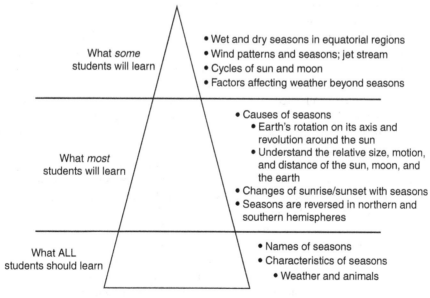

Differentiated content for seasons unit

FIGURE 7.2 Differentiated Content Instruction

that are necessary for accessing the lesson content? What type of activities or support might facilitate students with LLD accessing the content?

- ***Product.*** Students can be given multiple options for expressing what they know and understand. Do they do a drawing or produce an oral or written report? If written, is the report done by hand or on a computer? What is the level of complexity required for the product (does the task require knowledge, comprehension, application, analysis, synthesis, and/or evaluation?)?

This section of the chapter describes strategies for facilitating development of vocabulary and syntactic patterns associated with a literate language style and comprehension and production of content schemas and text structures.

Developing Linguistic Microstructures

DEVELOPING LITERATE VOCABULARY.   Compared to oral language, written literate-style language uses more specific vocabulary and more complex syntactic structures to specify the relationships among people, actions, and objects. A more literate style of language must be used any time the speaker and listener or reader and writer are not in the same time and space and do not share familiarity with the topic. To develop a literate language style, children must hear literate language and have the opportunity to use it in meaningful communicative contexts. Children can be exposed to a literate style in the language spoken by adults around them and in stories that are read to them.

Students must develop a literate vocabulary. Children's vocabulary in kindergarten and first grade is one of the best predictors of their language comprehension skills in middle school (Cunningham & Stanovich, 1997). Educators frequently try improving students' vocabularies by having them look up words in dictionaries, copy the definition, and then generate a sentence using the word. Such an approach to vocabulary teaching has little effect on increasing students' vocabulary. A traditional dictionary defines *devious* as: "(1) not sincere or candid, deceitful, underhand; (2) (of a route or course of action) rambling, indirect, roundabout; (3) going astray from a proper or accepted way, erring." In contrast, the *Collins COBUILD Dictionary* (Sinclair, 2006) provides user-friendly definitions of words. It defines devious as: "(1) devious describes people or plans and methods that are dishonest, often in a complicated way, but often also clever and successful. *You have to be a bit devious if you're going to succeed in business.* If you describe someone as **devious** you do not like them because you think they are dishonest and like to keep things secret, often in a complicated way; (2) not direct. *He took a rather devious route which avoids the city centre.*" When using traditional dictionaries, students are likely to produce sentences in which they use the words incorrectly or vaguely (so that one is uncertain if the student truly understands the meaning, e.g., *He was devious on his bike*).

Words are learned in context, but learning words from written contexts is not easy because written contexts lack the intonation, body language, and shared physical environment that supports word learning in oral language. Beck, McKeown, and Kucan (2002, 2008) proposed a strategy for selecting vocabulary to be taught. They suggested that one think of words in tiers. Tier 1 words are so familiar that they rarely require instruction. Tier 3 words are low-frequency words that are usually limited to a specific domain, for example, *isotope, peninsula,* and *meniscus,* and are best learned when needed in a content area. Tier 2 words are high-frequency words for mature language users and, hence, are valuable in adding productivity to students' language abilities. They add dimensions to a concept or idea that is already understood and can be worked with in a variety of ways. Tier 2 words are likely to occur in many contexts and are useful in describing experiences. Beck and colleagues recommend using student-friendly definitions, rather than traditional dictionary definitions when teaching vocabulary.

When reading *Esperanza Rising* in a fifth-grade class, a teacher chose to highlight the following Tier 2 words: *distinguished, capricious, devious, indignation, smirk, pungent,* and *stagnant.* *Esperanza Rising* is the story of a young girl from a wealthy Mexican family. When Esperanza's father is killed (supposedly by bandits), her uncle, Tio Luis, announces that he will marry Esperanza's mother so they can remain on the land. When the mother refuses, some buildings on the hacienda mysteriously burn. Under the cover of night, Esperanza and her mother flee to the United States hidden in a wagon with a false bottom. Understanding of the Tier 2 words is important for understanding the nature of the characters in the story and Experanza's perception of her experiences. On the hacienda, the grandmother is *distinguished* and *capricious.* These attributes serve her well in surviving and eventually making it to the United States. Understanding the *devious* nature of Tio Luis is critical to understanding why Esperanza and her mother flee. Although Tio Luis says his brother has been killed by bandits, he is now wearing his brother's belt buckle, leading one to believe that he may have been involved in the death. The mother feels *indignation* when Tio Luis asks to marry her, and Esperanza *smirks.* They know that Tio Luis is not to be trusted. As they flee, they cope with the *pungent* smells of overripe fruit covering them in the wagon and the *stagnant* air filled with the smell of body odor. Understanding these words is important for students to develop the mental models necessary for "reading between the lines" in the story.

Before teaching the words, the teacher presented them in a chart (as in Table 7.4) and asked the students to judge the level of their knowledge. Students could also be asked to classify the words as green light words (if they completely understand a word), yellow light words (if they have an incomplete understanding of the word or cannot use the word in more than one context), or red light words (if the student has no knowledge of the word; Lubliner, 2005). If a word is a green light word, students can read at the speed limit. If it is a yellow light word, the student will need to slow down and check comprehension. And if it is a red light word, the student needs to stop and seek clarification. As students read the story, they look for the words. When teaching the words, the teacher implemented the following steps:

- Explained the meaning of the word
- Contextualized the word for its role in the story
- Had children repeat the word so they create a phonological representation
- Gave examples in contexts other than the story
- Asked children to provide their own examples
- Had children say the word again to reinforce its phonological representation

TABLE 7.4   Judging Vocabulary Knowledge

Word	Know It Well, Can Explain It, Use It	Know Something About It, Can Relate It to a Situation	Have Seen or Heard the Word	Do Not Know the Word; Have Never Heard It
capricious				
distinguished				
devious				
indignant				
smirk				
pungent				
stagnant				

Some books are particularly useful for vocabulary learning or study. In *The Weighty Word Book* (Levitt, Burger, & Guralnick, 2000) the authors use an A-to-Z compendium of short stories to help students remember the definitions and pronunciations of tricky vocabulary words through the use of puns and mnemonic devices. For example, the word for E is *expedient*. The authors present a story of an ant who is very speedy. In fact, he is the quickest ant in the anthill, running everywhere to collect food and bringing back three times as much food as any other ant. Then one day he discovers a picnic table. With such a rich food supply, he decides there is no need to run any more. He comments, "Once I was a speedy ant, but now I'm happy to be called an ex-speedy ant" (p. 20). So whenever someone takes the easy way out, or takes the practical or convenient path, think of the ant who was content to be an ex-speedy ant, and you'll remember the word *expedient*.

Good vocabulary learners know multiple meanings for words. In-depth semantic knowledge increases readers' fluency as well as comprehension (Wolf, Miller, & Donnelly, 2000). Most common words, even those used in preschool and early elementary school, have multiple meanings. Ideally, educators should present the multiple meanings of words and, when possible, use the multiple meanings within a context (Nelson & Marchand-Martella, 2005). For example, consider the word *innocent* in the book *Holes* (Sachar, 1998). It can have at least three meanings, and each of these meanings has words that function as synonyms. See Figure 7.3. In the story, Stanley is accused of stealing a pair of shoes. He is found guilty and sent to Camp Green Lake, a juvenile detention camp in west Texas. Stanley is naive, whereas many of the other boys have a history of being in trouble and threatening other boys. Stanley tries to cope and to be accepted by the boys. The multiple meanings for "innocent" can be used in relation to this particular story, rather than in the abstract, for example,

- Not guilty of an offense: Stanley's parents knew Stanley was *innocent* of stealing the shoes.
- Not experienced or naive: Stanley was really a good kid; he was too *innocent* to be with boys who were real bullies.
- Not dangerous or harmful: Stanley thought his comment was *innocent*, but it made Zero very angry.

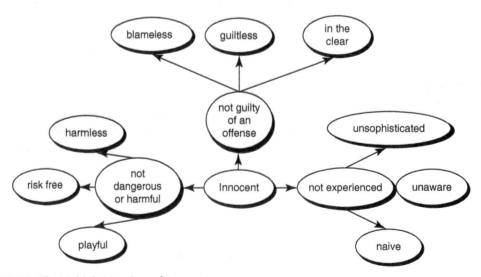

FIGURE 7.3 Multiple Meanings of *Innocent*

Students are asked to match the meaning of the word *innocent* to particular sentences in which it is used, and they are asked to judge if the word is used as intended in sentences, for example,

- The social worker knew Stanley was *innocent* because he was in school when the shoes were taken. (intended)
- When Zero confessed to stealing the shoes, he proved he was *innocent*. (not intended)
- Stanley's teaching Zero to read was an *innocent* activity. (intended)
- X-ray really knew how to survive at Camp Green Lake. He was the boy's leader because he was so *innocent*. (not intended)

Literate language makes frequent use of figurative language—idioms, analogies, metaphors, for example, *boils down to, read between the lines, sidestep the issue, that answer doesn't hold water, a thin argument,* and *crux of the matter*. Figurative language is used in all domains. In social studies, one talks about waves of immigrants; in science one speaks of the greenhouse effect. Zwiers (2010) suggests a strategy called FigFigs (Figuring our Figurative Language). Rather than simply saying that "waves of immigrants" means there were large groups of people coming from other countries; one explains what the author is trying to emphasize—in this case, how a wave and a large group of immigrants are similar. A wave is a large amount of water that comes in all at once; this is like a group of people who come in a short period of time. Figure 7.4 shows an example of a FigFig chart based on figurative language from *The Invention of Hugo Cabret*.

Lemony Snicket's *A Series of Unfortunate Events* explicitly teaches many words, including words with multiple meanings and figurative language. The series follows the adventures of

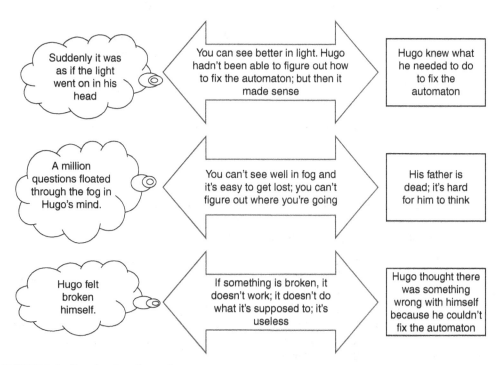

FIGURE 7.4 Figuring Out Figurative Language

three siblings—Violet, Klaus, and Sunny Baudelaire—after their parents were killed in a fire at the family mansion. In *Book of the Thirteenth* (Snicket, 2006), Violet meets Ishmael, the facilitator on the island where the children have washed ashore after a violent storm. Ishmael's feet are encased in mud, which he claims will heal his sore feet. " 'It's nice to meet you Ishmael,' said Violet, who thought heal clay was of dubious scientific efficacy, a phrase which here means 'unlikely to heal sore feet.'" Ishmael asks the children to tell him their whole story. Snicket writes, "But if the Baudelaires had told Ishmael the whole story, they would have had to tell the parts that put the Baudelaires in an unfavorable light, a phrase which here means that things the Baudelaires had done that were perhaps as treacherous as Olaf." He then describes the types of actions that would put them in a bad light.

Snicket begins Chapter 3 by stating that many words in our language are confusing because they can mean two completely different things. He begins with familiar examples. For instance, the word *bear* can refer to "a rather husky mammal found in the woods as in the sentence, 'The bear moved quietly toward the camp counselor, who was too busy putting on lipstick to notice,' but it can also refer to how much someone can handle, as in the sentence 'The loss of my camp counselor is more than I can bear.'" Or *yarn* can refer both to a colorful strand of wool as in the sentence, "'His sweater was made of yarn,' and to a long and rambling story as in the sentence 'His yarn about how he lost his sweater almost put me to sleep.'" He then returns to the story. The children are following Friday, a woman who has found them, through the shallow waters to the island. Snicket comments, ". . . they experienced both definitions of the word 'cordial,' which can refer both to a person who is friendly and to a drink that is sweet, and the more they had of one the more they were confused by the other. 'Perhaps you would care for some coconut cordial,' Friday said, in a cordial tone of voice."

It is not possible to teach children each of the words they need to know—and, in fact, children do not need to be explicitly taught every single word. Of 10,000 unfamiliar words an American fifth grader will encounter in reading, 4,000 will be derivatives of more frequent words. Between first and fifth grades, the increase in number of derived words is over three times greater than the increase in number of root words (Anglin, 1993). Teaching morphology can be a way to promote children's vocabulary development. The teaching of morphology can be divided into three components (Ebbers, 2004):

- Prefix study: Word initial morphemes such as: re-; un-; -in (im-; il-, ir-); pre-; sub-; anti-, -dis-; -de-; -mal-; -bene-; -pro-
- Suffix study: Word endings such as: -y; -er, -est; -ly; -hood; -ful; -less; -able, -ible; -some; -ish; -ness, -cide; -ment
- Root word study:
  - Greek combining forms such as: astro, bio, geo, therm, auto, homo, hydro, phone, scope, micro, macro, graph, photo, tele, meter, metry, path, psych
  - Latin roots such as aqua, prot, rupt, cript, tract, cept, spect, struct, ject, dict, mort

Teaching of common prefixes and suffixes can begin in mid-elementary school and the study of Greek and Latin roots in middle school. For each affix and root, the instructor explains the function of the morpheme and how it affects a part of speech. For example, the suffix -y changes a noun to an adjective (e.g., brat [a noun] becomes bratty [an adjective]). The meanings of the morpheme are explained and examples given, for example, the suffix -ly has three possible meanings (see Table 7.5). Reading the Harry Potter series provides numerous opportunities to teach Latin roots (Nilsen & Nilsen, 2006). (See Table 7.6.)

TABLE 7.5	-ly Definitions and Examples		
"In a Manner that Is" (Adverb)	**"Like a (Noun)" (Adjective)**	**Time-Related Adverbs**	**Time-Related Adjectives**
kindly ("in a manner that is kind") speaks kindly	sisterly ("like a sister") a *sisterly* hug	suddenly suddenly faints	daily (once a day) vitamins
quietly firmly sweetly courageously	friendly kingly motherly beggerly	periodically instantly eternally constantly	weekly monthly annually

DEVELOPING COMPLEX SYNTACTIC STRUCTURES.   Children can also be introduced to the literate style of texts through familiar stories that have repetitive or cumulative organization. Listen to the language style of *The Three Billy Goats Gruff* (Asbjornsen & Moe, 1957):

> Once upon a time there were three billy goats who were to go up to the hillside to make themselves fat, and the name of all three was "Gruff." On the way up was a bridge over a river they had to cross, and under the bridge lived a great ugly troll with eyes as big as saucers and a nose as long as a poker. So first of all came the youngest Billy Goat Gruff to cross the bridge. "Trip, trap! trip, trap!" went the bridge.

or from *Millions of Cats* (Gag, 1928):

> Once upon a time there was a very old man and a very old woman. They lived in a nice clean house which had flowers all around it, except where the door was. But they couldn't be happy because they were so very lonely.

The beginnings of these stories have relative clauses (introduced by *who* and *which*), literate conjunctions (*because, but, except*), inverted sentence structure (*on the way up was a bridge over the river they had to cross*), and descriptive vocabulary (*eyes as big as saucers, nose as long as a poker*).

A number of books highlight connectives. A list of such books is in Appendix 7.1.

TABLE 7.6	Latin Roots in *Harry Potter*		
Root	**HP use**	**HP meaning**	**English Derivations**
pes, pedis	Impedimental	spell to slow down/stop attacker	centipede, expedite, impede, peddler, pedometer, pedestrian, pedicure
mens, mentis	Dementors Legilmency Occulumency	Creatures who suck out human souls Mind reading Method of closing out mind reading	demented, dementia, Mensa, mental, mentality
malum, mali	Malfoy	Surname of "bad" characters	malady, malaria, malcontent, malevolent, malicious, malignant, malpractice

As an example, *Just Me and 6,000 Rats: A Tale of Conjunctions* (Walton, 2007) is the story of a boy and his 6,000, rats that visit a city. In describing the adventures of the boy and his rats, the author uses 14 different conjunctions. They go to the top of a skycraper:

> At the top I could see the entire city. But the rats had trouble seeing through the windows *until* some very nice people helped them out. From the top, we saw a parade. We hurried down and joined the march. It was fun, *even though* we were soon the only ones in the parade. After all that marching, we were hungry. We had lunch at a very fine restaurant. We ate just what we wanted *since* we served ourselves.

The boy is oblivious to the fact that people are screaming and running away. He is ordered out of town and decides he could *either* go home *or* visit your city.

Understanding and use of these connective words (and their associated dependent adverbial clauses) are particularly critical in social studies, math, and science. Rather than first teaching these connectives in abstract science and social studies contexts, however, I have begun by first teaching them in the contexts of familiar personal experiences, then teaching them in narratives or literature, and finally teaching them in social studies and science contexts. Students are much more likely to be able to understand the connectives when they refer to familiar contexts. The following are examples of adverbial dependent clauses in each of these three contexts.

- Personal:
  — My brother had to go to summer school *because* he failed in English.
  — *If* I have $10, I'll buy that new CD.
  — I won't get to go to the movies *unless* I clean my room. Or, I'll go to the movies *unless* I don't clean my room.
  — I'll take the Hershey bar, *although* it's not my favorite.
- Narrative (sentences based on the book *Holes* (Sachar, 2000):
  — Zero dug Stanley's holes *because* Stanley was teaching him to read.
  — *If* Stanley finds something valuable, he'll get a day off.
  — Stanley won't get a day off *unless* he finds something the warden wants.
  — Stanley said he had taken the sunflower seeds *although* he had not.
- Theoretical/expository:
  — The ice melted *because* the temperature was above 32°F.
  — *If* it's attracted to the magnet, it's metal.
  — Take the blocks that are on the table *unless* they are wooden.
  — Migrant workers work hard *although* they are not paid much.

If students are to comprehend written texts, they must understand and be able to use the complex syntactic structures used by authors. Like the United States, Australia struggles with a literacy gap between mainstream and minority students. In an effort to improve the literacy skills of children, Dr. Brian Gray and Wendy Cowey at Charles Darwin University developed a program called Accelerated Literacy (AL) that is now being used with many children who often have not been successful literacy learners. One goal of AL is to enable students to identify and use the text patterns of authors, and in so doing to teach the academic/literate discourses of the classroom. Using AL strategies, adults make the nature of academic/literate discourse explicit.

Several components of AL address microstructure and macrostructure aspects of text. A component called *Transformations* directs students' attention to the syntactic patterns an author has chosen. The goal is to change the student's orientation from that of a reader looking for meaning from the text to that of a writer learning how the author used vocabulary and structures to achieve a particular effect or purpose. The teacher selects sentences from a text to analyze, using the following steps:

- The teacher reads the text.
- Working together, students and the teacher segment a sentence into its component words or phrases, looking for cues (such as commas) that may help them determine how to group the words into phrases. They discuss the author's word choices and how the words affect their interpretation of the text. They note the word order and syntactic patterns and discuss why the author ordered the ideas as he or she did. What was the author trying to highlight by the structure chosen?
- Students may reorder segments of the sentence.
- Students identify key words to describe and find similar meanings.
- Students rewrite the text in their own words.

While in Australia, I observed a group of seventh-grade students engaged in an accelerated literacy lesson. The students had been reading the novel, *Rowin of Rin* (Rodda, 1993) a fantasy-adventure of the people of Rin, who live in the shadow of the Mountain ruled by a fierce but unseen dragon. The people of Rin are strong and brave, except for young Rowan. He spends his time caring for the bukshah, the gentle beasts that the villagers depend on for their survival. When their stream suddenly stops flowing and the bukshah are in danger of dying, six of the strongest, bravest villagers decide to climb the Mountain, hoping to avoid the Dragon that lives there, to find out what has happened. However, Sheba the Wise Woman is the only one who knows the way, and she has decided that Rowan must accompany the party, so she gives them a magic map that can only be read if he is holding it. Rowan starts off as fragile and a little whiny, but improves steadily, especially as he begins to realize that he plays an important role in the expedition.

The teacher selected the following sentence near the end of the book, which describes Rowan's thoughts as be returns to the village:

> He screwed his eyes shut, suddenly afraid that this was a dream, and he was still on the mountain top with the fire, the ice, the terror and the despair.

In the transformation activity, the students and teacher segmented the sentence and discussed ways to change words in the sentence. Table 7.7 shows the words the teacher highlighted and the content of the discussion.

Following the discussion, students were given this text pattern to follow:

He ____ (did something)

suddenly ____ (felt)

and ____ (imagined place)

with ____ (the elements of a hard life)

the ____ (how he felt, reaction)

Using this process, one student rewrote the passage as, "Rowan shut his eyes tightly, suddenly fearful that it was all an illusion and he was still stuck on the mountain top with the dragon, the freezing cold, the knowing that he would never see his mother, Annad, or Star again."

Children with language-learning impairments and students from cultures that do not use a decontextualized, literate style of communication experience difficulty comprehending the complex syntactic structures used in printed texts. Research has shown that teaching parts of speech or sentence patterns out of context does not promote syntactic development. AL helps students

TABLE 7.7   Accelerated Literacy Example

Rowan of Rin Text	Discussion
He **screwed** his eyes shut,	What physical actions could you do to show that you weren't sure this was real?
suddenly **afraid** that this was a **dream,**	What are other words for *afraid*? frightened, scared, fearful, terrified, anxious, troubled
	How could you say that this wasn't true? It was a **dream**—what different words could you use?
and he was still on the **Mountain top**	Where else could he be?—a different place or setting or the same idea
with the **fire**, the **ice,**	What could be with him that he didn't like or things that made his life difficult?
the **terror,** and the **despair.**	What are other words for the feelings of terror and despair?

comprehend syntactic patterns in context by understanding the meaning and the author's intent or reason for using the particular patterns. By "transforming" the author's writing into their own, they increase both their comprehension and their ability to make these structures their own.

Sentences in written text are sometimes syntactically quite complex, with multiple dependent clauses and prepositional and participial phrases that may be in unusual order. Students can easily get lost in such sentences. Consider the following sentence from *Harry Potter and the Order of the Phoenix* (Rowling, 2003):

> Indeed, from the tone of his voice when he next spoke, Harry was quite sure that Mr. Weasley thought Dudley was quite as mad as the Dursleys thought he was, except that Mr. Weasley felt sympathy rather than fear.

Flood, Lapp, and Fisher (2002) suggested a parsing strategy for complex sentences in which students determine the various ideas in the sentences, then restate the text in their own words. Table 7.8 shows how this sentence from Harry Potter can be parsed into its ideas.

TABLE 7.8   Parsing Sentences

Subject (who, what)	Verb (is do)	Object/Descriptor (who, what, when, where, how)
Idea 1: Mr. Weasley	speaking	in a concerned? tone
Idea 2: Harry	was	sure about what Mr. Weasley and the Dursleys thought
Idea 3: Mr. Weasley	thought	Dudley was crazy
Idea 4: Dursleys	thought	Mr. Weasley is crazy
Idea 5: Mr. Weasley	feels	sympathy for Dudley
Idea 6: Dursleys	were	afraid of Mr. Weasley

Developing Macrostructure Schemas

DEVELOPING CONTENT SCHEMA KNOWLEDGE.   The conceptual knowledge underlying narrative text involves awareness of temporal action sequences, cause–effect or reactive sequences (first physical causality and later psychological causality), planning, and understanding of the concept of trickery or deception. To learn to comprehend and produce narratives, children must hear a variety of well-structured narratives. Children with limited narrative abilities frequently do not enjoy listening to or reading complex stories. To ensure children's willingness to listen to or read stories, they must be provided with books that are comprehensible to them. By determining children's narrative abilities (using the guidelines presented earlier in this chapter), appropriate books can be made available.

Research has shown the critical role that early experience with books has on children's later school success (Clark, 1976; Durkin, 1966; Wells, 1986). For example, Wells (1986) documented that the amount children were read to during the preschool years was the language variable most related to academic success at fifth grade. As children gain language and book awareness skills, the types of books selected and the discussion about them should change (van Kleeck & Vander Woude, 2003).

Narrative facilitation can be done in language therapy sessions and in curriculum activities in classrooms. The language arts curricula can be developed around narrative production and comprehension, and stories can be selected to supplement other academic subjects. One begins the intervention based on the student's current narrative level. If one is working with a young preschool child or a student with a significant language impairment who does not produce a series of statements on a topic, one might begin by having the student describe activities in a picture in a book. They are then introduced to concepts about the nature of a story and asked to tell how the story begins and how it ends. The children are introduced to the idea that books present a sequence of activities about a character and that one begins at the front of the book and finishes at the back of the book. At this level, one does not want books with complex plots, but instead, books with straightforward temporal sequences. Books in this category include *The Very Hungry Caterpillar* (Carle, 1969), a story about a caterpillar who eats its way through a variety of foods; *The Snowy Day* (Keats, 1962), about Peter's activities in the snow; and *Charlie Needs a Cloak* (dePaola, 1974), about the sequence of events involved in making a wool cloak for Charlie. To facilitate relating a series of sequential activities, children can participate in activities similar to those in the story. For example, after reading *The Very Hungry Caterpillar*, children can sample the foods that the caterpillar ate. To extend children's experiences with *The Snowy Day*, a speech-language pathologist in Albuquerque took her ice chests to the mountain one weekend to fill them with snow so that on Monday the children in her class could make snowmen and throw snowballs. In another instance, children were studying a unit on early New Mexico. After the teacher read *Charlie Needs a Cloak*, weavers came to the classroom. They brought wool and showed the children how to spin it; then they threaded a small handloom and allowed the children to weave strips of cloth for scarves. Children can be encouraged not only to retell the stories in the books, but also to relate their own experiences. Stories of this type will result in action sequence narratives.

As children become able to deal with the beginning-to-end temporal action sequences, it is time to introduce cause–effect sequences, which give rise to stories of the reactive sequence type. In temporal sequence stories, the exact order of activities is not always critical. For example, in *The Snowy Day*, it is not important whether Peter first makes a snowball or an angel in the snow. Cause–effect (reactive sequence) stories, however, must have a set sequence of events. For example, in *Round Robin* (Kent, 1982), a small robin eats and eats until he becomes obese. When the other robins fly south for the winter, he must hop because he is too fat to fly. Because he is hopping along the snowy ground, a fox almost catches him.

Pourquoi tales that explain the origins of aspects of nature or the characteristics of certain animals are helpful to develop understanding of cause–effect because they make explicit links between actions and reactions. For example, in *Why Mosquitoes Buzz in Peoples' Ears* (Aardema, 1975), a mosquito annoys an iguana by buzzing in his ear. The iguana puts sticks in his ears so he can't hear the mosquito. A python talks to the iguana, who cannot hear him because of the sticks in his ears. The python thinks the iguana is angry with him and runs into a rabbit hole. The rabbits run from their hole because they think the python is coming to eat them. The birds see the rabbits running and sound an alarm because they think there is danger. Hearing the alarm the monkeys swing swiftly through the trees. One of the monkeys falls on an owl's nest, causing the death of an owlet. In *Why the Sun and the Moon Live in the Sky* (Dayrell, 1968), the water refuses to visit the sun and the moon because their house is too small. The sun responds by building a bigger house. The water comes to visit; the water gets deeper and deeper, causing the sun and the moon to climb to the roof of their house and eventually causing them to flee to the sky. Now, in addition to being asked to relate three things in sequence that happened in the story, the students are also asked questions that focus on the physical causality or the reason for the activity. Why questions are introduced, such as, "Why couldn't the robin fly?" "Why did the rabbits run from their holes?" or "Why did sun build a bigger house?"

Development of the abbreviated and complete episode structure requires understanding of psychological causality or an understanding of motivations for behavior. Students must become aware that characters have feelings that motivate behavior or that feelings can be elicited by events. By kindergarten, children can identify and give examples of situations eliciting the emotions happy, mad, sad, and scared (Harter, 1982). Stories that explicitly label or discuss feelings, such as *Feelings* (Aliki, 1984), *I Feel Silly* (Curtis, 1998), *What are YOU So Grumpy About* (Lichtenheld, 2003) or that report situations that elicit feelings, such as many of the Franklin Turtle stories and the Berenstain Bears stories for young children, can be used in activities. A story such as *Franklin in the Dark* (Bourgeois, 1986) is useful with young children for discussing the emotion of fear. Franklin is a young turtle who will not go into his shell because he is afraid of the dark. He visits a number of other animals who relate their fears, including a duck who wears water wings because he is afraid of deep water and a bird who wears a parachute because he is afraid of heights. In *Hetty and Harriet* (Oakley, 1981), two chickens set out to see the world. In the course of their adventures, they experience 33 different emotions.

For older elementary school and middle school students, the popular Goosebumps books by R. L. Stein are very useful for facilitating understanding of characters' emotions. Stein frequently uses adverbs and descriptive adjectives and verbs to describe characters' behaviors and thoughts. Consider some of the following examples from *Monster Blood* (Stein, 1992):

"Thanks," said Evan uncertainly. (p. 25)
"Hi," said Andy timidly, giving the man a wave. (p. 29)
"Poor Evan," Andy said, half teasing, half sympathetic. (p. 81)
"You been in a fight?" she asked, squinting suspiciously at him. (p. 86)

The book *Holes* (Sachar, 2000) does not explicitly describe emotions in words, but the experiences of Stanley and other boys at Camp Green Lake, a juvenile detention facility in a dry lake bed in west Texas, provide opportunities to discuss a range of emotions. Stanley, who lives under an old family curse, has unjustly been convicted of stealing a pair of shoes. At Camp Green Lake, Stanley and the boys spend their days digging holes in the sun, avoiding rattlesnakes and deadly spotted lizards, and dealing with the warden, who is seeking something in the holes. Gradually friendships and loyalty develop among the boys. Showing the *Holes* movie after reading the book provides students with additional visual cues to help them discuss the emotions the boys may be experiencing and why. Many students with language-learning impairments exhibit difficulty interpreting the emotional meanings of facial expressions, gestures, and tone of voice. The DVD set *Mind Reading* (Baron-Cohen, 2007) provides an excellent supplement for exploring emotions. This DVDs covers 412 emotions, with a wide range of emotional words associated with each emotion (33 words for sad, such as *lonely, tired, upset, distraught, gloomy, discouraged, devastated,* and *despairing*). Videos show persons of differing ages experiencing the emotions, and audio clips convey the vocal intonations associated with many of the emotions.

As students begin to attend to characters' emotions, they also become alert to common scripts and character traits. To further scriptal development and awareness of character traits, a series of books with the same character or theme can be presented. Younger children will enjoy books about pigs and wolves. After children are familiar with *The Three Little Pigs* (Galdone, 1970), they can read such books as *Mr. and Mrs. Pig's Evening Out* (Rayner, 1976), in which the babysitter turns out to be a wolf, and *Garth Pig and the Ice Cream Lady* (Rayner, 1977), in which the ice cream lady is a wolf. The children can be encouraged to predict what they think will happen when they see the wolf appear at the door as the babysitter, or when Garth Pig enters the ice cream lady's truck. Older students enjoy stories about giants, trolls, and dragons. Adolescents are into stories of vampires such as Stephanie Meyer's *Twilight* saga series (Meyer, 2005).

The temporal sequence, physical causality, and psychological causality of the earlier stages are further elaborated in the complete episode stage. The role of planning in meeting the character's goals becomes important at this stage. Children now understand secondary emotions, such as shame, guilt, embarrassment, and pride. These emotions are dependent on higher cognitive functioning and awareness of social sanctions (Lewis & Michalson, 1983). Books that describe situations that elicit these feelings can be read and discussed. Understanding emotions should lead to a better understanding of characters' intentions and their attempts or plans to cope with their problems and emotions. The majority of stories require understanding of psychological causality and planning of characters. Some examples of such stories are described next. Internal emotion charts can be used to focus students on characters' emotions, when the emotion occurred, and why it occurred. Table 7.9 shows a chart for the story *The Boy Who Lived with Seals* (Martin, 1993).

In *Farmer Duck* (Waddell, 1995), a duck has it hard because his owner is lazy and does no work. While the duck is out hoeing, ironing, and collecting the eggs, the farmer does nothing, occasionally calling out, "How goes the work?" One day, the duck grows so exhausted that the other animals make a plan to oust the farmer. They chase him away, and the animals take over the farm. In *Cross-Country Cat* (Calhoun, 1979), Henry, the cat, is left behind at his owner's winter cabin. To catch up with his owners, he sets out on skis and must cope with several dangers he encounters along the way. In *Fin M'Coul: The Giant of Knockmany Hill* (dePaola, 1981), Fin is being chased by a giant who is bigger and stronger than he is, and he and his wife must devise a plan to save themselves. In *Amazing Grace* (Hoffman, 1991), Grace is determined to be Peter Pan in the school play, even though classmates have told her she cannot be Peter Pan because she is a girl and she is Black. Grace practices and practices; at the tryouts there is no doubt that she should be Peter Pan.

Between ages 10 and 12, typical students produce stories that are elaborated in a variety of ways. Early elaborations involve multiple attempts in the characters' plans or multiple minichapters or episodes. Later elaborations involve stories told from the point of view of more than one character or stories embedded within stories. Underlying these narrative structures are

TABLE 7.9	Internal States Chart—*The Boy Who Lived with Seals*		
Characters	**When**	**Feeling**	**Why**
parents	they discover that their son is not in camp	sad; disconsolate, despondent	because they boy is gone and may have been carried off by wild animals
parents	when they learn that there is a boy living among seals	joyful	because they are sure it is their son
boy	when he hears the seals calling	melancholy	because he misses his life with the seals
parents	when the boy returns to live with the seals	sad but empathetic	because they didn't want to loose him but they understand his need to be with the seals
boy	when he was back with the seals	joyful and grateful/ appreciative	joyful because he was back with the seals who were his family; and appreciative for the skills he learned from his human parents

perception of character growth and change, awareness of deception, awareness of cyclical time, and understanding of figurative versus literal word meanings.

Beyond third grade, attention should be given to developing students' understanding of the landscape of consciousness. Not only must they be able to perceive the emotions and thoughts of the protagonists in response to events in stories, but they must also be able to perceive how other characters in stories respond to these same events. *Voices in the Park* (Browne, 1998) provides a good introduction to perspective taking. The book has four brief chapters, each told by a different gorilla character who has gone to the park. Although the four gorillas encounter one another in the park, they report markedly different interpretations of their experiences. Interpretation of multiple landscapes of consciousness is critical for the story, *John Brown, Rose, and the Midnight Cat* (Wagner, 1977). Rose, a lonely and elderly woman, owns a large dog, John Brown. A black cat comes into her home. She dearly wants the cat to stay, but John Brown is jealous of the cat and sends it away. Understanding of multiple perspectives is also essential if students are to comprehend the conflict in *Passage to Freedom: The Sugihara Story* (Mochizuki, 1997). Mr. Sugihara, the Japanese ambassador to Lithuania at the beginning of World War II, must decide what to do when Jews fleeing from Hitler in Poland arrive at the Japanese embassy pleading for visas to leave the country, but his superiors refuse his requests to issue the visas. Emery (1996) suggested developing character maps to help students focus on both plot (landscape of action) and character (landscape of consciousness). Students identify the plot elements of the stories and perspectives of the various characters in the story of the events. Table 7.10 shows a character map for the story *John Brown, Rose, and the Midnight Cat* (Wagner 1977)."

Stories that rely heavily on characterization can be appreciated in the elaborated narrative stage. The book *Sarah, Plain and Tall* (MacLachlan, 1985) is an excellent introduction to this level. It contains several episodes but is short enough to be read in one long session or two short ones. This book is the story of a motherless pioneer family and the woman who answers papa's letter to come and be his wife. The changes in the emotional responses of each of the characters

TABLE 7.10	Character Perspective Map for *John Brown, Rose, and the Midnight Cat*	
Rose's Perspective	**Story Events**	**John Brown's Perspective**
Rose is curious and wants to see what it is.	**Initiating event**: Something moves in the garden.	John Brown does not want to look; he is hesitant and uncertain.
Rose decides there is a cat; she is lonely.	**Subsequent events**: Rose looks outside.	John Brown insists there is nobody therefore; he is jealous.
Rose is in bed and doesn't know what John Brown had done.	John Brown checks outside.	Feels for the cat it is not needed; is aggravated by its appearance.
Rose is disappointed that John Brown won't acknowledge the cat.	The next night Rose sees the cat again.	John Brown resents the cat and hopes it will go away.
Rose hopes the cat will come in and be her friend.	Rose puts out milk for the cat.	John Brown tips the milk; is irritated that the cat is around.
Rose is depressed/melancholy.	John Brown refuses to let the cat in.	John Brown is satisfied with himself that he has gotten rid of the cat.
Rose is despondent.	Rose stays in bed all day.	John Brown is concerned/worried/alarmed about Rose.
Rose is relieved by John Brown's change of heart; is comforted by the cat.	**Resolution**: John Brown lets the cat in the house.	John Brown remains apprehensive/suspicious of the cat, but relieved that Rose is better.

over the course of the story are critical to the events and outcome. Students can discuss the traits of each of the characters. For example, papa is lonely, thoughtful, industrious, and sad; Sarah, the mail-order wife, is homesick, independent, optimistic, joyous, and adventuresome; Caleb, the boy, is wistful, worrying, and loving; and Anna, the girl, is hopeful, understanding, and missing her mother. The story is told through the eyes of Anna. Students can be encouraged to retell the story through the eyes of the other characters.

The concept of deception may be introduced with trickery tales. Students must be assisted in understanding that what a person says is not necessarily what he or she intends to do. The concept can be introduced to middle school students through trickery tales from different cultures, such as the coyote tales of the Southwest Indians, Anansi the Spider tales from Africa, raven tales from the Northwest, the Uncle Remus tales from the South, and Juan Bobo tales from Puerto Rico as well as trickster tales from other cultures. Because these tales come from oral histories, they include frequent repetition and lend themselves to easy role playing. Students are given the roles of the characters in the stories, and initially the teacher takes the role of the inner thoughts of the trickster. For example, in the story, *The Crocodile's Tale* (Aruego & Aruego, 1972), a Philippino folktale, the crocodile is caught in a noose. He promises to give a boy a gold ring if he cuts him down. We know, of course, that the crocodile has no intention of giving the boy a ring, but rather intends to eat him. When a student playing the crocodile finishes saying he will give the boy a gold ring, the teacher snickers and in a loud whisper says, "I'm not really going to give him a ring. I'm just saying that. I'm really going to grab him and take him into the river and eat him." After several role-playing experiences with the teacher verbalizing the inner thoughts and actual intentions of the trickster, a student can be assigned this role. Stories of Ikotomi, the Plains Indian trickster, also provide a means of teaching the concept of trickery (e.g., *Iktomi and the Berries* [Goble, 1989]; *Iktomi and the Ducks* [Goble, 1990]. The Iktomi books use three types of discourse—the discourse of the narrator telling the story (printed in large, dark black print), the discourse of Iktomi's inner thoughts (printed in small, dark print by pictures of Iktomi), and the discourse of the narrator commenting on Iktomi's behavior and trickery (print in large, light gray print). These multiple discourses make explicit Iktomi's deceptions.

The final stage of narrative development, metaphoric, does not result in additional complexity of narrative structure. The complexity is at the content level. The entire story may be allegorical and can be read for two levels of meaning. For example, the Narnia stories by C.S. Lewis, can be read as exciting adventures of a group of children or as a theological statement on the conflict between good and evil. *The Giver* (Lowry, 1993), a story about the experiences of 12-year-old Jonas who lives in a utopian world, challenges readers to interpret the multiple meanings of words and the symbolism of things and people. "Release" refers to death, although the community is led to believe it simply means that old or different are going to another community; "stirrings" refer to the developing sensations of adolescents, which are quickly suppressed with medication. The river, which runs into the community and out to Elsewhere, symbolizes escape from the confines of the community; Gabrial, the newborn child, symbolizes hope and a starting over; the color red, which is the color Jonas first sees, symbolizes the exciting ideas and emotions he discovers. The story can also be read as an allegory for the process of maturation—Jonah rejects a society where everyone is the same to follow his own path.

Normally developing adolescents can think of abstractions of time and space, and as a consequence they will enjoy science fiction and fantasy tales that play with these concepts. Such stories frequently have multiple embedded plots that take place during different time frames. Susan Cooper's *The Dark Is Rising* (1973, and its four sequels) and Madeleine L'Engle's, *A Wrinkle in Time* (1962, and its two sequels) are excellent examples of stories that manipulate time and space. Both move back and forth between the present situation and other times and places. The 2010 Newbery award book *When You Reach Me* (Stead, 2009) is a complex mystery that moves 12-year-old Miranda in time all the while she is reading and trying to make sense of *A Wrinkle in Time*.

As students develop the ability to produce well-structured stories, they also develop a meta-awareness of narratives. They know what to expect from narratives and can compare and contrast narratives in terms of structure and theme. This ability to compare and contrast narratives can be furthered by having students read different versions of the same story or several books on a similar theme. One can begin with highly familiar stories and obvious variations. For example, *The Three Little Hawaiian Pigs and the Magic Shark* (Laird, 1981), *The Three Little Javalinas* (Lowell, 1992), *The Three Little Wolves and the Big Bad Pig* (Trivizas, 1993), and *The True Story of the Three Little Pigs* (Scieszka, 1989) are all variations of *The Three Little Pigs*. *Wili Wai Kula and the Three Mongooses* (Laird, 1983), *Somebody and the Three Blairs* (Tolhurst, 1994), and *Goldilocks and the Three Hares* (Petach, 1995) are variations of *The Three Bears*. Stories with the same goal from different cultures can be compared. For example, there are a variety of Native legends regarding how man or animals got the sun. A Cherokee version is *Grandmother Spider Brings the Sun* (Keams, 1995); for the Northwest Indians, it is *Raven* (McDermott, 1993) who gets the sun; and in an Inuit version (*How Snowshoe Hare Rescued the Sun*, [Bernhard, 1993]) Snowshoe Hare gets the sun from the demons' cave. Many cultures have variants of the Cinderella tale. (See the listing in Appendix 7.2.) Students can study the geography and history of regions and countries and discuss the reasons for the variations in some of these stories. Using their metanarrative skills, students can discuss the similarities and differences in these tales in terms of story grammar components such as settings, characters, problems (initiating events), type of magic, attempts to cope with the problem, and endings. Some story versions, such as *The True Story of the Three Little Pigs* (Scieszka, 1989), which is told from the wolf's perspective, or *The Untold Story of Cinderella* (Shorto, 1990), which is told from the stepsisters' perspective, or *Cinderella's Rat* (Meddaugh, 1997), told by a rat who became Cinderella's coachman, can assist students in developing the multiple perspective taking that is a critical component of the landscape of consciousness.

Activities that encourage students to visualize the texts can also facilitate the mental modeling essential for comprehension (Gambrell & Javitz, 1993). Sensory imaging strategy (SIS) is a multisensory strategy that combines imagery with story elements (Romero, 2002). Students are told SIS, an acronym for sensory imaging strategy, will help them use their senses—seeing, hearing, smelling, tasting, and feeling—when they are reading about characters, settings, and events. They are shown the senses labeled on a picture of a girl. As a teacher or speech-language pathologist reads from a text, he or she pauses to describe the images that the passage evokes. Then the adult reads further and asks the students to describe a sensory image and name the sense. Table 7.11 shows an SIS chart for some of the elements in *Esperanza Rising* (Ryan, 2000).

TABLE 7.11 Sensory Images for Comprehension Based on *Esperanza Rising*

	Seeing	Hearing	Touching/ Feeling	Tasting	Smelling
Setting: edge of grape field at beginning of harvest	fields of grapevines heavy with ripe grapes on the El Rancho de las Rosas; mountains in the distance; brightly colored shirts of field workers; vaqueros in baggy pants tied at ankles, long-sleeve shirts, bandanas on foreheads	whinnying of horses; rattle of wagon wheels taking grapes to barns	heat of the sun, heaviness of the grapes	sweet juiciness of grapes	smell of ripe grapes, horses, roses
Character: Tio Luis	tall, skinny, tiny mustache, white beard on tip of chin, Papa's belt buckle	loud voice, clearing throat	shiver at his touch		
Event: fleeing to the U.S. at night by hiding in the false bottom of wagon	wagon with false bottom, dark, boards close above her, awful yellow dress that didn't fit her	murmuring of Alfonso & Miguel driving the wagon, creaking of wagon	rocking like a bumpy cradle, guavas rolling around feet	dry mouth	sweet, fresh smell of guavas, not enough air, smell of bodies around her

Narratives can be used to provide students with some of the schema knowledge they will need to comprehend expository texts in social study and science lessons. For example, when learning about the Civil Rights Movement, students can read narratives such as *My Brother Martin* (Farris, 2003), *Through My Eyes* (Bridges, 1999), *Harvesting Hope: The Story of Cesar Chavez* (Krull, 2003), and *If a Bus Could Talk: The Story of Rosa Parks* (Ringgold, 1999) and complete an I-Chart (Inquiry Chart; Hoffman, 1992). The I-Chart provides students with a framework for asking important questions, comparing answers across multiple texts, and coming to their own conclusions about the questions. The chart includes a row for new questions or interesting information that does not the basic questions. Table 7.12 provides an I-Chart framework for Civil Rights.

Comprehension in social studies requires that students understand the historical context and be able to take the perspectives of those portrayed in the historical accounts (Zarnowski, 2006). They have to understand what it might have been like to live in the past. To do this well, students must also be able to have some sense of empathy with the persons and recognize that the various persons in the period may have differing perspectives. They must attempt to understand the motivations, beliefs, and feelings of people in the historical setting. This type of understanding can be difficult for all students, but it is especially problematic for students with language impairments, who are notoriously poor at taking the perspectives of others. A book series, *You Wouldn't Want to Be* . . . published by Franklin Watts, a division of Scholastic, could be useful in helping students understand the historical context and the perspectives of those who lived in the past. The appearance of these nonfiction books should appeal to upper elementary school students who are reluctant readers and should also prove useful for middle school students with language-literacy difficulties). Their appearance is somewhat like the popular graphic novels or manga. The books can be used to build the background students need to comprehend the social studies lessons in the general education classroom. The whimsical cartoon-style artwork in all the books helps to convey the feelings of the people at the time. For example, *You Wouldn't Want to Be an American Colonist: A Settlement You'd Rather Not Start* (Morley, 2009) recounts the history of the first English colony, Jamestown, in North America. One could discuss the pictures showing seasick colonists; cold, starving colonists; colonists surprised by strange creatures; and colonists sweating, beating off mosquitoes, and worn out from hard work. Each book provides practical "handy hints" for daily living from people of the period, for example,

- If you get really hungry, boil up your boots and eat them.
- Don't steal food from the natives, or you might end up dead.
- Build well-protected livestock pens—even your own people might steal from you.
- Grow tobacco in your settlement. You might make a fortune selling it!

The books' authors talk directly to the reader, for example, "With the stormy Atlantic Ocean threatening to sink the boat, you're already thinking it was a bad decision. If you're lucky, you will spend two months at sea. However, the trip can take up to six months if storms blow your ship off course" (p. 10). There are numerous titles in this series, so you should be able to find one or more that links to social studies content in elementary or middle school.

Another approach to assist students in understanding the multiple perspectives of people in history is to find books that describe experiences through the eyes of different persons. For example, the book *Voices of Ancient Egypt* (Winters, 2003) presents the voices of 13 individuals in various occupations ranging from scribe to herdsman. The author uses first-person, free-verse poems to describe the workers' duties and places in society. She gives voice to the birdnetter and marshman, whom other authors neglect or lump together under headings such as "peasants." Women are

TABLE 7.12 Civil Rights Inquiry Chart

	My Brother Martin (Martin Luther King)	If a Bus Could Talk (Rosa Parks)	Harvesting Hope (Cesar Chavez)	Through My Eyes (Ruby Bridges)	Summary/ Interpretation
What was this person's early remembered experience with racism?	Not being allowed to play with white friends	Ku Klux Klan riding by home & shooting rifles	Teacher hung sign on him, "I am a clown. I speak Spanish."	Hearing people shouting bad words when she went to school	Some experiences were scary; some made people feel bad about themselves; some just didn't make sense.
What was his/her response or the response of others to this event?	Parents had been shielding them; parents explained what Blacks could not do	Family slept in clothes so could flee	Liked to learn, but came to hate school	Mother told her to pray for the people. Ruby didn't really understand what was happening. She didn't question why she was alone in school.	Families often affected how the child responded to the events.
What childhood experiences contributed to his/her adult goals?	Listening to his dad preach about bigotry; remembering his mother's words that someday it would be better	Her mother seeing that she got a good education	Torment of working in the fields—spasms in back; wheezing and stinging eyes from chemicals; felt like a slave	For a long time she didn't think about goals. When her brother died at 19 she began to think about what she should do to help.	You can decide to do important things even when you're a kid; sometimes you don't understand what's happening at the time.
Name a major thing he/she did as an adult that had an effect on civil rights.	Led a march on Washington, DC. Gave the "I have a dream" speech.	Refusing to give up her seat to a white man on a bus	Started the National Farm Workers Association; led a march of farm workers to Sacramento, CA state capitol	She went back to her grade school to help; she travels and talks about her experience.	There are many things a person can do. Some led groups of people, and others did something brave by themselves.
What was the effect of the person's actions on civil rights?	He turned the world upside down; many people began to speak against segregation.	People organized a boycott of the buses in Birmingham; Court ruled segregation against the law	Better working conditions for farm workers	A lot of people were impressed with her bravery; if she could do it, they could.	Many were influenced by what these people did.
Other questions/ interesting information	How did his sister help him?	Why did she move to Detroit?	What is it like for migrant workers now?	What were Ruby's experiences with white kids after her first year in school?	Why did all these people use nonviolence to get what they wanted? Do we still have problems with civil rights?

205

represented in the occupations of farmer, dancer, and weaver. In *Voices of the Alamo* (Garland, 2000), the author speaks in the voices of 16 characters whose lives lead up to the present day. She begins with an Indian woman of 1500 gathering nuts beside a river (presumably the San Antonio). She then gives voice to anonymous armored Spaniards and cowled priests, Tejanos and Texans, and finally to individuals such as General Santa Anna and David Crockett. The final voice belongs to a contemporary boy who records his impressions of seeing the Alamo for the first time.

The 2008 Newbery Award book *Good Masters! Sweet Ladies! Voices from a Medieval Village* (Schlitz, 2007) comprises monologues and dialogues featuring young people living in and around an English manor in 1255. The author offers first-person character sketches that build on each other to create a finer understanding of medieval life. Historical notes appear in the margins, and some double-page spreads carry short essays on topics related to individual narratives, such as falconry, the Crusades, and Jews in medieval society. Although often the characters' specific concerns are very much of their time, their outlooks and emotional states will be familiar to young people today. The book could be used to introduce social studies of the medieval time period or to provide background for reading the 2003 Newbery winner, *Crispin: The Cross of Lead* (Avi, 2002). Set in 14th-century England, this is the story of a village outcast, whose adolescent son is known only as "Asta's son." The boy learns his given name, Crispin, from the village priest. Crispin is fingered for murder by the manor steward, who declares him a "wolf's head" wanted dead or alive, preferably dead. Crispin flees and falls in with a traveling juggler. He eventually learns his true identity (he's the son of the lord of the manor) and finds his place. When discussing a historical event, Zarnowski (2006) suggested that educators have students develop T-charts, on one side listing what in the account is familiar in the past and *present* and on the other side, what is unfamiliar in the past. Table 7.13 shows a T-chart for the story of Marion Anderson, a famous Black singer of the mid-20th century, who was denied the right to sing to mixed audiences. (Based on *When Marion Sang* [Ryan, 2002] for elementary school students or *The Voice That Challenged a Nation: Marian Anderson and the Struggle for Equal Rights* [Freedman, 2004] for middle school students.)

Narratives can also provide a context for science lessons. For example, when beginning a unit on weather for third-grade students, a teacher read the book, *The Storm in the Night* (Stolz, 1990), in which a grandfather and a grandson sit out a storm while the grandfather tells about his fear of storms as a child. Following the story, children can be encouraged to share their experiences with storms. Then the legend, *How Thunder and Lightning Came to Be* (Harrell, 1995) can be read. In this story, two birds are given the task of figuring out a way to warn people of storms. Students can be told that this is one explanation for thunder and lightning and that they will be

TABLE 7.13 T-Chart for Familiar/Unfamiliar

What's Familiar Past and Present	What's Unfamiliar Past Only
• The songs she sang in church were the ones I sing • Working hard to get good at something • The Lincoln Memorial • Feeling good when you've accomplished your goal	• The music teacher was for whites only • Blacks not being allowed to attend concerts with whites • There was less prejudice in Europe than the United States • Marion have to go to Europe to sing • Listening to a concert on the radio

learning other explanations for thunder and lightning and other ways to warn people of storms. The informational storybook *The Magic School Bus inside a Hurricane* (Cole, 1995) can be used to introduce students to scientific principles of weather (including a scientific explanation of thunder and lightning and methods used to predict weather) in a combined narrative-expository format. Informational storybooks such those represented by the popular *Magic School Bus* books by Joanna Cole have the purposes and benefits of both narrative and expository texts. They can be especially helpful in transitioning students into expository texts (Leal, 1996). Compared to narrative or expository texts, informational storybooks have been shown to elicit richer discussion in elementary school students in several ways: (1) students used more of their prior knowledge along with the information gained from the text in constructing an understanding of both the story and the information, (2) they continued their discussions longer, (3) they made predictions twice as often, and (4) they exhibited a greater level of comprehension and were more likely to make extratextual connections to interpret this text (Leal, 1994; Maria & Junge, 1994).

Students must be aware that their comprehension is dependent on reading between the lines. They must recognize what information is explicitly stated in the text and what information they must bring to the interpretation of the text. Encouraging students to reflect on relationships between questions that can be asked of texts and their answers can develop their understanding of when inferencing is necessary. The following types of question–answer relationships are possible (Raphael, 1986):

- *Right there*, in which the answer is explicitly stated in the text
- *Think and search*, in which the answer is in the text but the words in the question and the words in the text are not the same or the answer is not in just one location
- *You and the author*, which involves thinking about what you have learned from the text and using what you already know to answer the question
- *On my own*, in which the question is motivated by some information in the text, but the answer has to be generated from students' prior knowledge

The following are questions asked about the book, *My Brother Martin* (Farris, 2003), a reflection of Martin Luther King's childhood told through the eyes of his sister:

- Right there: What was the best prank that Martin, his sister, and brother played on people when they were children?
- Think and search: What couldn't Martin, his sister, and his brother do as children because they were Black?
- You and the author: Why were the stories Martin's father told to the family as nourishing as food?
- On my own: What would you do if you saw an example of bigotry?

The ability to use cues is critical for comprehension of landscape of consciousness because a character's thoughts and feelings are often implied rather than explicitly stated (Barton, 1996). The clinician or teacher can discuss the types of cues present in texts and assist students in finding the cues. Table 7.14 lists the types of cues and provides examples from the story *Chinye* (Onyefulu, 1994), a West African version of Cinderella.

When we think of students reading, we think of them reading traditional texts or print, but in this multimedia world, students "read" many other types of "texts." They view pictures and movies, they listen to music and watch dances, and they handle objects or artifacts (coins, bones, fossils). These multimedia "texts" provide opportunities for students to think more deeply about concepts. Through the use of these materials, students can practice making observations and inferences in a setting that is engaging, but perhaps less taxing than traditional reading materials.

TABLE 7.14	Clues about Characters' Emotions

Category Name	Example
Character statements	The stepmother says: "What took you so long?" she demanded, glaring.
Character actions	She stretched out a hand and touched Chinye tenderly on the cheek.
Plot events	The stepmother sends Chinye into the forest at night for water.
Text features	!(exclamation points) "My life is bad enough already, without making my stepmother angry!"
Emotional vocabulary	Nkechi's eyes gleamed greedily.
Story setting	"Look, Mother," she said proudly when she got home. To reach the stream, Chinye had to go through the forest. Wild animals prowled there, and even on moonlit nights the bravest villagers stayed at home.
Character thoughts	The stepmother thinks: Why couldn't it have been Adanma (her daughter) who met the old woman. . . . Maybe it was not too late!
Story's mood	Note shifts in tone.
Author's style	The author may use pauses or different sizes of print to convey emotions or attitudes.

Educators and speech-language pathologists (SLPs) can encourage students to transfer the strategies from nontraditional to traditional texts.

Nokes (2008) suggests the use of an observation/inference chart (O/I chart). Students divide a sheet of paper into two sections, drawing a line down the center of the page from top to bottom. On the left-hand side they will list the observations they make about the text they are studying, and on the right-hand side they list the inferences they make based on those observations. They then draw lines between their observations and the inferences made from these observations. Figure 7.5 is based on students watching the first 2 minutes of a YouTube video of Martin Luther King's "I Have a Dream" speech. The video shows throngs of marchers carrying signs and singing "We Shall Overcome," the Washington monument and Lincoln memorial, the reflecting pool, an aerial view of the many thousands of persons crowded on the mall, and Martin Luther King beginning his speech.

When using the O/I chart, begin by explaining how to make good observations and how to use observations and background knowledge to make appropriate inferences. Students can make observations about anything they can see, hear, smell, taste, and touch through their senses or through instruments that magnify their senses. Using the O/I chart, students make educated guesses that are based on their observations. They must activate background knowledge as they consider their observations. If the inference is to be appropriate, it must be based on information observed in the text (or picture, video, or music) and the reader's relevant background knowledge. Students are often unaware of the inferences they make—and when they are aware, they are likely to make inappropriate inferences. By making students more aware of the inferential process, they should be more likely to make necessary and appropriate inferences in social and academic situations. They draw arrows linking inferences with observations that support it, with the arrows pointing from the observations toward the inference. Students should be asked to explain the bases for their inferences. As the O/I chart is completed, a complex system of arrows can develop because certain observations lead to more than one inference, and an inference is often based on more than one observation.

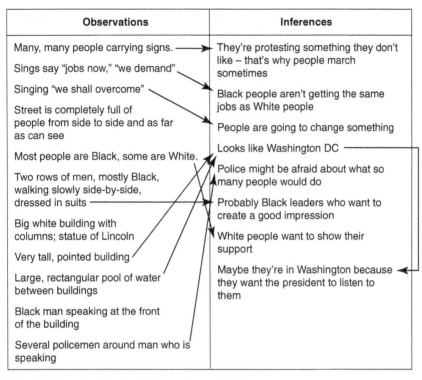

Observations	Inferences
Many, many people carrying signs.	They're protesting something they don't like – that's why people march sometimes
Sings say "jobs now," "we demand".	
Singing "we shall overcome"	Black people aren't getting the same jobs as White people
Street is completely full of people from side to side and as far as can see	People are going to change something
Most people are Black, some are White.	Looks like Washington DC
Two rows of men, mostly Black, walking slowly side-by-side, dressed in suits	Police might be afraid about what so many people would do
Big white building with columns; statue of Lincoln	Probably Black leaders who want to create a good impression
Very tall, pointed building	White people want to show their support
Large, rectangular pool of water between buildings	Maybe they're in Washington because they want the president to listen to them
Black man speaking at the front of the building	
Several policemen around man who is speaking	

FIGURE 7.5   O/L Chart for Intro to "I Have a Dream" Video

The students' observations and inferences can be evaluated by using a rubric such as the following:

- Observations
  1. Few observations
  2. Many observations but not specific or detailed
  3. Many observations, including ones that are specific and detailed
- Inferences linked to observations
  1. Some inferences, but they are not based on observations
  2. Bases inferences on observation, but does not show the relationship
  3. Bases inferences on observation and shows the relationship
- Inferences
  1. Makes few inferences or inferences that have no basis
  2. Several good inferences, but explanations may be fairly obvious
  3. Many good inferences, including ones that show depth of thinking

Using the evaluation rubric provides a means for documenting pre- and postintervention performance.

Students with language learning impairments may need support not only in inferencing, but also in making the initial observations. Bejos and colleagues (2009) differentiated the process of instruction on this activity by first having students label all the people, animals, and objects they saw in a picture; then label all the actions they saw; then write sentences with these observations; and finally make inferences. For example, students were shown Paul Revere's engraving of the Boston Massacre. Paul Revere used the incident to stir up the public's anti-British feelings. He made color prints from his engraving and distributed them around Boston. The prints did not paint an accurate picture of the event. On March 5, 1777, a mob of men and boys taunted a British soldier guarding the Boston Customs House. When other British soldiers came to his aid, there was a confused conflict in which the British fired shots into the crowd. Four Americans died, and a fifth died four days later. Six were wounded.

The students labeled what they saw: *British soldiers, dog, people, men and women, a man shot in the head.* The clinician elaborated, naming the people as colonists and noting that the men and women were unarmed. Next the students described the actions they saw: *British soldiers shooting people, a man was injured and people are picking him up, a dog is watching what's happening, the colonists are just standing there.* Next they were to write a summary interpretation of the picture by answering the question, "What happened on March 5, 1777?" For students with language learning disabilities, the SLP provided a cloze framework for them to complete. The words in parentheses were cues for the students. The underlined words are the words that were to be supplied by the students.

> The <u>British soldiers</u> (who) violently <u>shot</u> (verb) at <u>innocent</u> (what kind of) <u>villagers/colonists</u> (people). The <u>unarmed</u> (what kind of) men and women were <u>picking up</u> (doing what) the dead and <u>injured</u> (what kind of people). The dog was so <u>stunned</u> (how he felt) that he could not even <u>bark</u> (verb).

Finally they were asked: "According to the engraving who was at fault?" Why do you say this?

DEVELOPING TEXT GRAMMAR STRUCTURE.   In early elementary, a metanarrative approach can be incorporated into narrative activities to explicitly teach narrative structure. Narratives in Western tradition have a fairly characteristic structure. Explicit teaching of narrative structure has been shown to promote comprehension (Stetter & Hughes, 2010). Students can use story maps/graphic organizers as they identify the story elements: setting, initiating event, reaction, goal, attempts, consequences, and resolution. Because the narrative content drives narrative structure and narrative content typically centers on character goals, it is important that students be able to identify or make inferences about character goals (Lynch & van den Broek, 2007). To identify character goals, students must be able to recognize and understand the various plot elements of conflict and resolution (Macon, Bewell, & Vogt, 1991). To facilitate this identification, either during reading or after reading students can complete a chart that identifies a character, the character's goal or motivation, problems that the character faced, and how the character resolved (or failed to resolve) those problems. This strategy should help students generalize, recognize cause-and-effect relationships, and find main ideas.

The following example is based on the book *Percy Jackson & the Olympians: The Lightning Thief* (Riodan, 2005). This is the first of five books in the series that is popular among adolescents. Percy Jackson, the main character, is a 12-year-old boy diagnosed with dyslexia and ADHD. After being attacked by his math teacher, who is actually a Fury in disguise, he finds out that he is the son of Poseidon, the Greek god of the sea. He is brought to Camp Half-Blood (a camp for children with a Greek god and a human as parents) by his best friend, Grover, who turns out to be a satyr (half boy–half goat). He soon meets Annabeth, daughter of Athena, and they quickly become good friends. Percy is accused of stealing Zeus' masterbolt, the model for every lightning bolt made. He, Annabeth, and Grover are given 10 days to return the thunderbolt to Mount Olympus to prevent a war between the gods. (See

TABLE 7.15	Analyzing Conflict Resolution in Literature		
Somebody	**Wanted/Because**	**But**	**So**
Percy	to stop Medusa	if he looked at her when he swung his sword he would be turned to stone	he looked at her reflection in a mirror and swung his sword behind him
Grover	to get permission to go in search of Pan, the god of the fields because he has not been seen for many years	he had failed on his previous tasks	he had to prove himself by successfully protecting Percy
Annabeth	to leave Camp Half-Blood because she had not seen much of the real world	she could not live in the world with her stepfamily because she brought them into danger	going on the quest with Percy was a way to get out of camp

Table 7.15.) Because social studies' lessons often use narrative of historical figures, the strategy can also easily be adapted to social studies. (See Table 7.16.) Note that this activity also promotes the production of complex syntax.

A number of books published in the last 20 years do not follow the linear structure of a traditional story grammar. Such books can be classified as postmodern, a term used to describe attitudes, styles, and changes that have taken place in Western culture since World War II. Postmodern elements in books and movies include cynicism of traditional forms, reference to the process of producing the book or movie, encouraging the reader or viewer to coauthor the story, juxtaposing unrelated images, and creating nonlinear formats. These books represent a type of the new literacies that are increasingly common in the 21st century.

TABLE 7.16	Analyzing Conflict Resolution in Social Studies		
Somebody	**Wanted/Because**	**But**	**So**
President Thomas Jefferson	wanted to purchase a large amount of land in the middle of the continent because he felt uneasy about France and Spain having the power to block American trade	he did not know anything about the land he bought	he commissioned Lewis and Clark; the expedition was to explore the area and learn more about the Northwest's natural resources, inhabitants, and possibilities for settlement
Martin Luther King	wanted to end racial segregation and discrimination because Blacks were not treated fairly	he did not want to do this in a violent way	he used civil disobedience such as having people boycott riding buses

Postmodern picture books provide opportunities to develop these new literacies (Ansley, 2002). The following are common devices in postmodern picture books. Some books employ several of the devices.

- *Nontraditional ways of using plot, character, and setting, which challenge reader expectations and require different ways of reading.* Sometimes, this is a variation of a familiar story. In Wiesner's version of *The Three Pigs* (2001), the books begins predictably—the three pigs set out to seek their fortune, and when the first pig builds a house of straw, the wolf blows it down. But here the story changes. The wolf blows the pig right out of the picture and out of the story itself. In the following pictures, the story continues as expected: the wolf eats the pig and moves on to the other houses. But the pictures no longer match up. Pictures show the bewildered wolf searching hungrily through the rubble as first one, then all the pigs escape the illustrations and caper out into open space with the loose pages of the wolf's story swirling around them. After fashioning a paper airplane from one of these pages, the pigs soar off through blank white pages, then land and wander through other stories. The pigs eventually find and reassemble the pages to their own story and reenter to find the wolf still at the door. But here the story breaks down altogether, as the wolf flees, the text breaks apart, letters spill into a waiting basket, and the animals settle down to a bowl of alphabet soup instead of wolf stew.
- *Unusual uses of the narrator's voice to read the book in particular ways and through a particular character's eyes.* Sometimes the unusual use of voice raises issues of what is real—the story, the act of making the story, the characters, or the physical pages. The characters of the story may refer to themselves, the story, or the book. In *Aunt Isabel Tells a Good One* (Duke, 1992), a mouse named Penelope asks her aunt to tell a story. The aunt complies, but as she tells the story, she comments on elements of the story and asks for Penelope's assistance in deciding where and when the story happened, who would be in the story, what problem they would encounter, and what they should do about it. She explains to the reader how this transformation happened and pleads with readers to make her their pet.
- *A variety of genres in one text that require readers to employ a range of knowledge and grammars.* Content area textbooks and some nonfiction trade books are often a mixture of genres and picture representations. Pages in social studies and science books have text, pictures, graphs, and highlighted vocabulary. The student can read the material in any order, but they must integrate all elements if they are to comprehend the content fully. Each book in the *Magic School Bus* series by Joanna Cole includes three different genres on a page. There is the narrative story about the children's adventure (e.g., a trip through the waterworks, a volcano, or a hurricane), expository information about each of the topics (that generally appears in small notebook pages in the corner of each page of the book), and conversations among the children and Ms. Frizzle, their teacher, that appear in conversation bubbles. *The Pot That Juan Built* (Andrews-Goebel, 2002) combines factual information about Juan Quezada's life story in rural Mexico and his development as a renowned potter with a rhyme in the format of "This Is the House That Jack Built."

> *These are the flames so sizzling hot*
> *That flickered and flared and fired the pot,*
> *The beautiful pot that Juan built.*

- *New and unusual design and layout, which challenge the readers' perceptions of how to read a book.* The story may not progress in a logical sequential pattern. The text may be read left to right, right to left, or up and down. Some books have more than one story occurring simultaneously. Jan Brett has several books that involve multiple stories (e.g., *Trouble with Trolls,* 1992; *Gingerbread Baby,* 1999; *The Three Snow Bears*, 2007). In *Gingerbread Baby*, the reader follows the main story line of the escapades of the runaway Gingerbread Baby, while in the sidebars of pages, the reader observes a child making a gingerbread house, which he eventually uses to recapture the Gingerbread Baby. The book *Black and White* (Macaulay, 1990) appears to tell the story of an interruption in commuter train service and the impact on people's lives—or it is the story of a little boy's train ride, a burglar, or playful parents. Each double-page spread is divided into four sections. The first double-page spread shows what may be four titles—Seeing Things, Problem Parents, A Waiting Game, and Udder Chaos. How should the reader approach this book—should the reader approach it as one story, reading left to right and top to bottom, or should each story be read separately?

Changes in society and technology have produced new literacies. For example, computer media require students to master hypertext; that is, they must be able to integrate pieces of visual and print data within a single page and across multiple Web sites. Postmodern picture books have many of the textual features that have emerged as a result of changes in society and technology. These books require readers to process various representational forms, cope with unexpected structures, and consider multiple meanings. Students with specific language impairment (SLI) or learning disabilities (LD) experience difficulties acquiring an understanding of the stories that have a traditional structure. They will require guidance to discover the structure and meaning in postmodern texts. Although prediction and sequencing questions are useful for helping students comprehend traditional stories, they may not be equally successful for postmodern reading experiences. SLPs should consider using questions that provide students with an opportunity to think about the features of postmodern stories such as:

- Is there more than one story in this book? How do the two stories interrelate? Do the characters move from one story to another?
- Is there anything hidden from the characters that the readers know about? How does this make the student feel? How does this affect the story?
- Do the characters talk about the book, pages, or process of making a book? Do characters play with the pages of the book? What is real in the story?
- Are there any holes in the story? What is missing? How can the reader fix it?

Content does not guide the structure in expository texts—content on the same or similar topics can be presented in texts having a variety of structures. For example, the topic of global warming may be presented in terms of comparison/contrasts of theories of weather changes, a sequence of changes in the last century, causes and effects of global warming, or problems as a result of global warming and solutions to those problems. To facilitate comprehension of expository texts, teachers can explain the functions of different types of expository texts, identify the different types of texts, the organization of the types, the key words that students can look for, and complete graphic organizers that show the relationships between elements in the texts (DiCecco & Gleason, 2002; Finley & Seaton, 1987; Gajria, Jitendra, Sood, & Sacks, 2007; McGee & Richgels, 1985; Piccolo, 1987). Some examples of characteristics of expository texts are shown in Table 7.17.

TABLE 7.17 Expository Text Types and Characteristics

Text Type	Function	Key Words
Descriptive	Does the text tell me what something is?	for example, such as, to illustrate, characteristics
Sequence/Procedural	Does the text tell me how to do something or make something?	first . . . next . . . then, second . . . third, following this step, finally, before, after, previously, since
Cause/Effect	Does the text give reasons for why something happens?	because, since, reasons, then, therefore, for this reason, results, effects, consequently, so, in order, thus, then
Problem/Solution	Does the text state a problem and offer solutions to the problem?	a problem is, a solution is, if/then, so that
Comparison/Contrast	Is the text showing how two things are the same or different?	different, same, alike, similar, although, however, on the other hand, but, yet, still, rather than, instead of, in contrast, in comparison, nevertheless
Enumerative	Does the text give a list of things that are related to the topic?	an example is, for instance, another, next, finally

Summary

Comprehending text is essential if students are to become independent learners. There are many tests available to measure text comprehension, but only recently have attempts truly been made to teach comprehension. We cannot teach comprehension unless we understand what cognitive and linguistic abilities underlie the comprehension process. For many years it was assumed that if students were able to decode rapidly, comprehension would automatically follow. Although this does indeed appear to be the case for many typically developing students, it is not the case for students with language-learning disabilities.

In this chapter, procedures to assess and facilitate text comprehension were described. Adequate assessment would include evaluation of students' (1) literate language style, (2) physical and social world knowledge, and (3) ability to organize this conceptual knowledge into coherent texts. To assist students with learning disabilities in developing their reading comprehension abilities, we must facilitate students' development of text microstructures (literate vocabulary and syntactic patterns) and text macrostructures (content schemas and texts grammars). To do this, texts must be presented that are interesting and comprehensible to the students, and instruction must be differentiated to meet the needs of individual students. When differentiating instruction, educators and speech-language pathologists consider

- The specific aspects of the content to teach
- The process or strategies to use in teaching
- The products students will be asked to produce to demonstrate their learning and comprehension

References

Abrams, D., & Sutton-Smith, B. (1987). The development of the trickster in children's narrative. *Journal of American Folklore, 90*, 29–47.

Anderson, R. (1994). Role of the reader's schemata in comprehension, learning and memory. In R. B. Ruddell, M. Rapp, & H. Singer (Eds.), *Theoretical models and processes of reading* (4th ed., pp. 469–482). Newark, DE: International Reading Association.

Anglin, J. (1993). Vocabulary development: A morphological analysis. *Monographs of the Society for Research in Child Development, 58*(10), 1–166.

Ansley, M. (2002). "It's not all black and white": Postmodern picture books and new literacies. *Journal of Adolescent and Adult Literacy, 45*(6), 444–457.

Applebee, A. (1978). *The child's concept of story.* Chicago: Chicago University Press.

Baron-Cohen, S. (2007). *Mind reading.* Philadelphia: Jessica Kingsley.

Bartlett, F. (1932). *Remembering: A study in experimental social psychology.* Cambridge: Cambridge University Press.

Barton, J. (1996). Interpreting character emotions for literature comprehension. *Journal of Adolescent & Adult Literacy, 40*(1), 22–28.

Beaugrande, R. (1980). *Text, discourse, and process.* Norwood, NJ: Ablex

Beaugrande, R. (1984). Learning to read versus reading to learn: A discourse processing approach. In H. Mandl, N. Stein, & T. Trabasso (Eds.), *Learning and comprehension of text* (pp. 159–191). Hillsdale, NJ: Erlbaum.

Beck, I. L., McKeown, M. G., & Kucan, L. (2002). *Bringing words to life: Robust vocabulary instruction.* New York: Guilford.

Beck, I. L., McKeown, M. G., & Kucan, L. (2008). *Creating robust vocabulary.* New York: Guilford.

Bejos, K., Montano, C., & Westby, C. E. (2009). Differentiated academic language instruction for middle-school students. American Speech-Language-Hearing Convention.

Black, J. (1985). An exposition on understanding expository text. In B. Britton & J. Black (Eds.), *Understanding expository text* (pp. 249–267.) Hillsdale, NJ: Erlbaum.

Botvin, G., & Sutton-Smith, B. (1977). The development of structural complexity in children's fantasy narratives. *Developmental Psychology, 13*, 377–388.

Bower, G., Black, J., & Turner, J. (1979). Scripts in memory for texts. *Cognitive Psychology, 11*, 177–220.

Bransford, J. D. (1994). Schemata activation and schema acquisition: Comments on Richard C. Anderson's remarks. In R. B. Ruddell, M. Rapp, & H. Singer (Eds.), *Theoretical models and processes of reading* (4th ed., pp. 483–495). Newark, DE: International Reading Association.

Britton, B., Glynn, S., & Smith, J. (1985). Cognitive demands of processing expository text: A cognitive workbench model. In B. Bruce & J. Black (Eds.), *Understanding expository text* (pp. 227–248). Hillsdale, NJ: Erlbaum.

Brown, A. (1982). Learning how to learn from reading. In J. Langer & M. Smith-Burke (Eds.), *Reader meets author/Bridging the gap: A psycholinguistic and sociolinguistic perspective* (pp. 26–54). Newark, DE: International Reading Association.

Bruce, B. (1980). Plans and social action. In R. Spiro, B. Bruce, & W. Brewer (Eds.), *Theoretical issues in reading comprehension* (pp. 367–384). Hillsdale, NJ: Erlbaum.

Bruce, B., & Newman, D. (1978). Interacting plans. *Cognitive Science, 2*, 195–233.

Bruner, J. (1985). Narrative and paradigmatic modes of thought. In E. Eisner (Ed.), *Learning and teaching the ways of knowing* (pp. 97–115). Chicago: University of Chicago Press.

Bruner, J. (1986). *Actual minds, possible worlds.* Cambridge, MA: Harvard University Press.

Cain, K., & Oakhill, J. (Eds.). (2007). *Children's comprehension problems in oral and written language: A cognitive perspective.* New York: Guildford.

Chambliss, M. (1995). Text cues and strategies readers use to construct the gist of lengthy written arguments. *Reading Research Quarterly, 30*(4), 778–807.

Clark, M. (1976). *Young fluent readers.* London: Heinemann.

Cook-Gumperz, J., & Gumperz, J. (1981). From oral to written culture: The transition to literacy. In M. F. Whiteman (Ed.), *Variation in writing: Functional and linguistic differences* (pp. 90–109). Hillsdale, NJ: Erlbaum.

Cunningham, A. E., & Stanovich, K. E. (1997). Early reading acquisition and its relation to reading experience and ability 10 years later. *Developmental Psychology, 33*(6), 934–944.

DePaulo, B., & Jordan, A. (1982). Age changes in deceiving and detecting deceit. In R. Feldman (Ed.),

Development of nonverbal behavior in children (pp. 140–180). New York: Springer-Verlag.

Dewitz, P., & Dewitz, P. K. (2003). They can read the words, but they can't understand: Refining comprehension assessment. *The Reading Teacher, 56*(5), 422–435.

DiCecco, V., & Gleason, M. M. (2002). Using graphic organizers to attain relational knowledge from expository text. *Journal of Learning Disabilities, 35*, 306–320.

Dixon, C. (1979). Text type and children's recall. In M. Kamil & A. Moe (Eds.), *Reading research: Studies and applications.* Clemson, SC: National Reading Conference.

Durkin, D. (1966). *Children who read early.* New York: Teachers College Press.

Ebbers, S. M. (2004). *Vocabulary through morphemes: Suffixes, prefixes, and roots for intermediate grades.* Longmont, CO: Sopris West.

Eisenberg, S., Ukrainetz, T. A., Hsu, J. R., Kaderavek, J. N., Justice, L. M., & Gillam, R. B. (2008). Noun phase elaboration in children's spoken stories. *Language, Speech, and Hearing Services in Schools, 39*, 145–157.

Emery, D. W. (1996). Helping readers comprehend stories from the characters' perspective. *The Reading Teacher, 49*, 534–541.

Feagans, L., & Short, E. (1984). Developmental differences in the comprehension and production of narratives by reading disabled and normally achieving children. *Child Development, 55*, 1727–1736.

Feldman, C. F., Bruner, J., Renderer, B., & Spitzer, S. (1990). Narrative comprehension. In B. K. Britton & A. D. Pelligrini (Eds.), *Narrative thought and narrative language* (pp. 1–78). Hillsdale, NJ: Erlbaum.

Fillion, B., & Brause, R. (1987). Research into classroom practices: What have we learned and where are we going? In J. Squire (Ed.), *The dynamics of language learning* (pp. 291–225). Urbana, IL: ERIC.

Finley, C., & Seaton, M. (1987). Using text patterns and question prediction to study for tests. *Journal of Reading, 32*, 124–142.

Flood, J., & Lapp, D. (1987). Reading and writing relations: Assumptions and directions. In J. Squire (Ed.), *The dynamics of language learning* (pp. 9–26). Urbana, IL: ERIC.

Flood, J., Lapp, D., & Fisher, D. (2002). Parsing, questioning, and rephrasing (PQR): Building syntactic knowledge to improve reading comprehension. In C. C. Block, L. B. Gambrell, & M. Pressley (Eds.), *Improving comprehension instruction* (pp. 181–198). Newark, DE: IRA.

Ford, J. A., & Milosky, L. M. (2003). Inferring emotional reactions in social situations: Differences in children with language impairment. *Journal of Speech, Language & Hearing Research, 46*, 21–30.

Freedle, R., & Hale, G. (1979). Acquisition of new comprehension schemata for expository prose by transfer of a narrative schema. In R. Freedle (Ed.), *New directions in discourse processing* (pp. 121–134). Norwood, NJ: Ablex.

Fuchs, D., Fuchs, L. S., & Vaughn, S. (2008). *Response to intervention.* Newark DE: International Reading Association.

Gajria, M., Jitendra, A. K., Sood, S., & Sacks, G. (2007). Improving comprehension of expository text in students with LD: A research synthesis. *Journal of Learning Disabilities, 40*, 210–225.

Gambrell, L. B., & Javitz, P. B. (1993). Mental imagery, text illustrations, and children's story comprehension and recall. *Reading Research Quarterly 21*, 264–273.

Gillam, R., & Pearson, N. A. (2004). *Test of narrative language.* Austin, TX: Pro-Ed.

Glenn, C., & Stein, N. (1980). *Syntactic structures and real-world themes in stories generated by children* (Tech. Report). Urbana: University of Illinois.

Glod, M. (2008). Study questions "No Child" Act's reaching plan. *Washington Post*, Friday, May 2, 2008. Retrieved April 10, 2010, from http://www.washingtonpost.com/wp-dyn/content/article/2008/05/01/AR2008050101399.html

Graesser, A., & Goodman, S. (1985). Implicit knowledge, question answering and the representation of expository text. In B. Britton & J. Black (Eds.), *Understanding expository text* (pp. 109–171). Hillsdale, NJ: Erlbaum.

Graybeal, C. (1981). Memory for stories in language impaired children. *Applied Psycholinguistics, 2*, 269–283.

Hall, M., Ribovich, J., & Ramig, C. (1979). *Reading and the elementary school child.* New York: Van Nostrand.

Halliday, M. A. K., & Martin, J. R. (1993). *Writing science: Literacy and discursive power.* Pittsburgh, PA: University of Pittsburgh Press.

Hansen, C. (1978). Story retelling used with average and learning disabled readers as a measure of reading comprehension. *Learning Disability Quarterly, 1*, 62–69.

Harter, S. (1982). Children's understanding of multiple emotions: A cognitive developmental approach. In W. Overton (Ed.), *The relationship between social and cognitive development* (pp. 147–194). Hillsdale, NJ: Erlbaum.

Hoffman, J. (1992). Critical reading/thinking across the curriculum: Using I-charts to support learning. *Language Arts, 69*, 121–127.

Horowitz, R. (1985a). Text patterns: Part 1. *Journal of Reading, 28*, 448–454.

Horowitz, R. (1985b). Text patterns: Part ll. *Journal of Reading, 28*, 534–541.

Horowitz, S., & Samuels, S. J. (1987). Comprehending oral and written language: Critical contrasts for literacy and schooling. In R. Horowitz & S. J. Samuels (Eds.), *Comprehending oral and written language* (pp. 1–52). San Diego, CA: Academic Press.

Hunt, K. (1965). *Grammatical structures written at three grade levels.* Champaign, IL: NCTE Research Report 3.

Kalmar, I. (1985). Are there really no primitive languages? In D. Olson, N. Torrance, & A. Hildyard (Eds.), *Literacy, language, and learning.* New York: Cambridge University Press.

Kieras, D. (1985). Thematic processes in the comprehension of expository prose. In B. Britton & J. Black (Eds.), *Understanding expository text* (pp. 89–107). Hillsdale, NJ: Erlbaum.

Kintsch, W. (1998). *Comprehension: A paradigm for cognition.* New York: Cambridge University Press.

Lapp, D., & Flood, J. (1978). *Teaching reading to every child.* New York: Macmillan.

Leal, D. J. (1994). A comparison of third-grade children's listening comprehension of scientific information using an information book and an information storybook. In C. K. Kinzer & D. J. Leu (Eds.), *Multidimensional aspects of literacy research, theory, and practice* (pp. 137–145). Chicago: The National Reading Conference.

Leal, D. J. (1996). Transforming grand conversations into grand creations: Using different types of texts to influence student discussion. In L. B. Gambrell & J. F. Almasi (Eds.), *Lively discussions!* (pp. 149–168). Newark, DE: International Reading Association.

Leslie, L., & Caldwell, J. S. (2011). *Qualitative reading inventory–5.* Boston: Pearson.

Lewis, M., & Michalson, L. (1983). *Children's emotions and moods.* New York: Plenum.

Liles, B. (1985). Cohesion in the narratives of normal and language disordered children. *Journal of Speech and Hearing Research, 28*, 123–133.

Liles, B. (1987). Episode organization and cohesive conjunctives in narratives of children with and without language disorder. *Journal of Speech and Hearing Research, 30*, 185–196.

Lubliner, S. (2005). *Getting into words: Vocabulary instruction that strengthens comprehension.* Baltimore: Brookes.

Lucariello, J. (2004). New insights into the functions, development, and origins of theory of mind: The functional multilinear socialization model. In L. Lucariello et al. (Eds.), *The development of the mediated mind* (pp. 33–57). Mahwah, NJ: Erlbaum.

Lynch, J. S., & van den Broek, P. (2007). Understanding the glue of narrative structure: Children's on- and off-line inferences about characters' goals. *Cognitive Development, 22*, 323–340.

Macon, J. M., Bewell, D., & Vogt, M. (1991). *Responses to literature.* Newark, DE: International Reading Association.

Mandler, J. (1982). Some uses and abuses of a story grammar. *Discourse Processes, 5*, 305–318.

Mandler, J. (1984). *Stories, scripts, and scenes: Aspects of schema theory.* Hillsdale, NJ: Erlbaum.

Maria, K., & Junge, K. (1994). A comparison of fifth graders' comprehension and retention of scientific information using a science textbook and an informational storybook. In C. K. Kinzer & D. J. Leu (Eds.), *Multidimensional aspects of literacy research, theory, and practice* (pp. 146–152). Chicago: The National Reading Conference.

McGee, L., & Richgels, D. (1985). Teaching expository text structure to elementary students. *The Reading Teacher, 38*, 739–748.

Merritt, D., & Liles, B. (1987). Story grammar ability in children with and without language disorder: Story generation, story retelling, and story comprehension. *Journal of Speech and Hearing Research, 30*, 539–552.

Meyer, B. (1987). Following the author's top-level organization: An important skill for reading comprehension. In R. Tierney, P. Anders, & J. Mitchell (Eds.), *Understanding readers' understanding* (pp. 59–76). Hillsdale, NJ: Erlbaum.

Meyer, B., & Rice, G. (1984). The structure of text. In P. Pearson (Ed.), *Handbook of reading research* (pp. 319–351). New York: Longman.

Miller, J. (2010). Systematic analysis of language transcripts (SALT), English Version 2008 [Computer Software]. Madison, WI: SALT Software, LCC.

Morris, P. J., & Tchudi, S. (1996). *The new literacy: Moving beyond the 3Rs.* San Francisco: Jossey-Bass.

National Institute of Child Health and Human Development. (2000). *Report of the National Reading Panel. Teaching children to read: An evidence-based assessment of the scientific research literature on reading and its implications for reading instruction* (NIH Publication No. 00–4769). Washington, DC: U.S. Government Printing Office.

Nelson, J. R., & Marchand-Martella, N. (2005). *The multiple meaning vocabulary program.* Boston: Sopris West.

Nelson, K. (1985). *Making sense: The acquisition of shared meaning.* Orlando, FL: Academic Press.

New London Group. (1996). A pedagogy of multiliteracies: Designing social futures. *Harvard Educational Review, 66*(1), 60–93.

Nilsen, A. P., & Nilsen, D. (2006). Latin revived: Source based vocabulary lessons courtesy of Harry Potter. *Journal of Adolescent & Adult Literacy, 50*(2), 128–134.

Nippold, M. A., Hesketh, L. J., Duthie, J. K., & Mansfield, T. C. (2005). Conversational versus expository discourse: A study of syntactic development in children, adolescents, and adults. *Journal of Speech, Language, and Hearing Research, 48*, 1048–1064.

Nokes, J. D. (2008). The observation/inference chart: Improving students' abilities to make inferences while reading nontraditional texts. *Journal of Adolescent & Adult Literacy, 51*(7), 538–546.

Oakhill, J., & Yuill, N. (1996). Higher order factors in comprehension disability: Processes and remediation. In C. Cornoldi & J. Oakhill (Eds.), *Reading comprehension difficulties: Processes and intervention* (pp. 69–92). Mahwah, NJ: Erlbaum.

Obanya, P. (2003). Towards a reading society. In A. E. Arua (Ed.), *Reading for all in Africa* (pp. 2–6). Newark, DE: International Reading Association.

Otto, W., & White, S. (Eds.). (1982). *Reading expository material.* New York: Academic Press.

Owens, R. (2007). *Language development: An introduction.* Boston: Allyn & Bacon.

Paris, A. H., & Paris, S. G. (2001). *Children's comprehension of narrative picture books.* Ann Arbor, MI: University of Michigan. Retrieved April 1, 2010, from http://www.ciera.org/library/reports/inquiry-3/3-012/3-012.pdf

Pearson, P. D., & Fielding, L. (1991). Comprehension instruction. In R. Barr, M. L. Kamil, P. Mosenthal, & P. D. Pearson (Eds.), *Handbook of reading research* (pp. 815–860, Vol. II). White Plains, NY: Longman.

Perfetti, C., (1997). Sentences, individual differences, and multiple texts: Three issues in text comprehension. *Discourse Processes, 23*, 337–355.

Piccolo, J. (1987). Expository text structure: Teaching and learning strategies. *The Reading Teacher, 40*, 838–847.

Raphael, T. E. (1986). Teaching question/answer relationships, revisited. *The Reading Teacher, 39*, 516–522.

Reading First Impact Study: Interim Report. (2008). Retrieved 4/6/10 from http://ies.ed.gov/ncee/pdf/20084019.pdf

Richgels, D., McGee, L., Lomax, R., & Sheard, C. (1987). Awareness of four text structures: Effects on recall of expository text. *Reading Research Quarterly, 22*, 177–197.

Romero, L. (2002). At-risk students: Learning to break through comprehension barriers. In C. C. Block, L. B. Gambrell, & M. Pressley (Eds.), *Improving comprehension instruction: Rethinking research, theory, and classroom practice* (pp. 354–369). San Francisco: Jossey-Bass.

Roth, F., & Spekman, N. (1986). Narrative discourse: Spontaneously generated stories of learning disabled and normally achieving students. *Journal of Speech and Hearing Disorders, 51*, 8–23.

Rumelhart, D. (1980). Schemata: The building blocks of cognition. In R. Spiro, B. Bruce, & W. Brewer (Eds.), *Theoretical issues in reading comprehension* (pp. 33–58). Hillsdale, NJ: Erlbaum.

Saenz, L. M., & Fuchs, L. S. (2002). Examining the reading difficulty of secondary students with learning disabilities. *Remedial & Special Education, 23*, 31–42.

Scardamelia, M., & Bereiter, C. (1984). Development of strategies in text processing. In H. Mandl, N. Stein, & T. Trabasso (Eds.), *Learning and comprehension of text* (pp. 379–406). Hillsdale, NJ: Erlbaum.

Schank, R., & Abelson, R. (1977). *Scripts plans goals and understanding.* Hillsdale, NJ: Erlbaum.

Schumm, J. C., Vaughn, S., & Leavell, A. G. (1994). Planning pyramid: A framework for planning for diverse students' needs during content instruction. *The Reading Teacher, 47,* 608–615.

Scott, C. (1994). A discourse continuum for school-age students. In G. Wallach & K. Butler (Eds.), *Language learning disabilities in school-age children and adolescents* (pp. 219–252). New York: Merrill.

Sinclair, J. (2006). *Collins COBUILD learners' dictionary.* Glasgow, Scotland: HarperCollins.

Snow, C. (2002). *Reading for understanding: Toward an R & D program in reading comprehension.* Santa Monica, CA: Rand Corporation.

Spiro, R., & Taylor, B. (1987). On investigating children's transition from narrative to expository discourse: The multidimensional nature of psychological text classification. In R. Tierney, P. Anders, & J. Michell (Eds.), *Understanding readers' understanding* (pp. 77–93). Hillsdale, NJ: Erlbaum.

Stein, N., & Glenn, C. (1979). An analysis of story comprehension in elementary school children. In R. Freedle (Ed.), *New directions in discourse processing*, II (pp. 53–120). Norwood, NJ: Ablex.

Stein, N., & Policastro, M. (1984). The concept of story: A comparison between children's and teacher's viewpoints. In H. Mandl, N. Stein, & T. Trabasso (Eds.), *Learning and comprehension of text* (pp. 113–155). Hillsdale, NJ: Erlbaum.

Stetter, M. E., & Hughes, M. J. (2010). Using story grammar to assist students with learning disabilities and reading disabilities improve their comprehension. *Education and Treatment of Children, 33*, 115–151.

Tapiero, I. (2007). *Situation models and levels of coherence: Toward a definition of comprehension.* Mahwah, NJ: Erlbaum.

Thorndyke, P. (1977). Cognitive structures in comprehension and memory of narrative discourse. *Cognitive Psychology, 9*, 77–110.

Tomlinson, C. (2001). *How to differentiate instruction in mixed-ability classrooms* (2nd ed.). Alexandria, VA: Association for Supervision and Curriculum Development. ED 386 301.

Tough, J. (1981). *Talk for teaching and learning.* Portsmouth, NH: Heinemann.

Unsworth, L. (1999). Developing critical understanding of the specialised language of school science and history texts: A functional grammar perspective. *Journal of Adolescent & Adult Literacy, 42*(7), 508–521.

Vacca, J. A., Vacca, R. T., & Grove, M. K. (1991). *Reading and learning to read.* New York: Harper Collins.

van Dijk, T., & Kintsch, W. (1983). *Strategies of discourse comprehension.* New York: Academic Press.

van Kleeck, A., & Vander Woulde, J. (2003). Book sharing with preschool children with language delays. In A. van Kleeck, S. A. Stahl, & E. B. Bauer (Eds.), *On reading books to children* (pp. 58–92). Mahwah, NJ: Erlbaum.

Voss, J., & Bisanz, G. (1985). Knowledge and the processing of narrative and expository text: Some methodological issues. In B. Britton & J. Black (Eds.), *Understanding expository text* (pp. 385–391). Hillsdale, NJ: Erlbaum.

Watson, S., & Houtz, L. E. (2002). Teaching science: Meeting the academic needs of culturally and linguistically diverse students. *Intervention in School and Clinic, 37*, 267–268.

Weaver, P., & Dickinson, D. (1979). Story comprehension and recall in dyslexic students. *Bulletin of Orton Society, 28*, 157–171.

Wells, G. (1986). *The meaning makers.* Portsmouth, NH: Heinemann.

Westby, C.E. (1984). The development of narrative language abilities. In G. P. Wallach & K. G. Butler (Eds.), *Language learning disabilities in school-age children* (pp. 103–127). Baltimore: Williams & Wilkins.

Westby, C. E. (1985). Learning to talk—Talking to learn: Oral/literate language differences. In C. S. Simon (Ed.), *Communication skills and classroom success.* San Diego: College Hill Press.

Wilensky, R. (1978). Why John married Mary: Understanding stories involving recurring goals. *Cognitive Science, 2*, 235–266.

Williams, J. P. (1998). Improving the comprehension of disabled readers. *Annals of Dyslexia, 48*, 213–238.

Wolf, D., & Hicks, D. (1989). The voices of narratives: The development of intertextuality in young children's stories. *Discourse Processes, 12*, 329–351.

Wolf, M., Miller, L., & Donnelly, K. (2000). Retrieval, automaticity, vocabulary elaboration, orthography (RAVE-O): A comprehensive, fluency-based reading intervention program. *Journal of Learning Disabilities, 33*, 375–387.

Yuill, N., & Oakhill, J. (1991). *Children's problems in text comprehension: An experimental investigation.* New York: Cambridge University Press.

Zarnowski, M. (2006). *Making sense of history.* New York: Scholastic.

Zwiers, J. (2008). *Building academic language: Essential practices for content classrooms.* Newark, DE: International Reading Association.

Zwiers, J. (2010). *Building reading comprehension habits in grades 6–12: A toolkit of classroom activities.* Newark, DE: International Reading Association.

Children's Books

Aardema, V. (1975). *Why mosquitoes buzz in people's ears.* New York: Dial.

Aliki (1984). *Feelings.* New York: Greenwillow.

Andrews-Goebel, N. (2002). *The pot that Juan built.* New York: Lee and Low Books.

Aruego, J., & Aruego, A. (1972). *The crocodile's tale.* New York: Scholastic.

Asbjornsen, P., & Moe, J. (1957). *The three billy goats gruff.* New York: Harcourt Brace Jovanovich.

Avi (2002). *Crispin: The cross of lead.* New York: Hyperion.

Bernhard, E. (1993). *How snowshoe hare rescued the sun: A tale from the Arctic.* New York: Holiday House.

Bourgeois, P. (1986). *Franklin in the dark.* New York: Scholastic.

Brett, J. (1992). *Trouble with trolls.* New York: Scholastic.

Brett, J. (1999). *Gingerbread baby.* New York: Putnam.

Brett, J. (2007). *The three snow bears.* New York: Putnam.

Bridges, R. (1999). *Through my eyes.* New York: Scholastic.

Brown, A. (1998). *Voices in the park.* New York: DK Publishing.

Calhoun, M. (1979). *Cross-country cat*. New York: Mulberry Books.

Carle, E. (1969). *The very hungry caterpillar*. New York: Philomel.

Cole, J. (1995). *The magic school bus inside a hurricane*. New York: Scholastic.

Cooper, S. (1973). *The dark is rising*. New York: Atheneum.

Curtis, J. A. (1998). *Today I feel silly: And other moods that make my day*. New York: Joanna Cotler.

Dayrell, E. (1968). *Why the sun and the moon live in the sky*. New York: Houghton Mifflin.

dePaola, T. (1974). *Charlie needs a cloak*. Englewood Cliffs, NJ: Prentice Hall.

dePaola, T. (1981). *Fin M'Coul: The giant of Knockmany hill*. New York: Holiday House.

Duke, K. (1992). *Aunt Isabel tells a good one*. New York: Dutton.

Farris, C. K. (2003). *My brother Martin: A sister remembers*. New York: Simon & Schuster.

Freedman, R. (2004). *The voice that challenged a nation: Marion Anderson and the struggle for equal rights*. New York: Clarion Books.

Gag, W. (1928). *Millions of cats*. New York: Coward, McCann, and Geoghegan.

Galdone, P. (1970). *The three little pigs*. New York: Clarion Books.

Garland, S. (2000). *Voices of the Alamo*. New York: Scholastic.

Goble, P. (1989). *Iktomi and the berries*. New York: Orchard.

Goble, P. (1990). *Iktomi and the ducks*. New York: Orchard.

Harrell, B. (1995). *How thunder and lightning came to be*. New York: Dial.

Hoffman, M. (1991). *Amazing Grace*. New York: Dial.

Kasza, K. (1987). *The wolf's chicken stew*. New York: G.P. Putnam's Sons.

Keams, G. (1995). *Grandmother spider brings the sun*. Flagstaff, AZ: Northland.

Keats, E. (1962). *The snowy day*. New York: Viking.

Kent, J. (1982). *Round robin*. Englewood Cliffs, NJ: Prentice Hall.

Krull, K. (2003). *Harvesting hope: The story of Caesar Chavez*. Harcourt Brace.

Laird, D. (1981). *The three little Hawaiian pigs and the magic shark*. Honolulu: Barnaby Books.

Laird, D. (1983). *Wili Wai Kula and the three mongooses*. Honolulu: Barnaby Books.

L'Engle, M. (1962). *Wrinkle in time*. New York: Dell.

Levitt, P. M., Burger, D. A., & Guralnick, E. S. (2000). *The weighty word book*. Albuquerque: University of New Mexico Press.

Lichtenheld, T. (2003). *What are you so grumpy about?* Boston: Little Brown.

Lowell, S. (1992). *The three little javelinas*. Flagstaff, AZ: Northland Publishing.

Lowry, L. (1993). *The giver*. New York: Random House.

Macauley, D. (1991). *Black and white*. New York: Putnam.

MacLachlan, P. (1985). *Sarah, plain and tall*. New York: Harper and Row.

Martin, R. (1993). *The boy who lived with the seals*. New York: G.P. Putnam.

Mayer, M. (1974). *Frog goes to dinner*. New York: Dial.

Mayer, M. (2003). *A boy, a dog, and a frog*. New York: Dial.

Mayer, M., & Mayer, M. (1971). *A boy, a dog, a frog, and a friend*. New York: Dial.

Mayer, M., & Mayer, M. (1975). *One frog too many*. New York: Dial.

McDermott, G. (1993). *Raven: A trickster tale from the Pacific Northwest*. San Diego: Harcourt Brace.

Meddaugh, S. (1997). *Cinderella's rat*. New York: Houghton Mifflin

Meyer, S. (2005). *Twilight*. New York: Little, Brown.

Mochizuki, K. (1997). *Passage to freedom: The Sugihara story*. New York: Lee and Low Books.

Morley, J. (2009). *You wouldn't want to be an American colonist: A settlement you'd rather not start*. New York: Franklin Watts.

Oakley, G. (1981). *Hetty and Harriet*. New York: Atheneum.

Petach, (1995). *Goldilocks and the three hares*. New York: Grosset & Dunlap.

Rayner, M. (1976). *Mr. and Mrs. Pig's evening out*. New York: Atheneum.

Rayner, M. (1977). *Garth Pig and the ice cream lady*. New York: Atheneum.

Ringgold, F. (1999). *If a bus could talk: The story of Rosa Parks*. New York: Aladdin.

Riordan, R. (2005). *Percy Jackson & the Olympians: The lightning thief*. New York: Hyperion Books.

Rodda, E. (1993). *Rowan of Rin*. New York: Scholastic.

Rowling, J. K. (2003). *Harry Potter and the order of the phoenix*. New York: Scholastic.

Rowling, J. K. (2007). *Harry Potter and the deathly hallows*. New York: Scholastic.

Ryan, P. M. (2000). *Esperanza rising*. New York: Scholastic.

Ryan, P. M. (2002). *When Marion sang*. New York: Clarion.

Sachar, L. (2000). *Holes*. New York: Random House.

Schlitz, L. A. (2007). *Good masters! Sweet ladies! Voices from a medieval village*. New York: Candlewick Press.

Scieszka, J. (1996). *The true story of the three little pigs.* New York: Puffin.

Selznick, B. (2007). *The invention of Hugo Cabret.* New York: Scholastic.

Shorto, R. (1990). *The untold story of Cinderella.* New York: Citadel Press.

Snicket, L., (2006). *A series of unfortunate events: Book of the thirteenth.* New York: HarperCollins.

Soto, G. (1993). *Too many tamales.* New York: Putnam & Grosset.

Stead, R. (2009). *When you reach me.* New York: Wendy Lamb Books.

Stein, R. L. (1992). *Monster blood.* New York: Scholastic.

Stolz, M. (1990). *Storm in the night.* New York: Harper & Row.

Tolhurst, M. (1994). *Somebody and the three Blairs.* New York: Orchard.

Trivizas, E. (1993). *The three little pigs and the big bad wolf.* New York: Simon & Schuster.

Waddell, M. (1995). *Farmer duck.* New York: Scholastic.

Wagner, J. (1977). *John Brown, Rose and the midnight cat.* Scarsdale: Bradbury Press.

Walton, M. (2007). *Just me and 6,000 rats: A tale of conjunctions.* Salt Lake City, UT: Gibbs Smith.

Wiesner, D. (2001). *The three little pigs.* New York: Clarion.

Winters, K. (2003). *Voices of ancient Egypt.* Washington, DC: National Geographic Society.

Wood, A. (1996). *The Bunyans.* New York: The Blue Sky Press.

Appendix *7.1*

Books to Develop Connectives/Complex Clauses

RELATIVE CLAUSES

Aardema, V. (1981). *Bringing the rain to Kapiti plain*. New York: Dial.

Andrews-Goebel, N. (2002). *The pot that Juan built*. New York: Lee and Low Books.

Gag, W. (1928). *Millions of cats*. New York: Coward, McCann, & Geoghegan.

Rogers, J. (1968). *The house that Jack built*. New York: Lothrop, Lee, and Shepard.

Sierra, J. (1995). *The house that Drac built*. San Diego: Harcourt Brace.

Sloat, T. (2002). *There was an old lady who swallowed a trout*. New York: Henry Holt.

Taback, S. (1997). *There was an old lady who swallowed a fly*. New York: Viking.

BUT

Carle, E. (1969). *The very hungry caterpillar*. New York: Philomel.

Carle, E. (1990). *The very quiet cricket*. New York: Putnam.

Carle, E. (1995). *The very lonely firefly*. New York: Putnam.

Fox, M. (1995). *Wombat divine*. New York: Scholastic.

Mayer, M. (1975). *Just for you*. Racine, WI: Western Publishing Co.

Shulevitz, U. (1967). *One Monday morning*. New York: Scribners.

IF-THEN

Levine, E. (1990). *If you lived at the time of Martin Luther King*. New York: Scholastic.

Levine, E. (1993). *If you traveled on the underground railroad*. New York: Scholastic. (There are others in this series.)

Mayer, M. (1968). *If I had*. New York: Dial.

Most, B. (1978). *If the dinosaurs came back*. New York: Harcourt.

Numeroff, L. J. (1985). *If you give a mouse a cookie*. New York: HarperCollins.

Numeroff, L. J. (2000). *If you give a pig a pancake*. New York: HarperCollins. (There are others in this series.)

Paterson, D. (1977). *If I were a toad*. New York: Dial.

ADVERBIAL CONNECTIVES AND ADVERBS

Ahlberg, A. (2007). *Previously*. Cambridge, MA: Candlewick Press.

Feiffer, J. (1999). *Meanwhile*. New York: HarperCollins.

Mayer, M. (1983). *When I get bigger*. Racine, Wl: Western Publishing Co.

McNaughton, C. (2002). *Suddenly!* New York: HarperCollins.

Nobel, T. (1992). *Meanwhile back at the ranch*. New York: Puffin.

Rylant, C. (1982). *When I was young in the mountains*. New York: E. P. Dutton.

Walton, R. (2004). *Suddenly alligator: An adverbial tale*. Salt Lake City, UT: Gibbs Smith.

Appendix *7.2*

Cinderella Stories

Brown, M. (1954). *Cinderella*. New York: Macmillan. (French version)

Bernhard, E., & Berhard, D. (1994). *The girl who wanted to hunt: A Siberian tale*. New York: Holiday House. (A young girl uses her skills as a hunter to avenge her father's death and to escape her evil stepmother.)

Climo, S. (1989). *The Egyptian Cinderella*. New York: Harper Collins Publishers.

Climo, S. (1993). *The Korean Cinderella*. New York: HarperCollins.

Climo, S. (1996). *The Irish Cinderlad*. New York: HarperCollins. (An Irish version with a boy with big feet instead of a girl with small feet.)

Climo, S. (1999). *The Persian Cinderella*. New York: HarperCollins.

Coburn, J. R. (1996). *Jouanah: A Hmong Cinderella*. Arcadia, CA: Shen's Books.

Cobrun, J. R. (1998). *Angkat: The Cambodian Cinderella*. Arcadia, CA: Shen's Books.

Coburn, J. R. (2000). *Domitila: A Cinderella tale from the Mexican tradition*. Arcadia, CA: Shen's Books.

Delamare, D. (1993). *Cinderella*. New York: Simon & Schuster. (Italian version)

de la Paz, M. J. (2001). *Abadeha: The Philippine Cinderella*. Arcadia, CA: Shen's Books.

de Paola, T. (2002). *Adelita: A Mexican Cinderella story*. New York: G.P. Putnam's Sons.

Dwyer, M. (2004) *The salmon princess: An Alaskan Cinderella*. Sasquatch Books

Edwards, P. D. (1997). *Dinorella: A prehistoric fairy tale*. New York: Hyperion Paperbacks.

Ehrlich, A. (1985). *Cinderella*. New York: Dial. (French)

Grimm (1978). *Cinderella*. New York: Larousse. (German)

Han, O. S. (1996). *Kongi and Potgi: A Cinderella story from Korea*. New York: Dial.

Hayes, J. (2000). *Little Gold Star/Estrellita de Oro: A Cinderella story*. El Paso, TX: Cinco Puntos Press. (A Spanish Southwest version)

Hebert, S. (1998). *Cendrillon: A Cajun Cinderella*. Gretna, LA: Pelican.

Hickox, R. (1998). *The Golden Sandal: A Middle Eastern Cinderella story*. New York: Holiday House.

Jackson, E. (1994). *Cinder Edna*. New York: Lothrop, Lee & Shepard (Modern day version)

Jaffe, N. (1998). *The way meat loves salt: A Cinderella tale from the Jewish tradition*. New York: Henry Holt and Co.

Johnston, T. (1998). *Bigfoot Cinderrrrella*. New York: G.P. Putnam's Sons.

Lewis, S. (1994). *Cinderella: Lamb Chop's play along*. New York: Bantam Doubleday Dell.

Louie, A. (1982). *Yeh-Shen: A Cinderella story from China*. New York: Philomel.

Lum, D. (1994). *The golden slipper*. New York: Troll Associates. (Vietnamese Cinderella)

Macauley, D. (1991). *Black and white*. New York: Putnam.

Marceau-Chenkie, B. (1999). *Naya: The Inuit Cinderella.* Yellowknife, Yukon: Raven Rock Publishing.

Martin, R. (1992). *The rough-face girl.* New York: G.P. Putnam's Sons. (Algonquin Indian version)

Mayer, M. (1994). *Baba Yaga and Vasilisa the brave.* New York: Morrow Junior Books. (Russian Cinderella)

Meddah, S. (1997). *Cinderella's rat*. Boston: Houghton Mifflin.

Mehta, L. (1997). *The enchanted anklet: From India.* Toronto: Lilmur Publishing.

Minters, F. (1994). *Cinder-Elly*. New York: Viking. (An inner-city rap version of Cinderella)

Nhuan, N. (1995). *Tam Cam: A Vietnamese Cinderella story*. Arcadia, CA: Shen's Books.

Onyefulu, O. (1994). *Chinye: A West African folk tale*. New York: Viking.

Perlman, J. (1992). *Cinderella penguin*. New York: Puffin.

Pollock, P. (1996). *Turkey girl: A Zuni Cinderella*. Boston: Little, Brown. (A Southwest Pueblo Indian version)

San Souci, R. D. (1989). *The talking eggs*. New York: Scholastic. (Southern (Cajun or Gulluh) Cinderella story)

San Souci, R. D. (1994). *Sootface: An Ojibwa Cinderella story*. New York: Bantam Doubleday Dell.

San Souci, R. D. (1998). *Cendrillon*. New York: Simon and Schuster. (A Caribbean Cinderella)

San Souci, R. D. (2000). *Cinderella skeleton*. San Diego: Harcourt.

San Souci, R. D. (2000). *The Little Gold Star: A Spanish American Cinderella tale*. New York: HarperCollins.

Schroeder, A. (1997). *Smoky Mountain Rose: An Appalachian Cinderella*. New York: Dial Books.

Shorto, R. (1990). *The untold story of Cinderella*. New York: Citadel Press. (Told from the perspective of Cinderella's stepsisters)

Sierra, J. (2000). *The gift of the crocodile: A Cinderella tale*, New York: Simon & Schuster. (An Indonesian version)

Silverman, E. (1999). *Raisel's riddle*. New York: Farrar, Straus and Giroux. (Jewish version)

Spiegelman, A. (1997). *Open me . . . I'm a dog!* New York: HarperCollins.

Steptoe, J. (1987). *Mufaro's beautiful daughters*. New York: Scholastic. (African Cinderella)

Takayama, E. (1997). *Sumorella: A Hawaiian Cinderella story*. Honolulu: Bess Press.

Thaler, M. (1997). *Cinderella bigfoot*. New York: Scholastic.

Velarde, P. (1989). *Old father story teller*. Santa Fe: Clear Light. (A collection of tribal legends from Santa Clara Pueblo, including Turkey Girl, a version of Cinderella)

Walton, R. (2005). *Cinderella* CTR. Orem, UT: Halestorm. (Mormon version)

Wegman, W. (1993). *Cinderella*. New York: Hyperion Books. (Dog version of Cinderella)

Chapter 8

Spelling Assessment and Intervention: A Multiple Linguistic Approach to Improving Literacy Outcomes

Kenn Apel, Julie J. Masterson, and Danielle Brimo

. . . the English alphabet is pure insanity . . . It can hardly spell any word in the language with any degree of certainty.

—MARK TWAIN, N.D.

Twain's quote mirrors many individuals' feelings towards English spelling; spelling is a difficult, disagreeable task. They see spelling as an illogical, nonsensical activity in which one must engage on a daily basis and is a constant reminder of the dreaded "Friday Test" of their youth. One can hardly fault such feelings and thoughts. The traditional type of spelling instruction associated with the Friday Test involves repetitive, rote memorization activities to learn words that often have little in common with each other with the exception sometimes of meaning. In addition, there was no instruction on why words are spelled as they are. For some individuals, this type of spelling instruction was the linguistic equivalent of physical education class. Further, it often led to poor retention (e.g., Gill & Scharer, 1996) and, as evidenced by Twain's comments, ill feelings about spelling.

Spelling is not illogical; it is a language skill with a high degree of sense to its construction (Masterson & Apel, 2007). Indeed, only about 4 percent of English words are truly irregular or nonsensical (Hanna, Hanna, Hodges, & Rudorf, 1966; Moats 2005/2006). Unfortunately, the linguistic nature of spelling, and the language knowledge that leads to accurate spellings, remains relatively unknown to most teachers (e.g., Moats, 2009). The traditional spelling instruction approach, which remains the dominant teaching method (Fresch, 2003), does not expose children to the underlying language knowledge that contributes to accurate spelling. Inaccurate spelling and poor understanding of the language knowledge that supports it can negatively affect other literacy skills, such as reading (e.g., Ehri, 2000). In this chapter, we begin by providing an overview of the underlying language knowledge that supports spelling (and reading), evidence for the association between spelling and other literacy skills, and two theories for spelling development. We then discuss a spelling assessment approach we have advocated for over a decade that carefully assesses this language knowledge to aid in developing optimal instructional practices (e.g., Masterson & Apel, 2000). We conclude with instruction/intervention procedures, some of which are empirically validated, that collectively make up a multilinguistic instructional approach that leads to improvements in spelling, reading, and writing (Wolter, 2009).

THE LANGUAGE BASIS OF SPELLING

We often talk about the four "language knowledge blocks" that serve as the foundation for spelling as well as word-level reading (e.g., Apel & Masterson, 2001; Masterson & Apel, 2010a,b). These four blocks represent knowledge of how phonology, orthography, morphology, and semantics affect spelling. Awareness and use of these language blocks allow individuals to know why words are spelled the way they are and to spell new words for which they have no word-specific knowledge. When individuals use these language knowledge blocks successfully to spell and read new words, they then develop mental images of those words. These word-specific mental representations, which we label as mental graphemic representations (MGRs), can be applied later to spell and read words effortlessly and efficiently. In the following section, we describe the four foundational language knowledge blocks that support spelling, including word-specific MGRs.

Phonological Knowledge

As discussed earlier in this text (see Chapter 4), use of phonological knowledge, or phonemic awareness, involves a conscious, active ability to consider and manipulate the individual phonemes, or sounds, in words. A considerable body of empirical documentation for the importance of the use of phonological knowledge for early reading and spelling development exists (e.g., Ball & Blachman, 1991; National Institute of Child Health and Human Development [NICHD], 2000). When spelling unknown words, individuals use their phonological knowledge to segment words into their individual phonemes. Once this is done, they then can apply their orthographic and morphological knowledge to represent those sounds.

Orthographic Pattern Knowledge

Orthographic knowledge, in its broadest sense, is the knowledge required to represent spoken language in writing (Apel, in review). Orthographic knowledge is comprised of two separate knowledge sources or components. One of these knowledge sources, word-specific memories or MGRs, is discussed later. The other component of orthographic knowledge is orthographic pattern knowledge. Orthographic pattern knowledge is the knowledge of the set of patterns or conventions individuals apply when translating speech into print (e.g., Apel, in review; Masterson & Apel, 2000). Orthographic pattern knowledge encompasses several types of patterns, including letter–sound knowledge (i.e., knowing which letter or letters represent specific phonemes, such as using "c", "ck", "k", or "ch" for the /k/) and knowledge of allowable letter combinations (e.g., "dr" is an allowable letter combination; "jr" is not). It also includes knowledge of principles governing spelling of base words or roots (e.g., long and short vowel patterns) and knowledge for positional constraints for letters (e.g., "ck" can be used in the medial or final position of words, but not the initial).

For many individuals, explicit knowledge of orthographic patterns tends to be limited to letter–sound correspondence and some basic orthographic conventions learned via mnemonics (e.g., "when two vowels go walking, the first one does the talking"). This likely is the case because traditional spelling instruction does not focus on requiring children to actively think of orthographic principles. However, the ability to consciously consider orthographic patterns is associated with and predicts spelling abilities (e.g., Apel, Wilson-Fowler, Brimo, & Perrin, in review). When spelling a word for which a word-specific MGR does not exist, individuals can use their orthographic pattern knowledge to write an orthographically legal representation.

Morphological Knowledge

The use of morphological knowledge for spelling involves the explicit ability to consider the morphemic structure of words, how word spellings change as the result of adding a morpheme(s) to a base word, and the relationship between morphologically related words. It also includes overt knowledge of the spelling of prefixes and suffixes; in English, affixes have fixed spellings. Thus, when spelling words for which a clear, word-specific MGR does not exist, morphological knowledge allows individuals to consciously recognize and represent the correct number of morphemes in a word as well as to spell affixes added to a base word correctly. It also allows individuals to actively think about modifications to a base word when a suffix is added (e.g., dropping the "e" when adding "-ing" to "slope" or doubling the "p" when adding "ed" to "hop"). Finally, use of morphological knowledge permits individuals to recognize the relation between base words and their derived forms, leading to correct spellings when the derived forms are not necessarily transparent in their orthography or phonology to the base word or root (e.g., admit–admission).

Semantic Knowledge

The use of semantic knowledge for spelling involves an understanding of how meaning affects spelling. For example, anyone who has had experience with word processing on computers knows that spell-check tools only correct orthographic errors; they don't address correctly spelled words that are incorrect semantically. Thus, when a writer uses a homophone incorrectly (e.g., We went to *they're* house) or a real word that is incorrect semantically (e.g., Please *execute* my son from school), the spell-check tool will not alert the writer. However, when using semantic knowledge or explicitly considering the way in which meaning affects spelling and vice versa, writers can actively choose the correct word representation. Semantic knowledge, then, contributes to spelling when an individual consciously considers whether a word spelling accurately depicts the intended meaning.

Mental Graphemic Representations

Mental graphemic representations (MGRs) are the mental images of specific written words, or word parts (e.g., affixes), stored in the mental orthographic lexicon. The common notion is that specific MGRs are formed when individuals are confronted with a novel written word (e.g., phulovbaloney) and must use their orthographic pattern knowledge of letter–sound correspondence (i.e., alphabetic principle) and their phonological knowledge (phonemic blending skills) to decode or sound out the word. When this process is successfully completed, the specific sounds and letters of the novel word are bonded together to form a specific mental image of the word (e.g., Ehri, 2000; Share, 2004). Children in the initial stages of literacy development, before they have sufficient letter–sound knowledge and phonemic blending skills, also may develop initial, word-specific MGRs implicitly by "fast-mapping" or learning the orthographic representations via exposure (e.g., Apel, in press; Apel, Wolter, & Masterson, 2006; Wolter & Apel, 2010).

When MGRs are clearly constructed, they allow individuals to spell (and read) words fluently, with little to no thought of the words' written representations. When spelling words for which clear MGRs are available, writers can devote more mental energy to their composition. However, when an MGR is incomplete or "fuzzy" because of insufficient storage of the representation, spelling (and reading) of words is affected. Either the individual spells words incorrectly because she is using poorly constructed MGRs to guide her spellings, or she must tap into her phonological, orthographic pattern, and/or morphological knowledge to spell the words.

RELATION BETWEEN SPELLING AND OTHER LITERACY SKILLS

As a language and literacy skill, spelling is related to other language and literacy abilities. Specifically, growth in spelling ability is correlated highly with growth in word-level reading, written composition, and reading comprehension skills (e.g., Mehta, Foorman, Branum-Martin, & Taylor, 2005; Vellutino, Tunmer, Jaccard, & Chen, 2007). The associations between spelling and these other literacy skills are likely due to the shared reliance on the four "language blocks" outlined previously as well as the impact that attention to word spellings has on the cognitive/linguistic demands of other reading and writing activities (e.g., Bear, Templeton, & Warner, 1991; Ehri, 2000; Masterson & Apel, 2007).

Across multiple studies, researchers have reported that spelling and word-level reading are associated in children with and without literacy disabilities (e.g., Ball & Blachman, 1991; Bradley & Bryant,1985; Bruck & Waters, 1990; Ehri, 1991, 1997; Ehri & Roberts, 1979; Foorman, Francis, Novy, & Liberman, 1991). The relation between spelling and word-level reading is typically high (e.g., $rs = .68$ to $.86$; Ehri & Wilce, 1982; Greenberg, Ehri, & Perin, 1997). For example, spelling, an encoding task, can involve converting phonemes or morphemes to graphemes, which taps into phonological, orthographic, and morphological knowledge. Word-level reading, a decoding task, also may involve these three language knowledge skills as individuals sound out letters representing phonemes or morphemes to decode words. Successful spelling and word-level reading also can be accomplished when well-developed MGRs are available for use. In addition, as pointed out by Ehri (2000), the act of spelling words is a word-level reading task because most individuals read the words they have written to ensure their spelling is correct.

The relation of spelling to reading goes beyond the word level. Spelling also is associated with reading comprehension (Mehta et al., 2005). To obtain meaning from text (i.e., reading comprehension), readers must read in a fluent manner. Fluency in text comes from quick retrieval of MGRs, a part of orthographic knowledge that is shared by both word-level reading and spelling. Thus, the relation between spelling and reading comprehension is likely the result of both the shared reliance on MGRs and the fact that easy retrieval of MGRs frees up additional cognitive resources to comprehend text (Chall, 1996). Bruck and Waters (1990) distinguished good and poor spellers by analyzing word-decoding skills and reading comprehension. They found that students who were better readers (i.e., reading comprehension) also were better spellers. Furthermore, Lennox and Siegel (1996) found that students who scored below the 25th percentile on the spelling subtest of the Wide Range Achievement Test (WRAT-R) also were classified as poor comprehenders.

Written composition skills also are related to spelling ability. As writers compose, they must use their knowledge of spelling to produce meaningful text (e.g., Singer & Bashir, 2004). Moreover, writing requires the integration of various cognitive-linguistic and graphomotor abilities (Singer & Bashir, 2004). When students struggle in one area (i.e., spelling), the allocation of cognitive resources to spelling may be high, resulting in limited or less cognitive resources available for other aspects of written composition (e.g., word choice, sentence structure, cohesion, and genre requirements; Singer & Bashir, 2004).

DEVELOPMENTAL SPELLING THEORIES

As children develop their literacy skills, they must learn to consciously consider all four foundational language knowledge blocks that lead to correct spelling. For decades, researchers and theorists have discussed the manner in which spelling abilities, via the different language knowledge blocks, are acquired (e.g., Bear, Invernizzi, Templeton, & Johnston, 2003; Henderson, 1990; Masterson & Apel, 2000). For many years, stage theories of spelling abounded (Treiman & Bourassa, 2000). *Stage theory* suggests that children acquire the ability to use the language knowledge blocks in a stair step fashion; first, they acquire and use their phonological knowledge, then their orthographic pattern knowledge, and finally their morphological knowledge (e.g., Bear et al., 2003). Stage theory grew out of the early research that recognized spelling as a linguistic skill (e.g., Henderson, 1990). Researchers examined these influential language knowledge blocks at progressively later grades or ages and assigned their appearance and use to those ages.

As investigators delved more into the type of knowledge children use at different ages when spelling, they recognized that children of varying ages can apply, either explicitly or perhaps in a more implicit manner, their language knowledge when spelling. This led to a change in how spelling development was viewed (Apel & Masterson, 2001; Bourasssa & Treiman, 2009; Rittle-Johnson & Siegler, 1999; Siegler, 1996). Children were viewed as having a repertoire of language knowledge blocks to spell early in development. For example, Siegler's (1996) overlapping waves theory posits that children have access to and utilize their knowledge of phonology, orthography, and morphology for spelling at different ages; the flexibility of that use is dictated by the demands of the task and the children's overall level of literacy ability. Students in kindergarten or first grade may rely more on their phonological and orthographic pattern knowledge when spelling words for which no word-specific MGR exists, but they can utilize their morphological knowledge in some cases. Older students may tap more into their morphological knowledge when spelling words for which no MGR exists, partly due to the academic expectations to write (and read) more complex, multi-morphemic words. However, these children also tap into their phonological and orthographic pattern knowledge, when necessary, to accurately spell unfamiliar words. Thus, when children (and adults) attempt to spell, they have access to and use a repertoire of foundational language knowledge sources when spelling (Apel & Masterson, 2001).

Current developmental theories of spelling emphasize the importance of the foundational language knowledge used for spelling (e.g., Apel & Masterson, 2001; Bourassa & Treiman, 2009; Rittle-Johnson & Siegler, 1999). Researchers have applied the notion of these multiple language skills involved in spelling to assessment and intervention or instructional approaches. In the next two sections, we outline multilinguistic assessment and intervention procedures that are based on current theory and, in many cases, are backed by empirical research that suggests the benefits of using these approaches (Wolter, 2009).

MULTILINGUISTIC APPROACH TO ASSESSMENT

The purpose of assessment will determine the best tools used to test a student's spelling skills. Standardized tests, such as the *Test of Written Spelling-4* (Larsen, Hammill, & Moats, 1999), are sometimes needed to document that a student's performance is below grade-level expectations so that services can be provided. Although useful when such data are required for eligibility decisions, these tests do not facilitate treatment planning and documenting the effects of instruction or intervention. Instead, educators[1] should measure the skills and deficiencies students have in each of the foundational language knowledge blocks.

Determining Goals

Use of the multilinguistic approach to determine what areas to target in intervention has been described in several articles and book chapters (e.g., Apel, Masterson, & Wilson-Fowler, in press; Cron & Masterson, 2011; Masterson & Apel, 2000; 2007; 2010a,b; Wolter, 2009). The key elements of this prescriptive approach include (1) eliciting a sufficient sample of words, (2) identifying orthographic patterns that are misspelled, and (3) describing the nature of those spelling errors.

Moats (1994) observed that the domain of English spelling is comprehensive. Thus, the words that adequately sample skills in the four language knowledge blocks will vary across developmental (grade) levels. To elicit an appropriate sample, some may choose to take words from the language arts curriculum for the desired grades or create lists based on state grade-level expectations. We prefer to collect spellings for words that have been arranged hierarchically to represent increasing complexity in the four language knowledge blocks. To meet this challenge, we use the *Spelling Evaluation for Language and Literacy-2*[2] *(SPELL-2;* Masterson, Apel, & Wasowicz, 2006) because it administers one of four levels of spelling words based on a student's spellings for a selector list that is provided at the beginning of the assessment. Level 1 contains words with simple consonant and consonant digraph targets and short and long vowels. Level 2 contains these targets plus more complex base word structures, such as consonant blends, syllabic *r* and *l*, and consonant doubles. Level 3 adds inflected words and multisyllabic words containing unstressed schwas, and Level 4 adds derived words. Another possibility for obtaining words for a spelling assessment would be to select words from the school's language arts curriculum, while keeping in mind this developmental progression.

Once an appropriate sample has been collected, the student's spellings for each target structure (i.e., orthographic pattern) should be analyzed to determine accuracy level. For those patterns that are in error more than 40 percent of the time, we suggest additional analyses to determine which language knowledge block may be deficient and contributing most to the errors. When a pattern is not represented within a spelling (e.g., RN for *rain*) or by a spelling with a referent that is incorrect but acoustically similar to the target (e.g., PIG for *peg*), the spelling error is classified as a potential deficiency in the use of phonological knowledge because the error suggests the student may not be aware of the sound or not discriminating the sound accurately from another. Follow-up segmentation or phonemic discrimination (identification) tasks are given to determine whether there is indeed a problem in phonemic awareness. When the pattern is spelled with a spelling that is rarely, if ever, correct (e.g., RAN for *rain*), the error is classified as a problem with the use of orthographic pattern knowledge. If the target pattern is spelled with a spelling that is incorrect yet plausible or legal, (e.g., RANE for *rain*), the misspelling is classified as

---

[1]In the following sections, for sake of brevity, the term *educators* will be used to denote any adults, such as clinicians and teachers, whose goal is to assess and improve children's spelling abilities.

[2]The first two authors of this chapter are coauthors of SPELL and the later revisions, SPELL-2, and SPELL-2G, and have a financial interest in the software programs. The analyses and recommendations provided are based on the multilinguistic model and could be done by hand. They are not contingent on use of the software.

representing an inadequate MGR. Spellings for juncture modifications (i.e., when a suffix is attached to a root or base word, such as in *bussed*) and affixes (e.g., *bussed*) are scored separately. Errors for these structures are classified as either difficulties using phonological (for omissions such as BANG for *banged*) or morphological knowledge (for illegal misspellings such as TALKT for *talked*) or inadequate MGRs (for legal misspellings of affixes such as POTATOS for *potatoes*). In the next section, methods tailored to address deficiencies in each of these specific language blocks are presented.

Measuring Progress

A final purpose of assessment is to document baseline performance and monitor progress, or Response to Intervention (RtI; Fuchs & Fuchs, 2006). As with monitoring the effects of any type of treatment, the first step is to construct a list of words with the spelling elements that will be targeted across the instructional period. This list should contain words that will not be part of treatment activities. Students' spellings for these words can be collected prior to beginning intervention and then at intervals (e.g., every 2 or 3 weeks) deemed appropriate by the educator. Students also can be given story stems to elicit short written narratives, or samples of students' classroom work can be collected at various points to document the spellings for the specific orthographic or morphological targets being addressed in intervention. As an aside, with this latter option, the educator should ensure that no other individual or tool (e.g., spell-check) has helped in writing the sample. Although spelling accuracy is traditionally measured by determining percent words correct (PWC), we suggest the use of a metric that represents skills in each of the foundational language knowledge blocks. The *Spelling Sensitivity Score* (*SSS*) system has been shown to better identify differences within and across grade levels as well as between groups of students than the simple PWC (Apel, Wilson-Fowler, Brimo, & Perrin, 2008; Masterson & Apel, 2010b; Masterson, Lee, & Apel, 2008; Williams & Masterson, 2010). This measure is calculated by first parsing all probe words into base word, juncture, and affix elements. The student's spelling for each element (i.e., phoneme or morpheme) is aligned with the corresponding target orthographic representation and scored on a 0 to 3 scale. Omitted elements are scored as 0, elements misspelled illegally are given 1 point, elements misspelled legally are given 2 points, and elements spelled correctly are awarded 3 points. The spellings for entire words are coded similarly. Words with omissions are given no points, words that contain illegal misspellings are given 1 point, words that are misspelled legally are given 2 points, and correct spellings are given 3 points. Parsing target words and aligning and scoring the spellings using the *SSS* system are illustrated in Table 8.1. Metrics based on this scoring system include the *SSS-Elements*, which is calculated by summing the points and dividing by the number of elements, and the *SSS-Words*, which is calculated by summing the points and dividing by the number of elements.

The use of the *SSS* procedure has proven useful in several contexts. For example, Williams and Masterson (2010) compared spellings in Aboriginal and non-Aboriginal first graders. The effect sizes associated with the differences between groups were large for all three measures (PWC, *SSS-E, SSS-W*). However, their mean *SSS-Elements* was 1.47, which suggested that their spellings were characterized by adequate use of phonological knowledge (because the score was at least 1.00) and developing use of orthographic pattern knowledge (because the score was between 1.00 and 2.00). This information was missed by use of their simple average PWC, which was 11 percent. The *SSS* system also can be used to calculate the relative occurrence of each type of misspelling (i.e., percent omissions, percent illegal spellings, percent legal spellings). Maturing skills would be indicated by relatively lower omissions and illegal spellings over time.

TABLE 8.1	*SSS* Parsing and Scoring Examples								Juncture Elements	Affix Elements
					Base Word Elements					
Target	attitude	a	tt	i	t	u-C(onsonant)-e	d			
Child's spelling	attitude	a	tt	i	t	uCe	d			
Points		3[a]	3	3	3	3	3			
Target	bussed	b	u	s					s	ed
Child's spelling	bust	b	u	s					-	t
Points		3	3	3					0[b]	1[c]
Target	chain	ch	ai	n						
Child's spelling	chane	ch	aCe	n						
Points		3	2[d]	3						
Target	halves	h	a						lv	es
Child's spelling	halfs	h	a						lf	s
Points		3	3						1	2

Separate percentages for the error categories can be calculated for base word elements, juncture elements, and affix elements to determine the development of skills in monomorphemic and multimorphemic words.

Regardless of whether the main purpose of assessment is to determine intervention goals or document RtI, the multilinguistic approach can offer clinicians and teachers maximum information (see Masterson & Apel, 2010a). This information is useful for planning instruction for an entire classroom, intervention for small groups, and treatment for individual students. In the next section, we describe how this detailed information can be used to determine optimal methods for instruction and intervention.

MULTILINGUISTIC APPROACH TO SPELLING INSTRUCTION AND INTERVENTION

Assessment drives intervention. Having described a multilinguistic assessment approach, it should be intuitive that any classroom instruction or clinical intervention should target goals derived from such a prescriptive assessment. Typically, a multi-linguistic approach to instruction and intervention is exactly that; learning goals and objectives are tied directly to the needs of the student(s). In some cases, a prescriptive, multilinguistic assessment may not be possible. For example, it may be that a classroom teacher does not have the time to individually assess the language knowledge strengths and weaknesses evidenced in each student's spellings. Although tools exist to allow teachers to assess and group students by language knowledge block ability (i.e., Masterson, Apel, & Wasowicz, 2009) and teachers are highly interested in tailoring spelling instruction to their students' needs (e.g., Invernizzi & Hayes, 2004), spelling instruction continues to be provided mostly at the class level with very little individualization (Graham et al., 2008). However, even with whole-classroom, nondifferentiated instruction, educators can provide lessons based on a multilinguistic approach. We begin this final section by discussing how specific goals that are the outcome of a multilinguistic, prescriptive assessment can be implemented in small-group or individual-student settings. We then conclude this discussion by describing how educators could provide multilinguistic instruction at the classroom level. Although not tailored to the specific needs of the students, such an approach can lead to improvement in literacy skills (e.g., Apel, Masterson, & Hart, 2004; Wolter, 2009).

Regardless of whether an educator is providing lessons based on prescriptive assessment of individual needs or more general classroom-based instruction, the assumption is that the intervention/instruction is being provided because the students lack the specific, required foundational language knowledge required for spelling. To facilitate student learning, we advocate for a scaffolding approach suggested by Ellis (1999) that includes four steps: I do, We do, Y'all do, and You do. In the first step, a newly introduced strategy is strongly and repeatedly modeled by the educator (*I do*). Once several models have been provided, the educator then engages the student in the use of the strategy by requiring the student to imitate or repeat the strategy along with the educator (*We do*). After sufficient practice along with the educator, the students are required to take more control of the use of the strategy. If there is more than one student, the educator can encourage pairs or groups of students to practice the new strategy together (*Y'all do*), facilitating and guiding their strategy use as they implement the strategy. If there is only one student, or after completing the *Y'all do* step, students then are required to utilize the strategy on their own (*You do*). With this series of instructional prompts and facilitation, students progress in their strategy learning from maximum scaffolding to minimal or no scaffolding.

Prescriptive, Multilinguistic Spelling Intervention

Along with others (e.g., Kirk & Gillon, 2009; Wolter, 2009), we have promoted a multilinguistic intervention approach to spelling (e.g., Apel et al., in press; Apel et al., 2004). In this intervention approach, students' spellings provide guidance on the specific underlying foundational language knowledge blocks that need strengthening. Activities target specifically one of the language knowledge blocks with the goal of bringing students' language knowledge to an explicit level and applying that knowledge to their spellings. Because of the interrelatedness of spelling and reading, not only is one expectation that spelling activities will involve some aspect of reading, but it also is expected that the outcomes of spelling intervention will have an impact on reading skills. Initial evidence supports this latter assumption (Wolter, 2009). Next we present suggestions for working on each of the four foundational language knowledge blocks, including a strategy for strengthening word-specific MGRs. Other sources, such as SPELL-Links to Reading and Writing (Wasowicz, Apel, Masterson, & Whitney, 2004), can be consulted for additional activities. With each activity given here, a key component is to tie the explicit awareness and use of the foundational language knowledge block to the act of spelling.

Improving Orthographic Pattern Knowledge

Educators may need to improve students' orthographic pattern knowledge for two reasons: (1) students are omitting a letter(s) for a phoneme present in a word, or (2) they are using an illegal or incorrect letter(s) to represent a phoneme. In the former example, attention to students' use of phonological knowledge must be targeted as part of the orthographic pattern knowledge activity.

ACTIVITIES INCORPORATING PHONOLOGICAL AND ORTHOGRAPHIC PATTERN KNOWLEDGE USE. Intervention focused on strategies for using phonological knowledge for spelling typically are conducted when assessment of a student's spelling suggests he or she is consistently omitting letters for phonemes present in a word. Suggestions for improving deficient phonological knowledge abound (e.g., Gillon, 2005; Kaderavek, 2007; also see Chapter 5 in this text). What these suggestions have in common is a focus on facilitating students' ability to blend phonemes into words and to break down or segment words into their individual phonemes. This latter skill is the phonological knowledge skill directly tied to spelling; one must be aware of each phoneme to represent it orthographically. The important point when conducting activities targeting use of phonological knowledge to improve spelling is to explicitly tie the students' emerging knowledge and use of phonemes to the act of spelling. Years of research suggest that optimal outcomes occur when activities targeting the use of phonological knowledge include letter–sound correspondence (i.e., orthographic pattern knowledge) instruction (e.g., Troia, 2004).

To facilitate students' ability to consider all phonemes in a word and represent all those sounds with letters, we advocate the use of Sound Strings (Wasowicz et al., 2004). Sound Strings are simply strings or cords knotted on each end with approximately eight bright, different-colored beads on them. Use of the Sound String activity involves three steps. The first step is to segment a word into its individual phonemes. To do this, the educator provides a word and models moving one bead per phoneme. The educator also encourages the student to do the same with his Sound String. Once the student has moved the correct number of beads across the string, the second step involves the educator modeling and/or encouraging the student to place the sound string on his paper and write the word using at least one letter per bead. Requiring students to write at least one letter allows for instances where a sound is represented with more than one letter, such as in the case of consonant (e.g., ch, th) or vowel (e.g., ea, oa) digraphs (or tri- and quadgraphs, e.g., igh and eigh). Given that the goal of the activity and strategy is to be aware of each phoneme in the word and represent it orthographically, correct spellings are not the focus. For example, if a student moves three beads for the word "head" and then writes "hed" on his paper, the educator acknowledges that the student used the strategy correctly; he noted the correct number of sounds in the word and wrote at least one letter for each sound. The educator still can show the student how the word is "written in books" but the objective of the activity is the use of phonological knowledge to represent orthographically all sounds in the word, not correct spelling of the word, an MGR goal. The final step requires the student to read his spelling of the word that was segmented. The purpose of this final step, as mentioned previously, is to demonstrate the connection between spelling and reading.

Students who require instruction on the use of phonological knowledge as part of their instruction on orthographic patterns often may have difficulties specific to certain classes of phonemes. For example, it is not uncommon for students to have particular difficulty segmenting consonant clusters into individual phonemes (e.g., showing awareness for the three phonemes in a "str" cluster). In the prescriptive, multilinguistic intervention approach, the stimuli used within the lesson are representative of the student's specific difficulties. Using the preceding example of a Sound String activity, once the first two steps are explained and understood, educators likely would use words with "s" and/or "r" clusters. Initially, the clusters would be in the initial position of words, given children's inclination to demonstrate use of phonological knowledge for initial sounds of words first (e.g., Troia, 2004). Subsequently, the target phoneme(s) could be located in the final and then medial position of words.

Students of all ages may demonstrate spelling difficulties related to poor use of phonological knowledge (e.g., Apel & Masterson, 2001). In addition to the advantage of making use of their phonological knowledge more overt by moving beads across a string, there is an additional benefit to the use of Sound Strings with older students (students above third grade), particularly when they are seen in small groups. Educators can provide the students with Sound Strings that contain the same differently colored beads in the same order (e.g., red, blue, green, yellow, orange, pink, purple, white). When completing the first step of the activity, the students can hold the strings in their hands in a manner that does not reveal the color beads they have moved to their peers on either side of them. This technique allows the educator to note a student who may not have segmented a target word correctly without peers drawing negative attention to an inaccurate attempt.

OTHER ORTHOGRAPHIC PATTERN KNOWLEDGE STRATEGIES.   Students typically receive little focused teaching on specific orthographic patterns for spelling (e.g., Moats, 2009). Without active knowledge of orthographic patterns used across words, students are not able to explicitly think about orthographic conventions when spelling unfamiliar words (i.e., words for which they do not have a clear MGR). Researchers have determined that providing instruction that increases students' active use of orthographic pattern knowledge, as part of a multilinguistic instructional approach, leads to improved spelling abilities (e.g., Wolter, 2009; Zutell, 1998). Perhaps the most highly validated activity to improve orthographic pattern knowledge is word sorts (Zutell, 1998). Word sorts require students to consciously note differences in word spellings and then deduce the convention for why those differences exist. In word sort activities, the educator provides a set of word cards that contains words that represent two contrasting patterns (e.g., final /dz/ sounds in words written with a "ge" or a "dge," as in "huge" and "age" versus "hedge" and "badge"). Through modeling and scaffolding, the student is encouraged to separate the word cards into two piles, with each pile containing words that appear to be following an orthographic pattern (see Figure 8.1 for pre- and postsorting example).

After the student has sorted the word cards successfully, she is encouraged to verbalize the orthographic principle she believes is causing the words to be written differently. The key to this portion of the activity is to have the student deduce the pattern, not necessarily to verbalize it using the same words the educator might use. Any description that meets the basic premise of the orthographic principle should be accepted. The student then is encouraged to write the pattern in

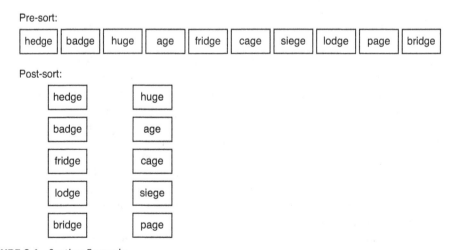

FIGURE 8.1   Sorting Example

her spelling journal. Follow-up activities to this basic word sort practice are many. For example, students can apply their newly learned orthographic pattern knowledge as the educator dictates a series of words, some of which contain the new pattern. The educator and students also can search for words that follow the same orthographic pattern in a familiar text and then write these words down next to their descriptions of the pattern. This latter activity increases the students' awareness of the tie between spelling and reading.

Word sorts encourage students to become "minilinguists," to seek out and discover the principles that govern the majority of English spelling. As students become accustomed to the notion of word sorts, they can be encouraged to apply the strategy spontaneously when they are confronted with spelling a word for which no clear MGR exists. When thinking about spelling a word, they can either refer to their spelling journal for a previously learned spelling pattern or conduct an impromptu word sort with a group of words to deduce why a word might be spelled a specific way.

Improving Morphological Knowledge

Word sorts not only are useful for improving orthographic pattern knowledge, but they also can be used to improve the use of morphological knowledge for spelling. For example, students must become knowledgeable of the regularity of affix spellings (e.g., the regular past tense is spelled with "ed" regardless of whether it sounds like /t/, /d/, or /Id/); word sorts can be used to improve use of this knowledge for spelling. In this case, the educator would have the student sort word cards with words that are either one or two morpheme words yet have final sounds that are identical (e.g., backed, fact, hiked, act). Other sorts involving word pairs can be used to help students deduce rules that modify a base word when an affix is appended (e.g., hop–hopping vs. pack–packing).

As students move through the elementary school years, more and more of the novel words they read or write are multimorphemic, derived words (e.g., Anglin, 1993). An explicit awareness of the morphological relation between base words, or roots, and their one or more derived forms is crucial for spelling, reading, and inferring the meanings of new derived words because these words typically share form and meaning. For example, the word "mnemonic" is often on individuals' lists of most difficult words to spell. The first three letters are not used in the initial position of other words, at least those typically read and spelled. Indeed, individuals typically question why the "m" is present when it is unheard. However, when these same individuals discuss the meaning of "amnesia" and then compare the overlap in meaning between amnesia and mnemonic (both have to do with memory) and identify the common segment representing the root (in this case, the "mne"), then the spelling of mnemonic no longer seems arbitrary or "irregular." Actively thinking about related derived words often will lead to more accurate spelling.

The notion of consciously thinking about morphologically related words is the basis for the Word Relatives strategy (Wasowicz et al., 2004). This strategy helps students use their explicit understanding for how to use their MGRs of words to spell (and read) related words for which an MGR does not exist. Specifically, the strategy enables students to recognize the relations among words, even when those words do not necessarily share identical phonological and/or orthographic features.

The Word Relative strategy has three general steps. The first step is used to help students understand the notion of relatives and their "resemblance" to each other. The educator asks the students about relatives in their family and encourages a discussion about how some family members look and sound alike, some look alike but don't sound like their relatives, and some are dissimilar in looks and sound, but are nonetheless relatives. For the second step, the educator then uses that relative scheme as an analogy for morphologically related words. Some derived words contain the identical phonological and orthographic features of their base word (e.g., bare–barely) and others differ both phonologically and orthographically (e.g., commit–commission). Word relatives also may only differ from their base phonologically (e.g., act–action) or orthographically (e.g., use–usually). The second step concludes with brainstorming activities of base words and their various derived forms.

After the students understand the concept of word relatives, the educator initiates the third step, which is using knowledge of word relatives to attempt spellings of words for which no MGR exists. For example, the educator chooses a base word for which the student has an MGR (e.g., oppose) and then asks or provides prompts to think of related derived words (e.g., opposition). The student then is prompted to use the base word to attempt the spelling, adding any other morphological knowledge of specific affixes that might contribute to the word (in this case, the "tion"). The outcome is an attempt at spelling that includes the spelling of the base and an additional suffix. When a student writes a plausible yet incorrect spelling (e.g., opposeition), the educator can encourage the student to look at the spelling and determine if it "matches a picture" in her head. Overall, the strategy is used to increase conscious awareness of derived words, how they share spellings with less complex words, and the idea that one can use the less complex, related words to help spell the derived forms. When it appears the student has learned and is using the strategy within spelling activities, the educator then can require the student to search texts for morphologically related words.

When using the Word Relative strategy, educators should be aware of the research that suggests the ability to recognize the relation between base words and their derived forms is influenced by the amount of phonological and orthographic shift between the words (Carlisle, 2000; Carlisle & Stone, 2005; Mann & Singson, 2003). Derived words that represent no change in the phonological or orthographic features of the base when they are spelled and spoken (e.g., preach–preacher) typically are the easiest word pairs to identify as related. Derived words that change the phonological or orthographic elements of the base word are less easily identified. Those derived words that represent a shift both phonologically and orthographically from the base word appear the most challenging to identify as related to their base form.

SUPPLEMENTING LANGUAGE KNOWLEDGE STRATEGIES WITH WORD-SPECIFIC LEARNING TACTICS

Activities such as those outlined earlier teach students strategies for using their language knowledge to spell words. These strategies are not word specific; they can be used for all words that follow a certain orthographic pattern or are morphologically related to other words. Educators can use the multilinguistic approach to teach students to spell using strategies representing the foundational language knowledge blocks, a teaching approach that differs substantially from the typical instruction students receive in school. With the traditional Friday Test spelling instruction approach, students are taught that spelling improves simply by memorizing more and more words (e.g., Graham et al., 2008). Unlike the multilinguistic approach, the traditional approach focuses on learning word spellings one at a time. Perhaps not surprisingly, the Friday Test approach does not always lead to a well-formed MGR, an outcome often lamented by teachers (Gill & Scharer, 1996).

Although a multilinguistic spelling instruction best fits current research and theory about spelling development, at times its focus on the use of phonological, orthographic pattern, and morphological knowledge may not lead to accurate spellings. For example, a student may use phonological and orthographic pattern knowledge strategies to spell a word, with the outcome being a plausible yet incorrect spelling (e.g., spelling "seed" as "sead"). In a case such as this, or when a student writes one homophone for another (e.g., "two" for "to"), direct attention to specific word spellings may be needed. We suggest using a strategy called "Picture This" (Wasowicz et al., 2004), which directs students' attention to all letters of a word to avoid developing an MGR based on only certain portions of a word.

Like the initial step of the Word Relative strategy, instruction for the Picture This strategy begins with the use of an analogy. The student is encouraged to picture a familiar scene (e.g., his bedroom, the family den) and describe the room to the educator, starting with the left side of the room and moving across his mental image of the room. When completed, the educator points out how the student's well-formed and easily retrieved mental image led to myriad details about the room. The educator then asks the student to describe the room starting from the right and moving to the left across the room image. After completing this task, the educator points out that the image was solid enough that the student could view it in his mental eye both forward and backward.

The second step of the Picture This strategy involves words for which at least a portion of the word requires word-specific knowledge (MGR) because use of phonological, orthographic pattern, and morphological knowledge only lead to plausible spellings. Initially, the educator looks at the word, describing various features (e.g., number of letters, number of vowels, number of consonants). To aid this process, the educator may wish to color code consonants and vowels. Both the educator and student take turns verbally spelling the word from left to right. After a series of practices and discussions about the word, the word is turned over and the student is asked to spell the word from memory. If the student can spell the word accurately, he then is asked to spell the word backward, as he did for his description of the familiar scene. If the student can do so correctly, it provides some indication that the word-specific MGR has been formed. Extension activities for this strategy involve writing the word in dictated sentences or searching for the target word in text.

MULTILINGUISTIC INSTRUCTION AT THE CLASSROOM LEVEL

Ideally, a multilinguistic approach to improving spelling occurs after a prescriptive, multilinguistic assessment so that instruction is optimally tailored to the needs of the student(s). Such an assessment, however, may not always be feasible for large groups of children. If assessment is not possible, educators can still provide students with multiple strategies for using their language knowledge to spell. Like other learning activities in the classroom, the specific lessons may be known information for some students and far advanced for others. Nevertheless, by implementing a multilinguistic instructional approach within the classroom, improved outcomes in spelling are obtained (e.g., Apel et al., 2004).

One approach to providing nonprescriptive multilinguistic spelling instruction is to introduce language knowledge strategies via curriculum units. Units typically are two to four weeks in length. A program we have implemented contains three units. The first unit focuses on using phonological knowledge to ensure orthographic pattern knowledge is represented. The Sound String strategy discussed previously is an example of a lesson provided in this unit. We then move on to our second unit, which targets use of orthographic pattern knowledge to spell. Lessons in this unit emphasize learning specific orthographic patterns. In these lessons, we choose one pattern and provide instruction that allows the students to deduce or discover the pattern through guided or scaffolded teaching. Word sorts, as discussed earlier, can be used at the classroom level to accomplish this task. Our third unit typically focuses on use of morphological knowledge, with lessons individually emphasizing the knowledge and spelling of specific inflectional or derivational markers (i.e., prefixes and suffixes), how base words are modified when specific suffixes are added, or the morphological relations among words that share the same base word or root. Typically, after each curriculum unit, we provide a summary lesson that reviews the new strategies and patterns learned before moving on to the next unit. We also rotate back through the different units targeting progressively more advanced skills or strategies or increasing the complexity of the words on which strategies are applied.

Classroom-level multilinguistic spelling instruction is very different from the traditional Friday Test approach. Our experiences suggest that classroom teachers may have some initial concern about not following spelling word lists suggested by the reading curriculum and/or not conducting weekly spelling tests. To deal with these concerns, we often tell educators to examine reading curriculum-based spelling word lists and place words from those lists into the most appropriate curriculum unit (e.g., orthographic pattern knowledge, morphological knowledge) and administer weekly tests for each unit. Using these latter two strategies, the educators can implement a multilinguistic spelling instruction approach that follows the school curriculum and is somewhat aligned with past experiences with spelling instruction.

Summary

Spelling is not illogical as Twain's quote may have suggested. Although it may seem that spelling is random, when viewed through the lens of the four foundational "language knowledge blocks" (i.e., phonological, orthographic, morphological, and semantic knowledge), the logical structure of spelling is evident. Importantly, these language knowledge blocks are used across the age span, from beginning spellers to more mature ones. Given a shared reliance on these four foundational language knowledge blocks, it is not surprising that spelling ability is associated with and supports other areas of literacy, including word-level and text-level reading and written composition.

Using a multiple-linguistic approach to spelling assessment, educators can obtain specific information regarding the strengths and weaknesses students may display in the knowledge necessary for spelling performance. This information then can serve as a guide to developing individualized instructional goals and be used as a baseline measure for monitoring progress. By targeting spelling with a multilinguistic perspective, educators will be well prepared to meet the developing needs of their students and improve their literacy outcomes.

References

Anglin, J. M. (1993). Vocabulary development: A morphological analysis. *Monographs of the Society for Research in Child Development, 58*(10, Serial No. 238).

Apel, K. (in press). What is orthographic knowledge? *Language, Speech, and Hearing Services in Schools.*

Apel, K., & Masterson, J. J. (2001). Theory-guided spelling assessment and intervention: A case study. *Language, Speech, and Hearing Services in the Schools, 32,* 182–195.

Apel, K., Masterson, J. J., & Hart, P. (2004). Integration of language components in spelling: Instruction that maximizes students' learning. In E. R. Silliman & L. C. Wilkinson (Eds.), *Language and literacy learning in schools* (pp. 292–315). New York: Guilford.

Apel, K., Masterson, J. J., & Wilson-Fowler, E. B. (in press). Developing word-level literacy skills in children with and without typical communication skills. In S. Ellis, E. McCartney, & J. Bourne (Eds.), *Insight and impact: Applied linguistics and the primary school.* London: Cambridge University Press.

Apel, K., Wilson-Fowler, E. B., Brimo, D., & Perrin, N. A. (in review). Linguistic contributions to reading and spelling in second and third grade students.

Apel, K., Wilson-Fowler, E. B., Conlin, C., Masterson, J. J., & Goldstein, H. (2008, July). *Assessing developmental changes in spelling in at-risk kindergarten and first grade children.* Poster presented at the XI International Congress for the Study of Child Language, Edinburgh, Scotland.

Apel, K., Wolter, J. A., & Masterson, J. J. (2006). Orthotactic and phonotactic probability factors in fast mapping in children's spelling. *Developmental Neuropsychology, 29*(1), 21–42.

Ball, E. W., & Blachman, B. A. (1991). Does phoneme awareness training in kindergarten make a difference in early word recognition and developmental spelling? *Reading Research Quarterly, 26*(1), 49–66.

Bear, D. R., Invernizzi, M., Templeton, S., & Johnston, F. (2003). *Words their way: Word study for phonics, vocabulary, and spelling instruction* (3rd ed.). Upper Saddle River, NJ: Pearson.

Bear, D. R., Templeton, S., & Warner, M. (1991). The development of a qualitative inventory of higher levels of orthographic knowledge. In J. Zutell & S. McCormick (Eds.), *Learner factors/teacher factors: Issues in literacy research and instruction* (40th yearbook of the National Reading Conference). Chicago: National Reading Conference.

Bourassa, D., & Treiman, R. (2009). Linguistic foundations of spelling development. In D. Wyse, R. Andrews, & J. Hoffman (Eds.), *Routledge international handbook of English, language and literacy teaching* (pp. 182–192). London: Routledge.

Bradley, L., & Bryant, P. E. (1985). *Rhyme and reason in reading and spelling.* Ann Arbor: University of Michigan Press.

Bruck, M., & Waters, G. (1990). Effects of reading skill on component spelling skills. *Applied Psycholinguistics, 11*, 425–437.

Carlisle, J. F. (2000). Awareness of the structure and meaning of morphologically complex words: Impact on reading. *Reading and Writing, 12,* 169–190.

Carlisle, J., & Stone, C. A. (2005). Exploring the role of morphemes in word reading. *Reading Research Quarterly, 40,* 428–449.

Chall, J. S. (1996). *Learning to read: The great debate.* New York: McGraw-Hill.

Cron, D., & Masterson, J. J. (2011). Annie: Treating reading and spelling skills in an elementary student. In S.

Chabon & E. Cohn, *The communication disorders casebook: Learning by example* (pp. 303–309). Upper Saddle River, NJ: Pearson.

Ehri, L. C. (1991). Learning to read and spell words. In L. Rieben & C. Perfetti (Eds.), *Learning to read: Basic research and its implications* (pp. 57–73). Hillsdale, NJ: Erlbaum.

Ehri, L. C. (1997). Learning to read and learning to spell are one and the same, almost. In C. Perfetti, L. Rieben, & Fayol, M. (Eds.), *Learning to spell: Research, theory and practice across languages* (pp. 237–269). Mahwah, NJ: Erlbaum.

Ehri, L. C. (2000). Learning to read and learning to spell: Two sides of a coin. *Topics in Language Disorders, 20,* 19–36.

Ehri, L. C., & Roberts, K. T. (1979). Do beginners learn printed words better in contexts or in isolation? *Child Development, 50,* 675–685.

Ehri, L. C., & Wilce, L. S. (1982). Recognition of spellings printed in lower and mixed case: Evidence for orthographic images. *Journal of Reading Behavior, 14,* 219–230.

Ellis, R. (1999). *Learning a second language through interaction.* Philadelphia: John Benjamins North America.

Fresch, M. J. (2003). A national survey of spelling instruction: Investigating teachers' beliefs and practice. *Journal of Reading Behavior, 35,* 819–848.

Foorman, B. R., Francis, D. J., Novy, D. M., & Liberman, D. (1991). How letter–sound instruction mediates progress in first-grade reading and spelling. *Journal of Educational Psychology, 83,* 456–469.

Fuchs, D., & Fuchs, L. S. (2006). Introduction to response to intervention: What, why, and how valid is it? *Reading Research Quarterly, 41,* 93–99.

Gill, C. H., & Scharer, P. L. (1996). "Why do they get it on Friday and misspell it on Monday?" Teachers inquiring about their students as spellers. *Language Arts, 73,* 89–96.

Gillon, G. (2005). Facilitating phoneme awareness development in 3- and 4-year-old children with speech impairment. *Language, Speech, and Hearing Services in Schools, 36,* 308–324.

Graham, G., Morphy, P., Harris, K. R., Fink-Chorzempa, B., Saddler, B., Moran, S., et al. (2008). Teaching spelling in the primary grades: A national survey of instructional practices and adaptations. *American Educational Research Journal, 45*(3), 796–825.

Greenberg, D., Ehri, L, & Perin, D. (1997). Are word reading processes the same or different in adult literacy students and 3rd–5th graders matched for reading level? *Journal of Educational Psychology, 89,* 262–288.

Hanna, P. R., Hanna, J. S., Hodges, R. E., & Ruforf, H. (1966). *Phoneme–grapheme correspondences as cues to spelling improvement.* Washington, DC: U.S. Office of Education Cooperative Research.

Henderson, E. H. (1990). *Teaching spelling* (2nd ed.). Boston: Houghton Mifflin.

Invernizzi, M., & Hayes, L. (2004). Development spelling research: A systematic imperative. *Reading Research Quarterly, 39*(2), 216–228.

Kaderavek, J. N. (2007). Early literacy development. In A. Kamhi, J. Masterson, & K. Apel (Eds.), *Clinical decision making in developmental language disorders* (pp. 223–248). Baltimore: Brookes.

Kirk, C., & Gillon, G. T. (2009). Integrated morphological awareness intervention as a tool for improving literacy. *Language, Speech, and Hearing Services in Schools, 40,* 341–351.

Larsen, S. C., Hammill, D. D., & Moats, L. C. (1999). *Test of Written SPELLing-4.* Austin, TX: PRO-ED.

Lennox, C., & Siegel, L. S. (1996). The development of phonological rues and visual strategies in average and poor spellers. *Journal of Experimental Child Psychology, 62,* 60–83.

Mann, V., & Singson, M. (2003). Linking morphological knowledge to English decoding ability: Large effects of little suffixes. In E. M. H. Assink & D. Sandra (Eds.), *Reading complex words: Cross-linguistic studies* (pp. 1–25). New York: Kluwer Academic.

Masterson, J. J., & Apel, K. (2000). Spelling assessment: Charting a path to optimal instruction. *Topics in Language Disorders, 20*(3), 50–65.

Masterson, J. J., & Apel, K. (2007). Spelling and word-level reading: A multilinguistic approach. In A. Kamhi, J. Masterson, & K. Apel (Eds), *Clinical decision making in developmental language disorders* (pp. 249–266). Baltimore: Brookes.

Masterson, J. J., & Apel, K. (2010a). Linking characteristics discovered in spelling assessment to intervention goals and methods. *Learning Disabilities Quarterly, 33*(3), 185–198.

Masterson, J. J., & Apel, K. (2010b). The Spelling Sensitivity Score: Noting developmental changes in spelling knowledge, *Assessment for Effective Intervention, 36*(1), 35–45.

Masterson, J. J., Apel, K., & Wasowicz, J. (2006). *Spelling evaluation for language and literacy-2 (SPELL-2)* [computer software]. Evanston, IL: Learning by Design.

Masterson, J. J, Apel, K., & Wasowicz, J. (2009). *SPELL-2g Spelling Performance Evaluation for Language and Literacy®–Second Edition with Grouping Tool workstation* [Computer software]. Evanston, IL: Learning By Design.

Masterson, J. J., Lee, S., & Apel, K. (2008, July). *The Spelling Sensitivity Score: A measure of children's developing linguistic knowledge.* Poster presented at the XI International Congress for the Study of Child Language, Edinburgh, Scotland.

Mehta, P. D., Foorman, B. R., Branum-Martin, L., & Taylor, W. P. (2005). Literacy as a unidimensional multilevel construct: Validation, sources of influence, and implications in a longitudinal study in grades 1–4. *Scientific Studies of Reading, 9*(2), 85–116.

Moats, L. C. (1994). Assessment of spelling in learning-disabilities research. In G. R. Lyon (Ed.), *Frames of reference for the assessment of learning disabilities* (pp. 333–350). Baltimore: Brookes.

Moats, L. C. (2005/2006). How spelling supports reading and why it is more regular and predictable than you may think. *American Educator, 29,* 12–22.

Moats, L. C. (2009). Knowledge foundations for teaching reading and spelling. *Reading and Writing, 22*(4), 379–399.

National Institute of Child Health and Human Development (NICHD). (2000). *Report of the National Reading Panel. Teaching children to read: An evidence-based assessment of the scientific research literature on reading and its implications for reading instruction* (NIH Publication No. 00-4769). Washington, DC: U.S. Government Printing Office.

Rittle-Johnson, B., & Siegler, R. S. (1999). Learning to spell: Variability, choice, and change in children's strategy use. *Child Development, 70,* 332–348.

Share, D. L. (2004). Orthographic learning at a glance: On the time course and development onset of self-teaching. *Journal of Experimental Child Psychology, 87,* 267–298.

Siegler, R. S. (1996). A grand theory of development. *Monographs of the Society of Research in Child Development, 61,* 266–275.

Singer, B. D., & Bashir, A. S. (2004). Developmental variations in writing composition. In A. Stone, E. Silliman, B. Ehren, & K. Apel (Eds.), *Handbook of language and literacy: Development and disorders* (pp. 559–582). New York: Guilford.

Treiman, R., & Bourassa, D. C. (2000). The development of spelling skill. *Topics in Language Disorders, 20,* 1–18.

Troia, G. A. (2004). Phonological processing and its influence on literacy learning. In A. Stone, E. Silliman, B. Ehren, & K. Apel (Eds.), *Handbook of language and literacy: Development and disorders* (pp. 271–301). New York: Guilford.

Vellutino, F. R., Tunmer, W. E., Jaccard, J. J., & Chen, R. (2007). Components of reading ability: Multivariate evidence for a convergent skills model of reading development. *Scientific Studies of Reading, 11*, 3–32.

Wasowicz, J., Apel, K., Masterson, J. J., & Whitney, A. (2004). *SPELL-Links to Reading and Writing.* Evanston, IL: Learning By Design.

Williams, C., & Masterson, J. J. (in press). Phonemic awareness and early spelling skills in urban Australian Aboriginal and non-Aboriginal children. *International Journal of Speech-Language Pathology.*

Wolter, J. (2009, June). Teaching literacy using a multiple-linguistic word-study spelling approach: A systematic review. *Evidence-Based Practice Briefs, 3*, 43–58.

Wolter, J. A., & Apel, K. (2010). Initial acquisition of mental graphemic representations in children with language impairment. *Journal of Speech, Language, and Hearing Research, 53*, 179–195.

Zutell, J. (1998). Sorting: A developmental spelling approach to word study for delayed readers. *Reading and Writing Quarterly: Overcoming Learning Difficulties, 14*(2), 219–238.

Chapter 9

Learning to Write

Cheryl M. Scott

A FRAMEWORK FOR WRITING

As children become readers, they also become writers. A chapter about learning to write seems like it should be straightforward enough, but in reality, it is a challenging topic. Some might think that if a child can talk—in other words "do" language and spell words, they can write. By this definition, writing would be only a matter of transcription—the act of getting words on paper. But writing is also a matter of composing text for a purpose, and as such it has additional and unique linguistic, cognitive, and social–pragmatic requirements. Moreover, the process of learning to write takes place almost entirely within a writing curriculum designed to turn nonwriters beginning in kindergarten into skilled writers who meet formal standards enacted by states. Although there are commonalities in the standards across states, there is also considerable variability from school to school on the specific goals and methods of teaching writing. In addition to these differences, children bring a variety of linguistic and cognitive abilities and different early literacy experiences to the kindergarten "writing center." And, children's intrinsic interest and motivation for writing will evolve and change over time. Thus, when examining texts that children write as evidence of what they've learned, it is a challenge to disentangle what the child brings to the task—the linguistic and cognitive resources intrinsic to the child—from the writing practices at school. The question is pertinent for educators and clinicians who want to do a better job of teaching children to write well.

The developmental course of writing is a long one; some would say it has a lifelong learning curve. Add to that the fact that many find writing to be difficult. Writing, for most adults at least, forces us to "face our thoughts" and, assuming a writing audience of one or more people, let others in on those thoughts. It leaves a permanent record that can be reexamined in the future. As adults, we "have a record" with our writing. Perhaps there was an instance when a superior wasn't happy about a piece of writing, or if we write in the academic setting, we see critiques of peer reviewers. How do people change from novices to individuals whose writing skills serve them well in their work and personal lives? Why do some individuals never get there?

Answering these questions has engaged scholars from many fields, including cognitive and developmental psychology, education, special education, speech-language pathology, and linguistics. The most direct way to study children's writing is to examine what they write—their *products*. The study of written products dominated the developmental literature until the 1980s, when novice–expert cognitive models were applied to writing (Hayes & Flower, 1980). Adult writers were asked to "think out loud" about what was going on in their minds as they wrote. Gradually, writing as a cognitive *process*, heretofore unobserved, became more transparent. This line of research revealed that the planning, generating, and revising stages of writing were far from linear/sequential for experienced writers; rather, they were better described as reciprocal and integrated processes that were going on somewhat concurrently. As the contribution of wider cognitive domains became more obvious, executive function, memory, attention, and motivational systems were incorporated into later iterations of the writing process model (Berninger, Garcia, & Abbot, 2009; Hayes, 1996, 2004).

Young children, however, who must grapple with transcription (spelling and writing words accurately) are novices by comparison. Young children find it difficult to plan and revise, and writing processes for them *are* more strictly sequential and much less global in scope. Observing and interacting with children as they plan, generate, and revise their writing provides another major source of developmental information. Researchers have also taken the ethnographic tact of asking children what they think about writing—what is writing good for and what makes for good writing.

This chapter reviews and summarizes what is known about writing development using these three types of information—examining writing products, observing writing processes, and interviewing children about their knowledge of writing. Because any one piece of writing serves a particular purpose, be it telling a story (narrative), informing (expository), or arguing a point (persuasive), writing development in these genres is of interest. The long course of writing development will be discussed in two periods: emergent through early elementary years, and later elementary and secondary years. Also addressed in this chapter are results of national writing tests and reading–writing connections. Although learning to transcribe words (spelling and handwriting) is a major part of learning to write that consumes major cognitive resources in the early years of writing (McCutcheon, 2006), this topic is covered separately in Chapter 8.

EMERGENT AND EARLY SCHOOL WRITING: AGE 4–8 YEARS

Researchers have used several approaches in studying the beginning of writing. One approach is to be an unobtrusive, sometimes quasi-interactive observer, exemplified in the work of Dyson (1989, 1993a, 2008). This approach yields rich descriptions of early writing in its social context and tentative interpretations about the individual psychological and larger sociocultural processes at work. In another approach, researchers interact more directly with children around instances of writing. For example, they might ask the children questions about what they are doing or what something "says" (e.g., Ferreiro, 1984), or even why they (and people in general) write (e.g., Merenda, 1996). Additional paradigms involve asking children to "write" something "their own way" (e.g., Sulzby, Branz, & Buhle, 1993) or to dictate a story for an adult to write down (Zucchermaglio & Scheuer, 1996). Interactive protocols like these provide valuable insights into how children analyze the forms and functions of writing.

At the beginning of this period, one of the main contexts for writing is drawing. Of note, almost as soon as children pick up writing tools (crayons, pencils) and before the writing "part" of what they are drawing is discernable as writing, careful study of videotapes shows that drawing and writing have different arm/hand movement patterns (Brenneman, Massey, Machado, & Gelman, 1996, as cited in McCutcheon, 2006), indicating that 2- to 3-year-olds distinguish between the two at some level. Writing quickly becomes more distinguishable in ways studied extensively by Ferreiro (1984) and others (e.g, Tolchinsky & Teberosky, 1998). By the age of 4, across languages and socioeconomic strata, children produce writing marks that are arranged linearly with regular spacing, a finding that reinforces the notion that the developmental foundations of writing are laid independent of and prior to formal schooling.

Dyson's research (1993b) on draw/write texts picks up with the advent of school in an extensive observational study of an urban San Francisco K–1 classroom. She described draw–write instances as "multimedia productions" (p. 12) in which children talk, draw, write, and sometimes dramatize the stories they are communicating. At first, the writing may be only a small part of the production, for instance a few letters, or letterlike forms, or words. Eventually, a longer text is accompanied by smaller pictures that may be added after the text is finished. Many children continue to draw small pictures with their written work even beyond the mid-elementary years. Dyson (1993b) observed that children began to talk playfully (and critically) about each others' writing as a separate object from the drawing. Gradually, they began to differentiate the type of information conveyed in print versus picture, with writing conveying more of the narrative action and drawing illustrating key ideas. Writing also became more integrated into the children's social worlds; friends became characters in their writing, writing centered on fictional (perhaps desired) playdates, and the children would write specific words that they knew would amuse their friends. Dyson's (1993b) tentative conclusion is that children's writing changes from a type of social prop to a social mediator whereby writing is the platform for social activity (p. 28). Verbal interactions between children about their texts at the writing table frequently extended to recess.

The draw/write text as social mediator is best exemplified in Dyson's recent description (2008) of a first-grade classroom in a Midwest central city, where she spent a year doing twice-weekly observations. A daily writing activity in this classroom went as follows. The teacher first modeled the process of writing a personal narrative on a large chart tablet, where the children could see the product as it unfolded and hear her talk out loud about the process (e.g., "I know my sentence has to start with a capital letter after this period"). Narrative topics included family outings and activities. This activity was one of the main ways of implementing the state's standard that first graders should be able to write "personal narratives of three to four coherent sentences (properly worded with basic punctuation"; Dyson, 2008, p. 124). Then it was the children's turn to compose. They had special paper with blank space on the upper half and lines on the lower half. They wrote about upcoming plans (many of them fictional get-togethers that included their peers in the classroom), video game themes, and fictional sporting events. The children sat in groups where there was plenty of conversation about what they were writing. At the end of the writing period, the children shared their texts. Dyson was interested in the "unofficial" as well as the official webs being spun by the children—how the children learned to "stay within the curricular lines" of the task, and in some cases struggled against them. Although, like their teacher, the children wrote about events that had taken place or were going to happen, many of the events were fictional and served as platforms for interacting with peers that were included (or not) in their writing (the unofficial part their writing experience). Because so much of the children's writing was different from the teacher's modeled texts, it was not clear to Dyson that young children "take with productive ease to personal narrative" (p. 150), and particularly not in a solitary way. Rather, the children found ways to make the writing curriculum their own. Dyson is an advocate of finding

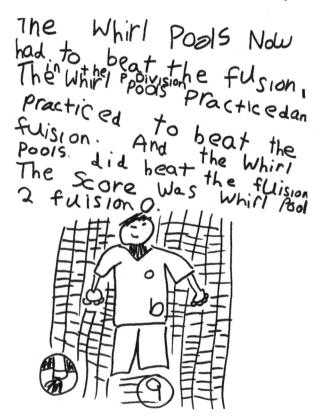

FIGURE 9.1   An Example of Conventional Writing Produced by Two First-Grade Children

ways to "marry" the official early writing curriculum agenda with the child-constructed unofficial agendas, a goal that, she fears, is increasingly difficult in today's atmosphere of tightly scripted writing standards.

At the end of the school year, many of the children observed by Dyson (2008) were conventional writers. Sulzby (1996) defined conventional writing as "connected discourse that another conventionally literate person can read without too much difficulty and that the child can read conventionally" (p. 27). To be a conventional writer, the child must have some understanding of (1) sound–symbol relationships; (2) words as stable, memorable units; and (3) text as a stable, memorable object (Sulzby, 1996, p. 27). Children who are conventional writers believe that they can write. This contrasts with younger, emergent writers, who often say they can't write even though they can usually be persuaded to "write" something by a researcher. The text in Figure 9.1 from two first grade boys is an example of convention writing. Spelling and basic sentence grammar are intact. Of the four sentences, one is complex (2 clauses), although both boys probably use greater sentence complexity when talking, a spoken-written form discrepancy that will be discussed later.

As the daily writing activity described by Dyson (2008) illustrates, most first-grade classrooms today provide opportunities for children to write at the text level. This contrasts with practices from the past, which were designed to teach children the *writing system*—

spelling, punctuation, and layout. Children copied spelling words and sentences from the board, wrote sentences that used certain words, and practiced forming letters and, later, penmanship. Today's textual writing opportunities in the first grade are often of the child's choosing. The self-sponsored nature of at least some portion of the writing curriculum in early elementary school has afforded the opportunity for researchers to study the early emergency of writing genre.

Chapman (1994) studied the emergence of genre in the writing of six first-grade children. She defined genre as a "typified form of discourse or way of organizing or structuring discourse, shaped by and in response to recurring situational contexts" (p. 352). In her study, the recurring context was the "Writing Workshop"—a time when children could write and draw about things of interest to them. Chapman constructed a typology and chronology of change in the production of 15 identified genres over the course of the school year. The raw data were 724 texts produced by the children throughout the year. The texts were first categorized as either *chronological* (action/event oriented) or *nonchronological* (object oriented). Chronological texts were based on the children's own experiences, either past or planned for the future, or imaginative. Distinctive forms in chronological texts included action verbs in past tense or future time, temporal connectives (e.g., *then, next*), and temporal adverbials (e.g., *yesterday, at Christmas*). There were two distinct strands of nonchronological texts. Descriptive texts provided information about a picture; interactive texts had as their goal some form of social action (e.g., a written question–answer dialogue between two children). Distinctive forms in nonchronological genres were verbs of attribution (e.g., *are, have, got*) or attitude (e.g., *like, want*) that took generalized present tense form.

Over the course of the year, there were dramatic changes in the children's writing. One major change was the gradual disassociation of drawing and writing. At the beginning of the year, almost all writing was associated with picture drawing; in the last third of the school year, this association had declined so that free-standing texts of several clauses were common. In addition, major changes occurred in both quantity (i.e., genre repertoire) and quality of genre writing. The children produced eight different genres in the first three months, adding an additional six in the next three-month period. *Labels* (a nonchronological type of writing) accounted for half of all texts at first, but were negligible in the last period. *Basic records* (chronological) declined from 18 percent to 1 percent, but *expanded records* increased from 6 percent to 31 percent. *Attribute series* (nonchronological, e.g., *This is an army base. I like it.*) increased from < 1 percent to 24 percent. Texts were usually single clauses (e.g., the label text *this is a soccer game*) at the start of the year, but texts of two or more clauses, rare at first, comprised 95 percent of all texts in the last period. In fact, at the end of the year, the average number of clauses per text ranged from 3.15 to 5.52. All six children, even those who were identified as delayed in language development by their teachers, wrote texts that could stand alone, without pictures, by the end of the year, thus meeting Sulzby's (1996) definition of conventional writing.

Where do these genres come from? Perhaps they are invented by the children, much like invented spelling (a cognitive constructivist position), or alternatively, they are appropriated from the environment (a social constructivist position). Chapman's (1994, 1995) observations of the larger classroom context for her subjects led her to believe that both origins contribute and interact. All children clearly used language experiences in the classroom as resources for their writing; however, they had individual genre preferences and unique styles.

Newkirk (1987) also studied self-sponsored school writing of young elementary school children, but restricted his sample to nonnarrative writing (100 different texts from children in grades 1 through 3). Like Chapman's much smaller group, the 100 children in Newkirk's study were in classrooms with teachers trained in the writing process approach, and they wrote regularly on self-chosen topics. The nonchronological genres identified by Chapman (1994) for first grade were also evident in texts examined by Newkirk, but were seen in a more developed form (for example, labels were now whole sentences, as in a list of sentences describing *10 Bad Things About My Brother* (Newkirk, 1987, p. 131). The general trend uncovered by Newkirk was one of redistribution. Several genres frequent in the texts of younger children were less frequent by the third grade, and vice versa. Attribute series texts were frequent in the first- and second-grade texts examined by Newkirk (21 percent and 26 percent of all nonchronological writing, respectively), but accounted for only 6 percent of third-grade texts. Notably, there were substantial increases in the length of texts: Only 15 percent of first-grade texts were more than one paragraph, but 49 percent of third-grade texts exceeded one paragraph. Newkirk interpreted his findings as support for the idea that young elementary children can write in genres that lay a foundation for later expository writing. The young child's labels, lists, and attribute texts are the tools of informational texts to come.

Figure 9.2 shows an example of a nonchronological text written by a second-grade child (the author's daughter Katie) describing a bearded seal. This text would be classified as an *attribute series* text in both the Chapman and Newkirk investigations. In this genre, facts are stated about a topic, but they are in no particular order and could be rearranged without affecting text coherence. Of note, at the time she produced the bearded seal text, Katie was capable of

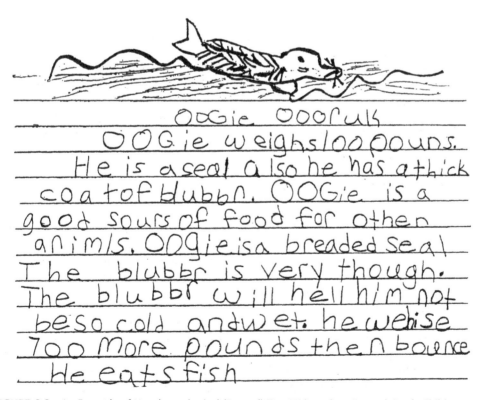

FIGURE 9.2 An Example of Nonchronological (Factual) Text Written by a Second-Grade Child

writing much longer fictional stories with identifiable macrostructure features (i.e., setting, initiating event). Some researchers argue that the well-documented developmental disparity between informational and narrative writing (in terms of overall length and text-level organization) is an artifact of the much greater exposure to narrative genre in early elementary grades (Christie, 1986; Duke, 2000; Martin, 1989), a point that is revisited later.

In addition to describing types of spontaneous emergent writing and their social contexts, researchers have been interested in the types of knowledge children may have about writing. Do young children know that written language has a distinctive lexicon and grammar? Can they talk about writing as an object, for example, why they wrote something a particular way, or why people write at all? Answers to these types of questions require researchers to interact with emergent writers in a more direct manner. Sulzby and her colleagues investigated what young children might know about the distinct form of writing by asking children to "read" their favorite storybooks and also to "write a story" and then to "read me your story" (Sulzby, 1996). Her research documents children's ability to use *written-like language* in both tasks (e.g., *once there was a bug. . . .*); in addition, children use *oral-like language* (quoted speech) in both activities. Sulzby's work is interesting because it demonstrates that spoken and written forms are potentially separable from the medium of delivery, or modality. Not only are preliterate children able to talk like a book, but they can also write like they talk. The ability to speak in a literate style while at the same time writing in a spoken style (if the need arises) has been touted as the highest level of literary style (e.g., Kroll, 1981). Sulzby's work indicates that the seeds for this literacy agility may be sown very early.

Merenda (1996, pp. 12–13) also talked with preschool and kindergarten children about writing. She asked them, simply, "Tell me why you write." Among the answers were (1) to tell a story, (2) to do homework, and (3) to warn people ("because we don't want anybody to touch it," referring to paint). These emergent writers had insights about writing that went deeper than what we can observe on the surface. These results, along with other studies summarized about emergent and early writing, show us that young children, as they are becoming conventional writers, have learned some things about genre, or types of writing (Donovan & Smolkin, 2006). In the following section about older writers, the topic of genre is encountered in more detail.

LEARNING TO WRITE GENRE-SPECIFIC TEXT: AGES 9+

Although in theory one can speak or write the same information, in practice discourse genres tend to be delivered in one or another medium but not both. Consequently, learning to write, particularly learning to write expository (informational) and persuasive (argument) genres, opens new avenues of making meaning for children. The familiar adage about *learning to read* versus *reading to learn* could also be applied to writing. Whereas transcription fluency (spelling and handwriting/keyboarding) takes up much cognitive space in the early school years, by late elementary years, writing should be a reliable means of knowledge-telling ("I know some things about dinosaurs—now I just have to get it all down on paper"). And, by the end of secondary school, for some students at least, writing has become a means for truly transforming knowledge (writing to learn). After writing about a topic, one's knowledge of the topic is far different—more advanced—*as a result of* having written about it (Bereiter & Scardamalia, 1987; McCutcheon, 2006). In a few cases, the process might actually result in *new* knowledge, for example uncovering a connection or devising a new theory. Writing in later school years needs to be seen not just as a basic literacy skill to be acquired, but also as a new way to communicate, a new tool for learning, and a productive way to discover and contribute new knowledge.

Learning the Macrostructure of Writing: Genre Development

Three written genres are typically recognized in state standards and assessments: narrative, expository (informational), and persuasive (argument). Researchers have studied children's writing development in single-genre and cross-genre designs (see reviews in Scott, 1994). Cross-genre designs compare children's ability to write in at least two genres (e.g., narrative writing is compared to expository writing). Evidence suggests that students first gain proficiency in narrative writing, followed by informative writing, with persuasive writing last (e.g., Crowhurst, 1987; Langer, 1985; McCutchen & Perfetti, 1982)—a sequence that matches the timing of genre work in school writing curricula, as noted previously. Proficiency has been measured in a variety of ways, including overall text length, types and frequency of cohesion markers, local and remote connections between sentences, and analyses of text structure. A review of cross-genre research shows that children write longer narrative texts and use more advanced systems of cohesion in narrative versus other types of texts (Scott, 1994). There is anecdotal evidence that children rely on narrative formats when other types of discourse are called for (Crowhurst & Piche, 1979). Likewise, Applebee (1984) found that adolescents beginning to write analytic texts sometimes start by embedding narrative stretches within a global analytic framework. Within any one genre, fine-grained analyses reveal content and form developments across the school years. McCutcheon and Perfetti (1982), for example, found that growth in cohesion patterns was evident in essays written in second, fourth, sixth, and eighth grades. Freedman's (1987) analysis of narratives written by 5th-, 8th-, and 12th-grade students revealed continuing change in text structure.

The fact that young children are more prolific writers of narratives in their early schooling has been explained in several ways. Narratives by nature are event based. They are about things that happen to people (and animals in children's literature) that unfold over time—about life, in other words. Temporal and causal relations are the main organizational frameworks, and children may have direct experience with some of the themes they write (and read) about. By the age of seven, children are capable of *telling* well-formed stories that have all or most of the story elements expected in a classic narrative (setting, initiating event, internal response, etc.). *Writing* well-formed stories may take a little longer because transcription (spelling and writing words) consumes cognitive resources. By the fifth grade, typically developing children are capable of writing well-formed, multiepisode narratives (Hidi & Hildyard, 1983). By comparison, children with language and learning disorders write shorter narratives, with more grammatical errors (Scott & Windsor, 2000).

The life-story nature of the narrative genre contrasts with expository text, which is logically based (e.g., relations such as condition, purpose, contrast). A robust literature has shown that the expository genre is more difficult for children to comprehend (Snyder & Caccamise, 2010). Much of the information encountered in expository text is new, with new vocabulary and new concepts. And, unlike narratives, which conform to one basic macrostructure, informational text is built on several different macrostructures (compare/contrast, description, problem/solution, causation, etc.), and one text might combine several of these. If students have difficulty constructing a mental representation of the gist of what they have read, it is unlikely they would be able to write a cogent summary of the same material.

With these caveats about the difficulties inherent in expository writing, investigators have established that texts written by many children in the mid-elementary years (third and fourth grades) show some hierarchical text structure. To illustrate, Scott and Jennings (2004) found that typically developing 11- and 12-year-olds wrote summaries of a descriptive video about desert ecosystems that contained both introductory statements (e.g., *To many the desert seems to be a lifeless community but really it has many different life forms that have adapted to the hot dry climate.*) and concluding statements. It is difficult to generalize conclusively about the development of text structure facility because findings vary according to the *particular* informational genre studied. As reported by Ward-Lonergan (2010), several investigators have found that compare/contrast essays about familiar people or places are better organized than explanation essays about how to do something. At present, we lack research leading to a complete longitudinal account of the development of textual organization of expository writing. Research has established a better picture of sentence-level features of expository writing, showing that syntax increases in complexity and meanings become more nuanced even beyond late adolescence (Berman & Nir, 2010; Nippold, 2010). If text development follows suit, it too would show improvements over the duration of formal schooling and beyond.

Several investigators have been interested in the development of persuasive writing. In a cross-sectional design, Knudson (1994) traced the development of persuasive writing in 3rd-, 5th-, 10th-, and 12th-grade students. Students were asked to write a letter to the school principal arguing that a school rule either should or should not be changed; types of arguments offered were categorized. Simple statements without supporting evidence decreased over time. The major developmental growth trend was a significant increase in the use of compromise. Whereas third-grade children never offered a compromise, 11 percent of the 12th-grade arguments were compromises. A similar developmental increment was found by Golder and Coirier (1994). They reasoned that the two most important processes in argumentative text writing are the supporting process (stating reasons to back a claim) and the negotiation process (convincing the reader to accept those reasons). Negotiation markers included (1) counterarguments (e.g., *even if, however*), (2) obligation and judgment (e.g., *one should, it's good*), (3) degree of certainty (*maybe, surely*), and (4) writer endorsement and accountability (*in my opinion*). Significant increase in the frequency of negotiation markers occurred between the ages of 10 and 16. Furthermore, for the oldest subjects, there was a strong association between negotiation in writing and the ability to judge the "argumentivity" of texts based on weak–strong argumentative text structure. Results were interpreted as lending support to the importance of text structure schema in genre writing. Golder and Coirier's study is particularly interesting because they presented subjects with several different tasks in an effort to explain as well as describe argumentative writing.

Durst, Laine, Schultz, and Vilter (1990) looked at factors that contributed the most to holistic scores of persuasive writing of high school seniors. Of the seven linguistic and rhetorical variables studied, four contributed the most: the use of logical appeals; the number of total words; degree of coherence (defined as "explicit interconnectedness of the various parts of the essay" including transitional sentences, cohesive ties, overall structure made explicit with an introduction, conclusion, and so on [p. 236]); and the use of the five-paragraph structure. There was no relationship between ratings and number of fragments, punctuation errors, agreement errors, and spelling errors.

In addition to measuring the ostensible products of genre knowledge as revealed in writing samples, researchers have also probed knowledge with direct questions (e.g., *What are the parts of a story? What kinds of things are included in a persuasive essay?*). Lin, Monroe, and Troia (2007) determined that clear genre distinctions were not provided by typically developing writers until middle school (grades 6 to 8) and not even then by struggling writers. Because students often show considerable genre knowledge in their written products before middle school years, it appears that there is a difference between implicit knowledge (being able to apply genre knowledge to one's writing, albeit perhaps not consciously) and explicit knowledge (being able to talk about one's knowledge).

Interpretation of Genre Studies: Effects of Task and Curriculum

Donovan and Smolkin (2006) summarized the numerous methods used to elicit writing samples analyzed in studies of genre and writing development along a continuum corresponding to the degree of scaffolding provided by the writing task. A task could be self-selected and self-generated (no scaffolding) or could be highly scaffolded with text structure supports and suggestions for revisions. In between were writing tasks such as recounting past experiences, daily journals, or writing with visual supports such as a wordless picture book. They were interested in how these methodological choices affect genre. The conclusion was that children produce more complex texts (that meet more of the micro- and macrostructure benchmarks associated with narrative and informational genres) when they write about things they are more familiar with (highly scaffolded). However, the researchers also found that one can go too far with familiarity and support. When an informational text used with upper elementary children was extremely simple, it seemed to constrain the children from demonstrating the full extent of their genre knowledge (Donovan & Smolkin, 2002). It would be important to scrutinize details of developmental genre research with an eye toward the potential effects of task. Evidence to date suggests that the specific task can help or hinder full expression of genre knowledge.

The question of how children and adolescents learn to write in specific genres is also complicated by the difficulty of separating intrinsic cognitive and linguistic developmental factors from the filter effects of school curricula and writing instruction, a problem noted earlier in this chapter. Thus, if a child writes a poor persuasive piece, is it because persuasion is too demanding cognitively and/or linguistically, or is it due to a lack of exposure to persuasive text and little or no instruction in the genre? Several studies of elementary school writing curricula confirm the domination of narrative writing, followed by informational writing, with persuasive writing addressed least frequently, if at all. Martin (1989) examined writing in an Australian suburban infants' and primary school in years 1 through 6. Only 15 percent of the texts were factual (13 percent reports, 2 percent procedural, and 0.5 percent explanations and expositions). Duke (2000) studied 20 U.S. first-grade classrooms in both low and high SES school districts. When instances of reading and writing were combined, Duke discovered that children were engaged with informational genres for only 3.6 minutes on average per school day. According to Burkhalter (1995), the rationale for the neglect of informational and persuasive texts is adherence to a Piagetian developmental model that reserves formal operational reasoning abilities until age 11. In practice, however, persuasive writing instruction and practice is further delayed beyond age 11 until late secondary school or even college (Applebee, Langer, & Mullis, 1986; McCann, 1989). There is evidence of increased interest in addressing the imbalance between narrative and nonnarrative text in the developmental literature (e.g., Nippold and Scott's [2010] book about expository discourse in children, adolescents, and adults).

There is also evidence that increased attention to informational writing standards, including those that are more discipline specific, is on the horizon (for a review, see Scott and Balthazar, 2010). Some educators and scholars have called for disciplinary literacy—the explicit teaching of the discourse forms of science, history, mathematics, and literature (Shanahan & Shanahan,

2008). The argument is that a "generalist" literacy curriculum fails to help students deconstruct the *content-specific linguistic features* unique to different subjects. What students need is more direct instruction and practice with these unique features (Heller & Greenleaf, 2007).

Research designed to develop content-specific knowledge and related academic language has been concerned mainly with the effects on reading comprehension (e.g., August, Branum-Martin, Cardenas-Hagan, & Francis, 2009). One notable exception, however, is a study on the effects of explicit teaching of science text properties on writing (Percell-Gates, Duke, & Martineau, 2007). This investigation is unique because it is truly experimental (comparison of two genre conditions with random assignment of conditions), longitudinal (growth curve modeling across six assessment periods spread over two years), and large N (420 participants). The study targeted young writers (and readers) who were second graders at the start. The two conditions compared were authentic writing practice of science text (45 minutes twice a week) and authentic writing plus explicit instruction in language features characteristic of science informational and procedures texts. Unexpectedly, the addition of an explicit curriculum did not predict writing growth (with the exception of second-grade growth in procedural writing); however, degree of authenticity was highly predictive of writing growth in both informational and procedural writing. The authors raise the possibility that perhaps the children were too young to benefit from the explicit genre methods. Taking into consideration the careful experimental methodology as described in this study, it is difficult to imagine what the essential elements of an ideal learning experience would look like. For younger or older writers, there is limited experimental work that would provide guidelines for fine-tuning the amount, sequence, or types of experiences to support content-related genre development over the long course of learning to write. If the call for discipline-specific literacy training continues, however, this should change.

Learning the Microstructure of Writing: Sentence Grammar

THE EFFECTS OF MODALITY ON SENTENCE FORM.   Children learning to write face several new grammatical challenges. Some stem from the requirements of genre and others from the nature of the medium (the written *modality*). Projects comparing written and spoken text provide insight into the development of a specifically "written" grammar. Several large-N investigations of speaking and writing have tracked syntactic changes throughout the school years (Harrell, 1957; Loban, 1976; O'Donnell, Griffin, & Norris, 1967). The focus of other investigations has been more limited in terms of age range or specific research questions (De Temple, Wu, & Snow, 1991; Golub & Frederick, 1971; Pelligrini, Galda, & Rubin, 1984). With one exception (Loban, 1976), these studies have compared written and spoken samples of the same genre, usually narrative (e.g., spoken and written versions of a film, two films in the same series, or similar pictures, and so on). As a result, the structures identified in writing can be assumed to reflect the influence of modality alone. The large-N studies in particular demonstrate that from mid-elementary through high school years, children's writing shows increasing frequency of later-developing syntactic forms such as relative clauses, expanded noun phrases, and nonfinite adverbial clauses (e.g., *looking out the window,* he could see they were in trouble), and that the frequency of these forms in writing is higher than in spoken language. Reviews of this literature are available in Perera (1986) and Scott (1988).

Kroll (1981) proposed four periods in the evolution of spoken/written form relationships. During a *preparation* phase in the early period of conventional writing, texts may not be up to the standard of spoken language. Sentences are shorter, and grammatical errors, usually omissions, occur that would be unusual in speech. Presumably spelling, punctuation, and layout decisions, being far from automatic at this early age, take up a large amount of the child's resources and attention. In a *consolidation* phase, writing more closely resembles speech. At the age of 9 or 10, many children enter a *differentiation* phase in which a more "written" grammar emerges, as shown by: (1) absence of distinctly oral structures (e.g., *well, you know*), (2) fewer coordinated main clauses with *and* and more subordinate clauses, and (3) structures more often found in written language such as passives and nonfinite verb forms. Further, patterns of written text organization appear, such as moving adverbial elements to the front of the sentence. Perera (1984) noted that this can be a somewhat awkward period; at times "spoken" and "written" grammar are mixed in the same text. The text in Figure 9.3, written at school by a third-grade child (Katie again, age 7 years 8 months) provides an example. The text is an imaginative narrative, written in the first person. There are several structures characteristic of mature writing, including (1) a series construction (lines 8–11) and (2) adverbial fronting and clefting, as in *there stood a little tiger cub* (line 13, also lines 1, 2, 6, 16, and 22). At the same time, Katie uses the spoken form *well* (line 19). Finally, in Kroll's (1981) last phase, the *integration* phase, writers move easily between oral and written form, adapting structure to fit the needs of a variety of text types. Using Sulzby's (1996) terminology for emergent literacy, a writer can now write *oral-like* if necessary (and is also able to speak *written-like*). Some writers may never reach an integration phase (Perera, 1984; Rubin, 1987).

An investigation by Scott (2002) lends credence to Kroll's developmental account of spoken/written form relationships. Scott examined structural differences in connectivity patterns in spoken and written discourse produced by 9- and 11-year-old children. Connectivity in this investigation referred to the ways in which clauses are combined within a sentence. Children spoke and wrote about the same content (a narrative content video and an expository content video)—a methodology that is particularly suited to reveal any independent effects of modality on sentence form. Sentences that were content matches were analyzed for syntactic structures, shown in previous research to distinguish written and spoken forms of language (Biber, 1986; Halliday, 1985, 1987; Perera, 1984). The writing of 9-year-olds contained many examples of a distinctive "written" clause connectivity grammar, but the writing of 11-year-olds contained significantly more instances (twice the number). The following three sentence pairs provide examples:

- (um um um) And then one day he's walking his sheep through the mountains/and (uh he) one of the goats got away (spoken)
- One day, when Yanis was walking his sheep through the mountain, one of the goats got loose (written)

- And once cactuses die animals move into the cactus to live (spoken)
- Animals make homes out of dead plants (written)

- And he doesn't really do anything with his friends or anything/and he doesn't listen to his dad as much/and his dad's realizing this (spoken)
- His father notices that he does not play with his friends or listen to his father anymore (written)

The first spoken–written comparison illustrates the replacement of coordination with subordination linkages. In the spoken version, two clauses are joined by the coordinator *and,* but the subordinate conjunction *when* connects the clauses in the written match. In the second comparison, two clauses in the spoken version are collapsed to one as the clause *cactuses die* is transformed to an attributive adjective *dead (plants)* in the written version. There is also a more specific lexicalization *(animals make homes)* in the written form, a wording that implies creating a place to live (which is explicitly stated in the spoken version). In the third example, a sequence of independent coordinated clauses (spoken) is reconfigured into an "umbrella" finite complement clause

TIGER CUB

One hot summer I was walking in the field
Just me, privace at last, Feeling
proud of myself I sat down with
a little sac lunch I had made.
I opend my thermas and set out
my blanket. as I ate mylunch
I planned what I was going to do.
I was going to: pick some wild
flowers, Swim in the field lake,
and biuld things in the fields
Sandpile I heard this little
new new. I looked behind me
there stood a little tiger cub.
he sat down beside me. new
new he said. I stroked his Soft
tiger fur After I hat done
my three tasks I noticed
the tiger cub had follod me.
Well I did the thing most
children would do I decied to
ask my folks if I could have him.
When I got home I asked
my dad why he was mewing?
My dad studeyd his mewing
for a minuit

... story continues

FIGURE 9.3   An Example of Narrative (Imaginative) Writing by a Third-Grade Child. The text
illustrates several "written" grammatical features as well as developing punctuation.

(notices that . . .) consisting of two clauses coordinated by *or,* with coreferential subject deletion *(. . . or* [null subject] *listen to his father anymore).* The three examples together illustrate the fact that written clause connectivity draws on a different set of structures. Clauses combined by coordination in speaking (a linear code) are reconfigured into a more hierarchical code (subordination and coordination combinations and nominalization of whole clauses).

THE EFFECTS OF GENRE ON SENTENCE FORM.   Cross-genre studies of children's writing show that genre has an impact on syntactic complexity, summarized by Rubin (1984) as follows:

> First, discourse function exerts a profound effect on syntactic complexity. Within-age style shifts are of a magnitude equal to or exceeding between-age contrasts. Second, there is a strong tendency for style-shifting in writing to increase with age. That is, more mature writers are sensitive to the differential stylistic demands of the various functions to a greater degree than younger writers. (p. 220)

When children are asked to write in several genres, narratives show the least amount of syntactic complexity, with reports showing more complexity, and persuasion the most (Langer, 1985; Rubin, 1984). Persuasion brings about the highest degree of syntactic complexity because of the interdependence of subordination operations and the expression of logical relationships (Rubin, 1984). Syntactic complexity in cross-genre studies has usually been measured in terms of sentence length and/or subordination ratio (subordinate/main clauses). These effects are not usually obvious before the late elementary or early secondary years, however, when children have sufficient fluency in factual as well as narrative writing. Kress (1982, pp. 100–101) published two texts written by a 7-year-old that illustrate this point quite well. An imaginative story written at home was 31 sentences with an average sentence length of 9.90 words; a factual piece from school, written at the same age, was eight sentences with an average sentence length of 7.00 words.

Recently published accounts comparing narrative and expository discourse offer finer-grained analyses of genre effects on microstructure in the writing of older children. In two separate studies with similar designs (Scott, 2003; Verhoeven et al., 2002), findings were in agreement on the following points: First, there was a significant genre effect on the distribution of major types of clause connectivity. Thus, in texts written by children in mid to late elementary grades (ages 9 to 12 years), narratives were characterized by a preponderance of coordination and complement clauses, whereas relative and adverbial clauses, particularly adverbials that signal conditional, purpose, and comparison relations, were more common in expository writing. Genre effects in written language were also observed for spoken language, indicating that the effect of genre is quite robust. Using average sentence length as a measure of overall syntactic complexity, both studies reported that expository texts are more complex than narrative texts. By the age of 11 to 12, children are capable of writing sentences that contain as many as five or six clauses connected via hierarchical as well as linear organizing principles, and these types of sentences are more often found in expository writing, with its greater variety of logical and textual structures.

Several research programs have provided additional detail about the development of genre-specific microstructure features of expository writing. Berman and Nir (2010) analyzed the special features of expository writing of students across a wide age span (9–10 years, 12–13 years, 16–17 years, and young adults) as part of a large-scale cross-linguistic project that compared narrative and expository written and spoken texts. The students wrote (and talked) about the topic of interpersonal conflict. Their results are categorized into four domains. The first of these is temporal expression via tense, aspect, and mood. Expository texts were characterized by generic present tense forms of verbs to match an "atemporal" (timeless) meaning (i.e., a generalization about a state of affairs, presumed true for "all time"). Modal auxiliary verbs were used frequently and shifted with development from deontic prescriptive statements about what people *should* do to *can* or *will*—epistemic forms expressing a more nuanced view of what is possible. Increased developmental flexibility and variety was also shown with greater use of past progressive and past perfect aspect rather than strict adherence to invariant present. Within clauses, expository writing features long and complex noun phrases, generic pronouns, and passive constructions, all of which allow for a depersonalized, evaluative stance, as illustrated in the following piece of writing by an 11th-grade student (noun phrases are underlined, and passive forms of verbs are in italics):

> Conflict is <u>a large problem</u> particularly in High School, although it never goes away. High school is <u>a major focal point of conflict</u> because of <u>the extreme amount of new tension that students</u> *are confronted with*. Coming from <u>a sheltered environment with the close supervision and intervention of parents and teachers,</u> students *are thrust into* <u>realization of the so called "real world" where you must not make choices and resolve problems on your own.</u> (Berman & Nir, 2010, p. 108)

As a third feature, expository writing links clauses and sentences with an array of lexical and phrasal connectives such as *however, but, although, while, thus, for example, in contrast,* and *on the other hand.* Expository writing depends on these types of connectors to link logical relations, whereas narratives have the "default" organizational scheme of event sequence in time. Berman and Nir noted that the explicit marking of logical relations between clauses and sentences increased in variety and depth with age and was not truly well developed until late adolescence. They also analyzed types of dependent clause-linking and report that three structures were particularly favored in their expository samples: relative clauses, conditional adverbial clauses, and nonfinite adverbial clauses (e.g., *many times the problem can be figured out by simply talking things out or getting to the root of the problem,* p. 110). Last, Berman and Nir reported on lexical characteristics of expository samples. Word length, lexical density (the relative proportion of nouns, verbs, and adjectives), register (formal vs. colloquial), and noun abstractness all showed significant increases with age.

To summarize, research confirms that with only a few years of writing experience, children's writing begins to take on a "written" grammar that is evident by comparing oral and written texts. They also begin to control the structural means to communicate different discourse schemas and content with the use of specific verb forms, clausal constructions, clause/sentence combining forms, and word types. Although these microstructure features make an early appearance, their full development takes many years, and changes are evident well into adolescence and beyond. Over time, genre effects on form are even more prominent, while at the same time there is less "canonical" application of one genre form over another as writers express multiple perspectives (e.g., evaluative as well as factual) on topics (Berman & Verhoeven, 2002; Verhoeven et al., 2002).

Learning the Process of Writing

The development of the writing process has been studied from several vantage points. Some studies have simply observed writers—for example, recording the time spent in initial planning or, once writing starts, the amount of time actually writing as opposed to pausing (see reviews in Faigley, Cherry, Joliffe, & Skinner, 1985). Other investigators have intervened at various points in the writing process. As an example of this type of paradigm, an experimenter might provide a model of planning before children begin to write or provide suggestions for revisions.

The seminal developmental work on processes involved in writing remains the work of Bereiter and Scardamalia, much of it summarized in their 1987 book, *The Psychology of Written Composition*. Children between the ages of 10 and 14 (students in the fourth, sixth, and eighth grades) were asked to generate factual text from information in a matrix; they also wrote an opinion piece in response to the prompt, "Should students be able to choose what things they study in school?" In a study of planning, Bereiter and Scardamalia (1987) provided specific planning instructions prior to writing the opinion text. In general, 14-year-olds were able to utilize planning prompts about audience and purpose, whereas the younger children used their planning time in a more constrained way to merely generate content. One analysis centered on a comparison of notes made before writing and the actual finished text. Whereas the 14-year-olds' written notes listed "gists" of ideas that were expanded into complete ideas in the text, the notes of the 10-year-olds were already complete sentences, which then recurred practically unchanged in the text. The product of planning for the younger children was the text itself, not an intermediate plan. As another indication of planning productivity, an analysis of think-aloud protocols from the planning period revealed that the number of idea units doubled between the ages of 10 and 13. Another sign of developmental change in planning was evident in the children's ability to recognize when planning, as modeled by an adult, took place. With age, then, there is an increasing differentiation of planning from content itself, or text production. Even though considerable planning development occurred by the age of 14, college undergraduates, by comparison, were more skillful planners (Burtis, Bereiter, Scardamalia, & Tetroe, 1983). Bereiter and Scardamalia stressed that more mature planning "consists of thinking *about* the composition rather than planning that consists of mentally rehearsing or creating the composition" (1987, p. 210).

One explanation of younger children's difficulty in planning is that they are still in a state of "cognitive overload" when they write (Gombert, 1992, p. 169). Specifically, energies devoted to transcription are thought to interfere with planning efforts. Perhaps it is no coincidence, then, that planning begins to show developmental change at about the same time that these competing processes are becoming more automatic.

The text generation phase of writing—turning ideas into words, sentences, and text—usually receives less attention in developmental reviews of writing. Perhaps this is because text generation is a mental process that is not very observable. One question frequently addressed for young writers, however, is the brevity of their writing. Bereiter and Scardamalia (1987) surmised that children may approach the writing task from their oral mode of a conversational "turn"; hence, they write very little. Several studies lend credence to this view because supplying a "conversational" partner to children while they write or just telling them to write more frequently increases text length (McCutcheon, 2006). The high processing costs of transcription for young children is frequently cited as a factor in brevity and quality of their writing (Berninger, 1999, 2000). By fourth grade, transcription is sufficiently fluent to allow for longer texts, but continues to contribute to writing quality into junior high and beyond. Other methods used to study text generation involve observing places where children pause when writing (not surprisingly, often at syntactic boundaries) and observing effects of working memory manipulations on text quality (e.g., increasing memory load leads to more grammatical errors). Bereiter and Scardamalia (1987) reported that children who could combine more information points about a topic into a single sentence were better able to defend ideas in expository writing.

Hayes and Flower (1987) reviewed developmental literature on the revision phase of writing. They noted that adult and more expert writers devote proportionally more time to revising.

Adults also view revising from a more global perspective, as a way of "molding the argument." On the other hand, high school and even some college students devote little time to revision, and when they do revise, changes are largely limited to the sentence level (correcting/changing grammar and punctuation), in other words "fixing up" the current version. Sometimes, the changes are harmful rather than helpful. Other studies confirm that high school and some college students avoid making major organizational and content changes in their texts, perhaps because major problems are not detected (e.g., Beason, 1993; Yagelski, 1995).

Being able to revise one's writing subsumes some type of an internal standard of comparison. Internal standards for writing are also shown in evaluations of others' writing. According to McCormick, Busching, and Potter (1992), the evaluation of a particular text involves "the conversion of multiple kinds of knowledge into specific criteria" (p. 314). A beginning literature on the development of internal standards of writing as revealed in evaluations of others' texts indicates that children between second and sixth grades frequently justify their evaluations with personal affective responses (e.g., *I didn't like it 'cause I'm scared of snakes*; McCormick et al., 1992). Toward the end of elementary school years, development is seen in the move from affective to objective responses and from simple to multiple criteria. McCormick and colleagues (1992) sought to provide a more detailed account of children's evaluation of writing. They studied 27 fifth-grade children identified as either high or low achievers, with follow-up one year later. The children were asked to rank-order four of their own pieces of writing and another four peer texts that were actually written by the researchers to capture degrees of topic interest and craft. The children's comments were assigned to one of five criteria categories (pp. 320–324):

- *Text-based:* Refers to characteristics, qualities, and content of the text itself (e.g., *that just isn't a good story to me; it's all right but it's not my favorite one; they don't tell when they seen the big creature and everything; it's just dull, . . . you don't think The pencil's all mine!; it sounds like a little kid wrote it*)
- *Nontext association:* Evaluations based on events and ideas from student's own experience (e.g., *'cause I love my dog . . . like to help my dog and he likes to help me*)
- *Surface qualities:* Refers to mechanics, spelling, or another aspect of linguistic correctness or image (e.g., *well I made a lot of obvious mistakes in that one; and it's neat and everything*)
- *Process:* Refers to processes of creating and sharing/publishing text (e.g., *I just kind of threw it down so that's why I put it last*)
- Not interpretable

Within each of these categories, further subcategories were created by the authors for a total of 31 distinct types of criteria.

Most fifth-grade students used at least 3 (of the 31) criteria to justify their rankings, and 70 percent were *text-based* in nature. For example, the students commented on features of the text that created (or failed to create) interest, or they commented on whether the text was easy or hard to understand. Interestingly, and at odds with some previous research, only 5 percent of the children's comments, on average, referred to *surface qualities* (but low achievers cited surface qualities more often than high achievers). There was considerable variation among children, with many struggling to articulate any criteria, some merely repeating parts of the text they liked, and others resorting to personal associations. High-achieving students voiced a mixture of personal and objective reactions, were able to state multiple criteria, and seemed to have a growing sense of awareness of the craft of writing. However, they did not use a "teacher's grid" (the same set of criteria) for each story; rather, each story was treated separately according to a unique template. In sum, the study showed that older elementary children are beginning to develop a meta-evaluative stance toward writing. An association between highly developed internal standards of writing and the ability to write well would be expected and has been demonstrated for college freshman (Johnson, Linton, & Madigan, 1994).

As we saw with genre knowledge, researchers have probed explicit process knowledge and general beliefs about writing by interviewing students and posing questions like: What constitutes "good" writing? What kinds of things can help a writer plan? Why do teachers teach writing? How can writing help in life? Why do some people have trouble with writing? What can a writer do if they have trouble with an assignment? Saddler and Graham (2007) interviewed fourth-grade skilled and less skilled writers and found positive relationships between the veracity of student responses to interview questions and both writing skill (group membership) and writing quality (measured independently). Examination of interview responses in children from second through eighth grade by Lin et al. (2007) revealed that typically developing middle school students showed a more sophisticated understanding of writing purpose than younger students, as shown in the following response:

- Middle school writer: *When we get our job, we need to know how to write and get our recommendations. To prepare everything for life, you need to write*
- Younger writer: *Because maybe one of us wants to be a writer when we grow up. . . .* (p. 215)

In terms of what they do when they plan, younger writers said they "just think about it" but by the fourth grade, many children mentioned using graphic organizers, and by middle school some even talked about when graphic organizers could provide the most help. When talking about revision, younger writers restricted their answers to items like spelling and punctuation changes, whereas older writers discussed content changes more readily. The overall developmental pattern is that, with time, student writers move from a "self-centered, local focus toward a more global, audience-oriented, self-aware, and self-regulated focus" (Lin et al., 2007, p. 226).

HOW WELL DO CHILDREN WRITE? INCIDENCE OF WRITING DISORDER AND NATIONAL ASSESSMENTS

Many children and adolescents have difficulty writing. Efforts to establish how many would first need to provide an operational definition of a writing disorder and then establish prevalence in a population. To my knowledge, there are few if any large-scale, population-based studies, with one notable exception. In a recently published study of a population-based birth cohort of school-age children followed from age 5 through 19, cumulative incidence rates varied from 6.9 percent to 14.7 percent, depending on the formula used, with boys two to three times as likely to be affected (Katusic, Colligan, Weaver, & Barbaresi, 2009). Written language disorders were at least as prevalent as reading disorders. The study included 5,718 children in a school district of Rochester, Minnesota. The authors defined a written language disorder according to *DSM-IV-TR* criteria, which uses four characteristics of poor writing, including grammatical or punctuation errors in sentences, poor paragraph organization, multiple spelling errors, and poor handwriting. They then searched for these characteristics in IEP goals and/or specific writing subtests scores available in school records to establish prevelance. By any standard, these numbers show that an alarming number of students have major problems writing—problems likely to affect vocational decisions and/or performance.

Another approach that addresses writing difficulty is to ask how well students perform on state and national writing tests. Almost any document about "the state of writing" in U.S. schools (e.g., foundations such as the Carnegie Corporation of New York or The Alliance for Excellent Education) begins by reporting the troubling statistics on the number of students that do not meet basic standards of proficiency. Writing capabilities in 4th-, 8th-, and 12th-grade students have been assessed periodically at the national level since NAEP (National Assessment of Education Progress) was established in 1969 under the auspices of the U.S. Department of Education. In the most recent 2007 administration of the test, 8th- and 12th-grade students (167,900) wrote in an *on-demand* format in response to prompts designed to elicit narrative, informative, and persuasive writing. Trained readers assign a holistic score based on a rubric that addresses content, organization, and language parameters. Results showed that only 33 percent of 8th-grade and 24 percent of 12th-grade students wrote at or above a proficient level (defined as solid academic writing), although the report noted that the 8th grade results were slightly higher than the previous 2002 scores (Salahu-Din, Persky, & Miller, 2008). Turning those numbers around, two-thirds of 8th graders and three-fourths of 12th graders are not meeting a standard of solid academic writing. The dire statistics about student writing give pause and certainly raise questions about writing standards, curricula, and teacher training, as well as student variables such as motivation, and even larger cultural factors and technological changes. The way that writing is tested on the NAEP and in state-level writing assessments is also not without critics, who question exams from the standpoints of content validity, scoring, and effect on what is taught in schools (Hillocks, 2002). For a review of these issues, see Scott (2010).

WRITING, READING, AND ORAL LANGUAGE

Like reading, writing is not an isolated language domain with a well-defined place in a developmental sequence that follows the acquisition of oral language. Despite the fact that speaking and listening emerge earlier than reading and writing, it would be too simplistic to restrict the role of the oral modalities to that of laying a foundation for literacy, although this is clearly an important part of the overall picture. Rather, Berninger (2000) encourages a view of the four language modalities—speaking, listening, reading, and writing—as developing in an overlapping and parallel manner. Few specific details of the association between oral language and writing have been investigated, however. We know that oral language ability is related to writing in a general way, as demonstrated in studies of children with language learning disabilities (e.g., Scott & Windsor, 2000), whose expository writing in particular compares poorly with typically developing age peers. Further, oral volubility (amount of talking) and verbal IQ are associated with writing quality (Shanahan, 2006). Writing also seems to be the last language frontier for adults with learning disabilities because writing difficulties will remain well after oral language and reading abilities have improved (Johnson & Blalock, 1987). Another perspective on the writing–oral language connection is that writing could also affect oral language. One possibility often mentioned is that writing could provide a more salient format for increasing knowledge of derived words (those composed of root forms and affixes, e.g., *adore/adorable, commit/commitment*; Carlisle, 1996).

Relationships between writing and reading have actually attracted more attention than writing and oral language (Shanahan, 2006). Fitzgerald and Shanahan (2000) identified four ways in which reading and writing depend on common cognitive domains. Clearly, both draw on content knowledge (although the influence of content knowledge on reading comprehension has been better researched). Writing, after all, has to be *about* something, and the more one knows, the more text one can produce. Content knowledge, then, provides a supportive framework for both reading and writing. Content knowledge can also be increased by reading (obviously) and writing (less obviously). The view of writing as a *tool* for learning, popularized by Bereiter and Scardamalia (1987) as the knowledge-transforming view of writing and discussed earlier, draws our attention to this additional similarity between writing and reading. A second common cognitive domain is conscious knowledge (meta-knowledge) about written language. For example, writers develop insights about how to assist their eventual readers to understand their perspective, and vice versa, readers could gain insight about how to be a better writer through their experiences (good or bad) with reading. A third shared domain is the common cognitive and linguistic subsystems that underlie writing and reading. These include features at the level of both word recognition/spelling and text comprehension/composition. As reported by Shanahan (2006), the amount of linguistic variance shared by writing and reading was rarely above 50 percent, but when researchers in recent studies have used multiple measures of linguistic variables, shared variance has increased substantially (to as high as 85 percent). Typically, shared variance is higher for word-level measures than for text-level measures. Of note, the relationships are bidirectional, with writing influencing reading and the reverse, reading influencing writing (Berninger, Abbott, Abbott, Graham, & Richards, 2002). The final area that writing and reading share is in the area of procedural knowledge, namely the "hows" of writing and reading. An example would be knowing that the strategy of summarizing is useful in both writing as well as reading.

Insights into writing–reading connections provided by correlations, although they are helpful, cannot provide data that establish either causation or sequence (which modality influences the other). Because writing and reading develop over a long period of time, both rely on many subsystems, and the nature of their relationship could change at different points along this developmental continuum, it is important to pursue other research designs. Shanahan (2006, 2009) summarized cross-modality instruction research, which is better suited to answer causality and sequence questions. Shanahan noted that the effect of writing instruction on reading achievement has received the most emphasis (as opposed to reading instruction effects on writing), a fact he attributes to the imbalance generally in the scientific study of reading and writing and the national sense of urgency to bolster children's reading achievement. In addition to Shanahan's work, a recently published report (*Writing to Read*, Graham & Hebert, 2010) has published results of a meta-analysis of instructional research on the effects of writing on reading. Several important findings from these sources include

- Writing about a reading passage (e.g., answering questions, summarizing, analyzing and interpreting, writing a personal reaction) improves comprehension above and beyond "just" reading, rereading, reading and studying, and reading and discussion.
- Reading comprehension is improved by explicit teaching of (1) text structure in exemplar passages (that are read), followed by writing passages using the same template, and (2) paragraph and sentence construction, including sentence-combining.
- Reading fluency is improved by explicit teaching of spelling and sentence construction.
- Word recognition is improved by explicit teaching of spelling.
- Increasing the amount of writing students do improves reading because the act of writing prompts more thoughtful engagement when reading others' writing.

Shanahan (2009) concluded that the best course of action is to teach reading and writing simultaneously in a much more integrated fashion than commonly occurs now and, because the connections between reading and writing differ across the long developmental continuum, to do so over the entire period of literacy learning. He would have teachers look for ways to exploit the relationship between writing and reading at the right time. For example, when the students' task is to compose more extended historical analyses, at that point they would be asked to read model texts, to explicitly analyze what makes those texts work well, and to reproduce those features in their own writing.

Summary

Writing well is a worthwhile goal given the critical role it plays in education, work, and personal lives. Learning to write well is a long and complicated process as detailed in this chapter. It involves learning about unique ways of making meaning with unique forms of language for unique purposes. It requires degrees of linguistic and cognitive awareness and control that transcend speaking and listening. While sharing many features with reading, writing often stands alone as a challenge for students of all ages, particularly those with language and learning disabilities.

Writing, like reading, has origins that precede entry into formal schooling. A preschool child experiments with "making writing"—marks that are unique and can be distinguished from drawing early on. As young children draw and write together in school, writing seems to be at the center of complex social interactions that are not entirely understood. By the end of the first grade, most children are conventional writers, creating short but coherent texts that can be read by others. Within a few years, their written texts can be distinguished from spoken discourse in terms of sentence structure and lexical choice. With several more years of school, the older elementary and middle school student should be able to write texts with good narrative and expository organization and content. By now writing is the main avenue for demonstrating learning (and reading comprehension) in all content disciplines. As a result, there is a strong association of writing ability with academic achievement. State and national testing reveals that more than half of all students are not writing proficiently.

Several changes in the way writing is taught have been suggested. One is to stress informational forms of writing earlier in the curriculum. Another is to revise literacy instruction to be more content specific—for example, teach students the ways that science and history texts utilize different language structures and patterns and provide practice writing in these distinctive ways. Another is combining instruction in reading and writing throughout the school years in ways that are mutually enriching. A challenge for writing researchers will be to demonstrate that these methods are effective, using designs with higher levels of experimental control.

References

Applebee, A. (1984). *Contexts for learning to write*. Norwood, NJ: Ablex.

Applebee, A., Langer, J., & Mullis, I. (1986). *The writing report card: Writing achievement in American Schools*. Princeton, NJ: Educational Testing Services.

August, D., Branun-Martin, L., Cardenas-Hagan, E., & Francis, D. (2009). The impact of an instructional intervention on the science and language learning of middle grade English language learners. *Journal of Research on Educational Effectiveness, 2*, 345–376.

Beason, L. (1993). Feedback and revision in writing across the curriculum classes. *Research in the Teaching of English, 27*, 395–422.

Bereiter, C., & Scardamalia, M. (1987). *The psychology of written composition*. Hillsdale, NJ: Erlbaum.

Berman, R. A., & Nir, B. (2010). The language of expository discourse across adolescence. In M. Nippold & C. Scott (Eds.), *Expository discourse in children, adolescents and adults* (pp. 99–121). New York: Psychology Press.

Berman, R., & Verhoeven, L. (2002). Cross-linguistic perspectives on the development of text-production abilities. *Written Language & Literacy, 5,* 1–43.

Berninger, V. (1999). Coordinating transcription and text generation in working memory during composing: Automatized and constructive processes. *Learning Disability Quarterly, 22,* 99–112.

Berninger, V. (2000). Development of language by hand and its connections with language by ear, mouth, and eye. *Topics in Language Disorders, 20,* 65–84.

Berninger, V. W., Abbott, R. D., Abbott, S. P., Graham. S., & Richards, T. (2002). Writing and reading: Connections between language by hand and language by ear. *Journal of Learning Disabilities, 35,* 39–56.

Berninger, V. W., Garcia, N. P., & Abbot, R. D. (2009). Multiple processes that matter in writing instruction and assessment. In G. A. Troia (Ed.), *Instruction and assessment for struggling writers* (pp. 15–59). New York: Guilford.

Biber, D. (1986). Spoken and written textual dimensions in English: Resolving the contradictory findings. *Language, 62,* 383–414.

Burkhalter, N. (1995). A Vygotsky-based curriculum for teaching persuasive writing in the elementary grades. *Language Arts, 72,* 192–199.

Burtis, J., Bereiter, C., Scardamalia, M., & Tetroe, J. (1983). The development of planning in writing. In B. Krolls & G. Wells (Eds.), *Exploration in the development of writing* (pp. 153–176). New York: Wiley.

Carlisle, J. (1996). An exploratory study of morphological errors in children's written stories. *Reading and Writing: An Interdisciplinary Journal, 8,* 61–72.

Chapman, M. (1994). The emergence of genres: Some findings from an examination of first-grade writing. *Written Communication, 11,* 348–380.

Chapman, M. (1995). The sociolinguistic construction of written genres in the first grade. *Research in the Teaching of English, 29,* 164–192.

Christie, F. (1986). Writing in the infants grades. In C. Painter & J. Martin (Eds.), *Writing to mean: Teaching genres across the curriculum* (pp. 118–135). Melbourne, Australia: Applied Linguistics Association of Australia, Occasional Papers, No. 9.

Crowhurst, M. (1987). Cohesion in argument and narration at three grade levels. *Research in the Teaching of English, 21,* 185–201.

Crowhurst, M., & Piche, G. (1979). Audience and mode of discourse effects on syntactic complexity in writing at two grade levels. *Research in the Teaching of English, 13,* 101–109.

De Temple, J. M., Wu, H.-F., & Snow, C. (1991). Papa pig just left for pigtown: Children's oral and written picture descriptions under varying instructions. *Discourse Processes, 14,* 469–495.

Donovan, C. A., & Smolkin, L. B. (2002). Children's genre knowledge: An examination of K–5 students' performance on multiple tasks providing differing levels of scaffolding. *Reading Research Quarterly, 37,* 428–465.

Donovan, C. A., & Smolkin, L. B. (2006). Children's understanding of genre and writing development. In C. A. MacArthur, S. Graham, & J. Fitzgerald (Eds.), *Handbook of writing research* (pp. 131–143). New York: Guilford.

Duke, N. (2000). 3.6 minutes per day: The scarcity of informational texts in first grade. *Reading Research Quarterly, 35,* 202–224.

Durst, R., Laine, C., Shultz, L., & Vilter, W. (1990). Appealing texts: The persuasive writing of high school students. *Written Communication, 7,* 232–255.

Dyson, A. (1989). *Multiple worlds of child writers: Friends learning to write.* New York: Teachers College Press.

Dyson, A. (1993a). *Social worlds of children learning to write in an urban primary school.* New York: Teachers College Press.

Dyson, A. (1993b). A sociocultural perspective on symbolic development in primary grade classrooms. In C. Daiute (Ed.), *The development of literacy through social interaction* (pp. 25–40). San Francisco: Jossey-Bass.

Dyson, A. (2008). Staying in the (curricular) lines: Practice constraints and possibilities in childhood writing. *Written Communication, 25,* 119–159.

Faigley, L., Cherry, R., Joliffe, D., & Skinner, A. (1985). *Assessing writers' knowledge and processes of composing.* Norwood, NJ: Ablex.

Ferreiro, E. (1984). The underlying logic of literacy development. In H. Goelman, A. Oberg, & F. Smith (Eds.), *Awakening to literacy* (pp. 154–173). London: Heinemann.

Fitzgerald, J., & Shanahan, T. (2000). Reading and writing relations and their development. *Educational Psychologist, 35,* 39–50.

Freedman, A. (1987). Development in story writing. *Applied Psycholinguistics, 8,* 153–170.

Golder, C., & Coirier, P. (1994). Argumentative text writing: Developmental trends. *Discourse Processes, 18,* 187–210.

Golub, L., & Frederick, W. (1971). *Linguistic structures in the discourse of fourth and sixth graders.* Wisconsin Research and Development Center for Cognitive

Learning, Technical Report No. 166. Madison: University of Wisconsin.

Gombert, J. E. (1992). *Metalinguistic development.* Chicago: University of Chicago Press.

Graham, S., & Hebert, M. (2010). *Writing to read: Evidence for how writing can improve reading.* Washington, DC: Alliance for Excellent Education.

Halliday, M. A. K. (1985). *Spoken and written language.* Oxford: Oxford University Press.

Halliday, M. A. K. (1987). Spoken and written modes of meaning. In R. Horowitz & S. J. Samuels (Eds.), *Comprehending oral and written language* (pp. 55–82). San Diego: Academic Press.

Harrell, L. (1957). A comparison of the development of oral and written language in school-age children. *Monographs of the Society for Research in Child Development, 22,* Serial No. 66, No. 3.

Hayes, J. R. (1996). A new framework for understanding cognition and affect in writing. In M. C. Levy & S. Ransdell (Eds.), *The science of writing* (pp. 1–27). Mahwah, NJ: Erlbaum.

Hayes, J. R. (2004). What triggers revision. In L. Allal, L. Chanquoy, & P. Largy (Eds.), *Studies in writing: Vol 13. Revision: Cognitive and instructional processes* (pp. 9–20). Norwell, MA: Kluwer.

Hayes, J. R., & Flower, L. (1980). Identifying the organization of writing processes. In L. Gregg & E. Steinberg (Eds.), *Cognitive processes in writing: An interdisciplinary approach* (pp. 3–30). Hillsdale, NJ: Erlbaum.

Hayes, J. R., & Flower, L. (1987). On the structure of the writing process. *Topics in Language Disorders, 7,* 19–30.

Heller, R., & Greenleaf, C. (2007). *Literacy instruction in the content areas: Getting to the core of middle and high school improvement.* Washington, DC: Alliance for Excellent Education.

Hidi, S., & Hildyard, A. (1983). The comparison of oral and written productions in two discourse types. *Discourse Processes, 6,* 91–105.

Hillocks, G. (2002). *The testing trap: How state writing assessments control learning.* New York: Teachers College Press.

Johnson, D. J., & Blalock, J. W. (1987). *Adults with learning disabilities: Clinical studies.* Toronto: Grune & Sratton.

Johnson, S., Linton, P., & Madigan, R. (1994). The role of internal standards in assessment of written discourse. *Discourse Processes, 18,* 231–245.

Katusic, S. K., Colligan, R. C., Weaver, A. L., & Barbaresi, W. J. (2009). The forgotten learning disability: Epidemiology of written-language disorder in a population-based birth cohort (1976–1982), Rochester, Minnesota. *Pediatrics, 123,* 1306–1313.

Knudson, R. E. (1994). An analysis of persuasive discourse: Learning how to take a stand. *Discourse Processes, 18,* 211–230.

Kress, G. (1982). *Learning to write.* London: Routledge & Kegan Paul.

Kroll, B. (1981). Developmental relationships between speaking and writing. In B. Roll & R. Vann (Eds.), *Exploring speaking–writing relationships: Connections and contrasts* (pp. 32–54). Urbana, IL: National Council of Teachers of English.

Langer, J. (1985). Children's sense of genre. A study of the performance on parallel reading and writing tasks. *Written Communication, 2,* 157–187.

Lin, S. C., Monroe, B. W., & Troia, G. A. (2007). Development of writing knowledge in grades 2–8: A comparison of typically developing writers and their struggling peers. *Reading & Writing Quarterly, 23,* 207–230.

Loban, W. (1976). *Language development: Kindergarten through grade twelve.* Champaign, IL: National Council of Teachers of English, Research Report No. 18.

Martin, J. R. (1989). *Factual writing: Exploring and challenging social reality.* Oxford, UK: Oxford University Press.

McCann, T. M. (1989). Student argumentative writing: Knowledge and ability at three grade levels. *Research in the Teaching of English, 23,* 62–76.

McCormick, C., Busching, B., & Potter, E. (1992). Children's knowledge about writing: The development and use of evaluative criteria. In M. Pressley, K. Harris, & J. T. Guthrie (Eds.), *Promoting academic competence and literacy in school* (pp. 311–335). San Diego, Academic Press.

McCutchen, D. (2006). Cognitive factors in the development of writing. In C. A. MacArthur, S. Graham, & J. Fitzgerald (Eds.), *Handbook of writing research* (pp. 115–130). New York, Guilford.

McCutchen, D., & Perfetti, C.A. (1982). Coherence and connectedness in the development of discourse production. *Text, 2,* 113–139.

Merenda, R. (1996). Writing: An adventure for young children. *Writing Teacher, 9,* 12–14.

Newkirk, T. (1987). The non-narrative writing of young children. *Research in the Teaching of English, 21,* 121–144.

Nippold, M. (2010). Explaining complex matters: How knowledge of a domain drives language. In M. Nippold & C. Scott (Eds.), *Expository discourse in children, adolescents and adults* (pp. 41–62). New York: Psychology Press.

Nippold, M., & Scott, C. (2010). *Expository discourse in children, adolescents, and adults*. New York: Psychology Press.

O'Donnell, R., Griffin, W., & Norris, R. (1967). *Syntax of kindergarten and elementary school children: A transformational analysis*. Champaign, IL: National Council of Teachers of English, Research Report No. 8.

Pelligrini, A., Galda, L., & Rubin, D. (1984). Context in text: The development of oral and written language in two genres. *Child Development, 55,* 1549–1555.

Percell-Gates, V., Duke, N. L., & Martineau, J. A. (2007). Learning to read and write genre-specific text: Roles of authentic experience and explicit teaching. *Reading Research Quarterly, 42*(1), 8–45.

Perera, K. (1984). *Children's writing and reading*. London: Blackwell.

Perera, K. (1986). Grammatical differentiation between speech and writing in children aged 8 to 12. In A. Wilkinson (Ed.), *The writing of writing* (pp. 90–108). London: The Falmer Press.

Rubin, D. (1984). The influence of communicative context on stylistic variations in writing. In D. D. Pellegrini & T. D. Yawkey (Eds.), *The development of oral and written language in social contexts* (pp. 213–232). Norwood, NJ: Ablex.

Rubin, D. (1987). Divergence and convergence between oral and written language communication. *Topics in Language Disorders, 7,* 1–18.

Saddler, B., & Graham, S. (2007). The relationship between writing knowledge and writing performance among more and less skilled writers. *Reading & Writing Quarterly, 23,* 231–247.

Salahu-Din, D., Persky, H., & Miller, U. (2008). *The nation's report card: Writing 2007.* NCES 2008-468. National Center for Educational Statistics. Institute of Education Sciences Washington, DC: U.S. Department of Education.

Scott, C. (1988). Spoken and written syntax. In M. Nippold (Ed.), *Later language development: Ages nine through nineteen* (pp. 49–95). San Diego: College-Hill Press.

Scott, C. (1994). A discourse continuum for school-age students: Impact of modality and genre. In G. Wallach & K. Butler (Eds.), *Language learning disabilities in school-age children and adolescents* (pp. 219–252). New York: Merrill.

Scott, C. (2002, June). *Speaking and writing the same texts: Comparisons of school children with and with-out language learning disabilities*. Paper presented at the 12th annual meeting of the Society for Text and Discourse, Chicago.

Scott, C. (2003, June). *Literacy as variety: An analysis of clausal connectivity in spoken and written language of children with language learning disabilities.* Paper presented at the 24th Annual Symposium on Research in Child Language Disorders, Madison, WI.

Scott, C. (2010). Assessing expository texts produced by school-age children and adolescents. In M. Nippold & C. Scott (Eds.), *Expository discourse in children, adolescents and adults* (pp. 191–214). New York: Psychology Press.

Scott, C., & Balthazar, C. (2010). The grammar of information: Challenges for students with and without language impairments. *Topics in Language Disorders, 30*(4), 288–307.

Scott, C., & Jennings, M. (2004, November). *Expository discourse in children with LLD: Text level analysis.* A paper presented at the annual meeting of the American Speech-Language-Hearing Association, Philadelphia, PA.

Scott, C., & Windsor, J. (2000). General language performance measures in spoken and written narrative and expository discourse in school-age children with language learning disabilities. *Journal of Speech, Language, and Hearing Research, 43,* 324–339.

Shanahan, T. (2006). Relations among oral language, reading, and writing development. In C. A. MacArthur, S. Graham, & J. Fitzgerald (Eds.), *Handbook of writing research* (pp. 171–186). New York: Guilford.

Shanahan, T. (2009). Connecting reading and writing instruction for struggling readers. In G. Troia (Ed.), *Instruction and assessment for struggling writers* (pp. 113–131). New York: Guilford.

Shanahan, T., & Shanahan, C. (2008). Teaching disciplinary literacy to adolescents: Rethinking content-area literacy. *Harvard Educational Review, 78*(1), 40–59.

Snyder, L., & Caccamise, D. (2010). Comprehension processes for expository text: Building meaning and making sense. In M. Nippold & C. Scott (Eds.), *Expository discourse in children, adolescents and adults* (pp. 13–40). New York: Psychology Press.

Sulzby, E. (1996). Roles of oral and written language as children approach conventional literacy. In C. Pontecorvo, M. Orsolini, B. Burge, & L. B. Resnick (Eds.), *Children's early text construction* (pp. 25–46). Mahwah, NJ: Erlbaum.

Sulzby, E., Branz, C., & Buhle, R. (1993). Repeated readings of literature and low socioeconomic status black kindergartners and first graders. *Reading and Writing Quarterly, 9,* 183–196.

Tolchinsky, L., & Teberosky, A. (1998). The development of word segmentation and writing in two scripts. *Cognitive Development, 13*, 1–21.

Verhoeven, L. Aparici, M., Cahana-Amitay, D., van Hell, J., Kriz, S., & Viguié-Simon, A. (2002). Clause packaging in writing and speech: A cross-linguistic developmental analysis. *Written Language & Literacy, 5*, 135–162.

Ward-Lonergan, J. (2010). Expository discourse in school-age children and adolescents with language disorders: Nature of the problem. In M. Nippold & C. Scott (Eds.), *Expository discourse in children, adolescents and adults* (pp. 155–190). New York: Psychology Press.

Yagelski, R. P. (1995). The role of classroom context in the revision strategies of student writers. *Research in the Teaching of English, 29*, 216–238.

Zucchermaglio, C., & Scheuer, N. (1996). Children dictating a story: Is together better? In C. Pontecorvo, M. Orsolini, B. Burge, & L. B. Resnick (Eds.), *Children's early text construction* (pp. 83–98). Mahwah, NJ: Erlbaum.

Chapter 10

Developing Knowledge and Skills for Writing

Carol E. Westby

Many students have strong feelings about writing, and these feelings, particularly for older students, are frequently not positive. Even though they may not exhibit any specific reading or writing difficulties, many students do not look forward to writing assignments. Like 6-year-old Calvin, in the *Calvin and Hobbes* comic strip popular in recent years, they find they must be in the right mood to write, and that mood is "last-minute panic." They wish they could jump into a time machine and return after the paper is completed. They complain of writer's block, although unlike Calvin, the block is not a chunk of wood you put on your desk "so you can't write there anymore."

Approaches to teaching writing have changed in the last four decades. Through much of the 20th century, the teaching of writing focused on handwriting, spelling, diagramming sentences, and evaluation of a final written product. Research conducted in the latter part of the 20th century (Graves, 1983; Emig, 1971) led to a focus on the process, rather than solely the product, of writing. Attention was given to stages in writing—prewriting, writing, editing, and revision. As teachers observed children engaged in the process of writing, they were to identify the difficulties students were having and provide appropriate instruction and support. In the writing process approach, mechanics and skills were de-emphasized. Specific skills were addressed as students exhibited a need for them in their writing. Educators/researchers supporting a writing process approach based their ideas on a constructivist theory in which students were expected to discover how to write by writing. They rejected the teaching of discrete skills such as handwriting, vocabulary, and grammar, as well as the belief that mastery of basic skills is a necessary prerequisite for more advanced learning. The advantages of a constructivist approach over a skill-and-drill or workbook approach are intuitively obvious. The constructivist writing activities are more authentic, and if students self-selected activities, they are more likely to be motivated to do them well. Difficulties, however, arise in practice. When the purist, constructivist philosophy is applied to writing, teachers are not to assume the role of experts either by requiring particular types of writing or by correcting students' writing. Although these practices work for some students, parents and teachers voiced concerns about students who do not learn to read naturally and students whose handwriting is illegible and labored and whose spelling remains poor long past the early grades. The purist constructivist approach is falling into disfavor and is being replaced by a more balanced approach to writing that integrates authentic writing activities and the stages of the writing process with explicit skill teaching.

Harris and Graham (1996a) have expressed concern about the use of a writing process or constructivist approach, particularly with students with learning disabilities. These students are likely to have difficulty generating ideas and content, translating the ideas into graphemes and sentence structures, organizing the ideas, monitoring their performance, identifying errors, and knowing how to correct those errors. Simply providing these students opportunities to write and addressing their skill deficits in "teachable moments" or minilessons is not likely to result in improvements in their writing. Important strategies might not be introduced because "teachable moments" are overlooked, and minilessons might not provide the explicitness and intensity of instruction required by students with disabilities. Many of these students will require more extended, structured, and explicit instruction to develop the skills and strategies essential for writing. Harris and Graham (1996a, b) advocate integrating explicit writing strategy instruction within the writing process. There is no reason that one cannot use the process stages (prewriting, drafting, revising, editing, publishing, and evaluation) while also providing students with direct teaching of components essential to carry out the writing process. This requires attention to the individual strengths and needs of the students and the requirements of the writing tasks.

Singer and Bashir (2004) proposed a framework that is intended to explain the variations and difficulties students exhibit in the production of written language. When writing, students must manage and coordinate multiple processes simultaneously. They must have what Singer and Bashir have termed the foundations for writing and the ability to carry out writing processes. The writing foundations comprise four elements:

- Production: The graphomotor skills to produce a written text whether by handwriting or keyboarding.
- Cognitive/linguistic: This includes linguistic skills (phoneme/grapheme match, vocabulary, syntax); conceptual understanding and content knowledge, including knowledge of the structures of various genres; metalinguistic and metacognitive knowledge; and processing speed/working memory.
- Social rhetorical knowledge of the rhetorical task: knowledge of when and how to use the various genres.
- Beliefs and attitudes regarding oneself as a writer.

The writing processes comprise five elements:

- Planning: Setting a goal.
- Organizing: Deciding how to structure and sequence the content of the text.

- Generating: Generating ideas that will be expressed in linguistic units; recruiting knowledge of discourse structure as the linguistic units are strung together.
- Revising: Making changes to text so that it conveys the writer's intended meaning.
- Executive functions and self-regulation: Executive functions subsume abilities such as selective, sustained, and divided attention; attention span; inhibiting; maintenance of cognitive set; and anticipatory processes. Self-regulation refers to behaviors that are used to guide, monitor, and direct the success of one's performance. All the elements of the writing processes are dependent on executing functioning/self-regulation.

Some degree of the foundational skills must be in place if students are to engage in the writing processes that involve using self-regulatory skills for planning, generating, organizing, and revising texts. Yet, the two components—writing foundations and writing processes—are interactive. The need or motivation to participate in the writing process provides a reason or purpose for developing the foundational skills. Students with writing disabilities exhibit deficits at multiple levels that impair their ability to produce cohesive, coherent written texts. Intervention programs to facilitate development of writing should address each of these components. Many writing intervention programs are beneficial for all students and can be carried out within regular education classrooms. Many students with writing disabilities, however, will generally require more time and more explicit instruction than can generally be given within the regular classroom (Nelson, Roth, & Van Meter, 2009; Scanlon, Deshler, & Schumaker, 1996). Such students will require support from speech-language pathologists and special educators to develop their writing abilities.

A meta-analysis of research on writing instruction by Graham and Perin (2007a, b) and Graham and Hebert (2010) provides guidelines for best practices in writing instruction. The focus of these reports was on all students, not just those who display writing difficulties. The premise is that all students need to become proficient and flexible writers. In the reports, the term *low-achieving writers* is used to refer to students whose writing skills are not adequate to meet classroom demands. Some of these low-achieving writers have been identified as having learning disabilities; others are the "silent majority" who lack writing proficiency but do not receive additional help. In the *Writing Next* report (2007b), Graham and Perin described a number of evidence-based approaches to writing instruction that include teaching students writing strategies for planning, revising, and editing their compositions; explicitly teaching students how to summarize texts; providing activities in which students collaborate to plan, draft, and revise their writing; assigning products with specific goals; using word processing; teaching students sentence combining as a way to produce more complex sentences; engaging students in prewriting activities and inquiry activities that help them generate and organize ideas; studying models of good writing; and using writing for learning content material. In the *Writing to Read* report, Graham and Hebert (2010) describe additional evidence-based practices that not only improve writing but also improve reading comprehension. They recommend having students write about texts that they read, take notes on texts, write summaries, and write personal reactions and analyses. They also recommend explicitly teaching students the skills that go into creating texts—teaching spelling, sentence and paragraph constructions, the structure of different types of texts, and the processes of writing (planning, drafting, revising, and editing). And finally, they advocate that students write more because reading comprehension is influenced by the amount of their own texts that students produce. This chapter describes strategies for developing writing foundations and writing processes based on the research that has documented the most effective educational practices.

DEVELOPING WRITING FOUNDATIONS

Production/Transcription Skills

Students must have some method for putting their ideas into print, either through handwriting or word processing. The Graham and Perin (2007a) meta-analysis indicated that the quality of students' writing was better when they used word processing rather than handwriting. The specific factors that contributed to this improved performance using word processing are uncertain. Word processing may reduce motoric effort and require less working memory skills for children (they do not have to remember how to produce letters), and hence they may be able to devote more attention to other aspects of writing. Alternatively, the use of computers may simply be more motivating than writing by hand. To develop keyboarding fluency, however, attention will need to be given to keyboarding skills.

In this multimedia world, students should be taught how to use computers for writing tasks, but this does not mean that handwriting should be ignored. There continue to be many instances where handwriting is necessary. Many students with writing disabilities have difficulty with the motor act itself of putting pencil to paper. For these students, the physical act of writing—putting graphemes on paper—disrupts the writing process before it begins. Attending to mechanics of writing may interfere with higher order writing in several ways (Berninger & Amtmann, 2003; Graham, 1992):

- Causes writers to forget already developed intentions and meanings
- Disrupts the planning process, resulting in writing that is less coherent and complex
- Takes time away from the time necessary to find expressions that precisely fit their intentions
- Prevents students from writing fast enough to keep up with their thoughts, thus causing them to lose ideas and plans
- Affects students' persistence, motivation, and sense of confidence for writing

If students are to be able to attend to the process and products of writing over the mechanics, the motor act of writing must become automatic or at least easier. As the role of fluent handwriting in the quality of spelling and text production has become recognized (Graham, Berninger, Abbott, Abbot, & Whitaker, 1997), schools are reintroducing structured writing programs such as *Writing without Tears* (Olsen, 1998).

Cognitive/Linguistic Skills

The cognitive/linguistic writing foundation elements involve knowledge of both text microstructure (syntax, connectives, vocabulary) and text macrostructure (the gist and organization of the text). The authors of the *Writing Next* and *Writing to Read* reports reviewed experimental studies that investigated the effectiveness of individual interventions or strategies addressing both microstructure and macrostructure aspects of writing. In practice, many of these interventions would be used in combination. For example, educators can provide models of good writing at all macrostructure and microstructure levels. Dorfman and Cappelli (2007, 2009) described the ways to teach the writing of narrative and expository texts by using children's literature as mentor texts.

The genre-based writing approach to teaching writing employs the use of mentor texts and teacher expertise to develop students' knowledge and use of microstructure and macrostructure elements in writing. Academic success in later elementary school and beyond requires that students be able to produce texts representing a variety of functions or genres. A genre-based approach to the teaching of writing arose in Australia influenced by Halliday's work in functional linguistics (Halliday, 1985). Halliday's work brought educators and linguists together in a transdisciplinary manner to enable teachers to see linguistics as a practical tool in their everyday work. A genre is defined as *a staged, goal oriented social process* achieved primarily through language (Martin, 1987, cited in Coe, 1994). Genres are ways that people make meaning with one another in stages to achieve their goals. Stages represent the components or structure of the genres (e.g., the beginnings, middles, and ends). Genres are considered social processes because members of a given culture have learned particular ways to use them in particular settings. Genres are designed for a variety of goals: to inform, to entertain, to argue a point, to persuade, to complain, to consult, etc. Different genres have different macrostructures and use different microstructures to convey their meanings. Three phases are employed in genre-based teaching.

PHASE 1: MODELING.   In the first phase, teachers introduce the genre to be studied. They discuss the social function of the genre, the schematic stages or components of the genre, and the linguistic characteristics of the genre. A model of the genre is introduced that is tied to a thematic unit in the curriculum. A text can be displayed on an overhead, and macrostructure elements and linguistic characteristics can be highlighted and the components of the text discussed. The teacher also notes particular grammatical structures and technical vocabulary that are important in building the case. It can also be useful for students to compare a good model with a model that fails to meet the criteria of the genre.

Many mentor texts are available that highlight the organization of particular genres and the use of particular syntactic patterns. In *Aunt Isabel Tells a Good One* (Duke, 1992), Aunt Isabel introduces the basic ingredients of stories—characters, problem, solution—as she tells a story and simultaneously teaches her niece how to create a story by combining elements such as a heroine, a hero, excitement, and romance. Narrative books can highlight structures that can not only be useful for narratives, but that can also provide an introduction to types of structures needed in expository texts. For example, *The Secret Shortcut* (Teague, 1996) can be used to focus on sequence. Wendell and Floyd tell a number of tall tales about why they are late for school. They decide to reform their bad habit, and to get to school on time, they take a shortcut. This shortcut turns into an adventurous series of experiences. Students can use the story as a frame to design their own "shortcut" to school. As they introduce each event, the teacher can ask that they use a new sequencing word that leads to a different event (e.g., *before, after, then, next, during, finally, first, second, third, earlier, later, last, meanwhile, simultaneously*).

I Wanna Iguana (Orloff, 2004) can be used to introduce the components and structure of persuasive texts. In *I Wanna Iguana*, a boy named Alex wants to adopt his friend's iguana. He decides to write this desire down in friendly letter form and give it to his mother. The book is told from both his and his mother's perspectives as they write friendly letters to each other. Alex doesn't beg—he formulates convincing arguments about why he and this iguana belong together. Alex is careful to address his mother's concerns through presenting facts, clarifying his ideas, and promising to be a great pet owner. Through Alex's skill in persuasion, he comes out the victor and receives a scaly surprise on his bedroom dresser.

PHASE 2: JOINT CONSTRUCTION OF A TEXT.   During this phase the teacher and students work together to produce a text. The teacher guides the students by asking questions that focus on the stages of the genre. Initially the students research the topic through reading, interviewing others, watching videos, using library books and computer resources, or going on field trips.

After they collect data, the class is brought together to summarize their information on the chalkboard/whiteboard. The teacher may assist the students to organize the information they have gathered in a semantic web. Once all the information has been gathered and organized, the teacher guides the students as a group in producing the text. The teacher asks questions and makes comments that point to the structure of the text or the possibility or reasonableness of a statement. The teacher writes the text on the board or overhead transparency so that the children can concentrate on the meanings they are formulating.

A popular way to begin the process is by teaching poetry or narratives. Templates can easily be provided for both of these genres. Educators may use a poem such as, "Where I'm from" (Lyon, 1999), to teach a structure and for giving students experience in writing what they know. A variety of templates is available for this poem. A fifth-grade teacher provided the following framework.

I'm from_____ (one or two objects in your home)

with _____ (something you eat)

with _____ (what someone does)

with _____ (what someone says)

_____ (what you are doing)

_____ (what you are doing)

If you ask me where I'm from, I'll tell you I'm from ____

Using this framework, an English-language learner (ELL) wrote the following poem.

I'm from my Grama's special dishes with pink flowers
With great posole and quesadillas for lunch.
With my grandpa's dragging feet
Dragging on the floor, wanting dinner, tired and worn out.
With my Grama yelling to my sisters and Mom,
"Enchiladas for dinner, come and eat!"
Well, dinner is before dishes
Anxious to start reading a book
"Hurry!" yelling to my sister.

Sitting on the tree calmly reading my book,
Looking at my Grama's colorful garden.

If you ask me where I'm from
I'll tell you

I'm from Mexico.

PHASE 3: INDEPENDENT CONSTRUCTION OF A TEXT.   Students choose a new topic for their writing. Students must conduct their background research more independently. They write a draft, referring to the model and jointly constructed text that had been presented. The students then consult with the teacher about their draft. The teacher's questions and comments focus in a constructive way on what the students have done and what they can do to further develop their piece. This strategy is different from simply telling the students what they did right or wrong. The feedback is explicit. It is not simply encouraging; it also offers advice or guidance on how to make the text more effective.

Numerous studies have shown that providing frameworks or templates for producing narratives greatly improves the quality of students' narratives. *The Story Grammar Marker* (SGM;

Moreau & Fidrych-Puzzo, 1994) is one system that has been used to increase students' awareness of narrative structure. Students use a braided yarn "critter" with small charms attached to it. A pom-pom head represents the story characters, a star below the head represents other elements of the setting (time, place), a boot represents the story kickoff or initiating event, a heart is the reaction to the initiating event, a hand represents a character's goal or plan to respond to the event, beads represent a series of attempts, bows near the end of the braid represent the consequences, and small hearts at the very end of the braid represent characters' reactions to the consequences. The SGM reduces the load on working memory by externalizing the global structure and sequence of components in stories. This allows students to concentrate on translating their ideas into words and sentences to convey the content of each element of the story. With the SGM, they do not also have to keep in mind where they are in the story.

In preparing to write a story, students can be encouraged to outline the elements of the story on a sheet that lists each of the story elements. Westby, Moore, and Roman (2002) incorporated the symbols from the SGM with the circular presentation of story elements proposed by Esterreicher (1994). A circle or wheel was divided into seven equal pies, representing the setting, initiating event, internal response, internal plan, attempt, consequence, and ending for a story. The SGM symbols were drawn in their respective pies. The circular format reminded the students that the end of the story should tie back to the beginning—a story should *come full circle*. A small version of this wheel was taped (using wide plastic tape) to the upper left-hand side of all third- through sixth-grade students' desks for reference when reading stories. When students were to write stories, they were given large wheels on 8 1/2-by-11-inch sheets of paper. They planned or outlined their stories on these sheets before writing them.

Exploring the Postmodern Genre

In postmodern books, the layout of the book is nontraditional. For instance, the layout might be comic-book style to tell a fairy tale or a series of pictures that tell two different stories, at the same time. This genre may ask the reader to become a part of the story, ending the traditional form of story reading, that of being outside characters' lives. Postmodernism asks the readers to impose their beliefs and prejudices onto the story. Another aspect of postmodernism is the element of the unreliable narrator. The readers do not know whether to believe the story or not. Readers have to suspend their disbelief throughout the story to get to the story's core. Many postmodern books require that students understand the content and structure or organization of traditional texts and recognize how the postmodern text plays with this content and structure. Postmodern books give students experience in playing with narrative structure. To fully appreciate such stories, students must recognize the structure and expectations in traditional narratives.

A fifth-grade class enjoyed sharing the postmodern book *Open Me . . . I'm a Dog!* (Spiegelman, 1997). In this book, a dog tries to convince the reader that he was turned first into a sheep herder by a mean witch, then into a frog by a magic maiden, and finally into a book by a wizard. The book comes complete with a leash and persuades the reader to take it home so he can become the reader's pet. After students read the book, they wrote they own stories following the structure of Spiegelman's book. In doing so, the students had to understand that this was a form of a fairy tale because it involved magic, remember that the main character changed forms many times during the book, and react to the persuasion that this was not a book they were holding but a dog. All the students wrote a piece reminiscent of the original, mostly using animals as their main character. The teacher provided a rubric for the elements that should be included in the

TABLE 10.1	Rubric for *Open Me . . . I'm a Dog!* (See Appendix 10.1 for the student stories referenced in this table)

	Open Me . . . I'm a Dog! (Spiegelman, 1997)	Read Me, I'm a Baseball	Open Me, I'm a Penguin
Replicate story structure			
Beginning	"What's that? You think I smell of paper and ink? You think I look like a book?"	**Author doesn't suggest that baseball was anything other than a baseball	Uses very similar opening ("What's that? You think I smell of paper and lead?")
Repetitive phrases	"get triple temper tantrum mad . . . said some words I don't even dare repeat". . . . "	**No repetitive phrases	Repeats phrases, e.g., "got really mad" "got super mad"
Ending persuades reader that the character is something other than a book	"I love sitting in your lap, but I want you to pet me not just turn my pages."	**The ball wins the world series. The ball was never turned into a book.	"But I can still squeak 'squeak, squeak' and cuddle in your lap. If you let me be your Arctic pet, I'll tell you my story anytime you like."
Tragic character	Dog experiences tragedies (e.g., turned into a shepherd, frog, and book)	**Baseball doesn't experience tragedy	Penguin experiences tragedies (e.g., turned into balloon, fish, and book)
Fairy tale characters	Witch, magic maiden, wizard	**No fairy tale characters	Wizard. Whale and albatross not fairy tale characters
Magic acts	Dog turned into shepherd, then frog, then book	*Baseball talks, but no indication how this happened	Penguin turned into flying balloon by whale, fish by albatross, and book by wizard
Character's typical behaviors trigger magic acts	Dog chews witch's broom, licks maiden	**No behaviors that trigger magic	Penguin hunts fish
Character behaviors fit its nature		**Never anything but a baseball	Penguin hunts fish, chased by whale, wants to do snow activities (ski, snowboard, and slide down ice)

*Student attempted to incorporate a component but did not do so *adequately.*
**The component was missing or did not fit the model.

students' stories. Table 10.1 shows the rubric and the components of the original story and of two stories written by students.

One student wrote a clever story from the point of view of Babe Ruth's special baseball titled, *Read Me, I'm a Baseball.* The story was imaginative, but did not include fairy tale characters and did not follow the prescribed framework. The baseball had always been a baseball—it had not magically been changed into a baseball, and it did not try to convince the reader that it was other than a baseball. The story did not use any of the syntactic patterns or repetitive phrases of the original story. In contrast, *Open Me, I'm a Penguin* incorporated many of the elements of the original story, including some similar syntactic patterns and repetitive phrases. The author adapted the events of the story to activities a penguin would do. The penguin experienced several magical tragedies that were triggered by typical penguin behavior. Children's books can be used to highlight different structures within and across genres. Dorfman and Cappelli (2007, 2009) provide detailed suggestion for ways to use literature and nonfiction texts to mentor students in writing.

Expository Texts

The genre approach to instruction becomes especially critical for expository texts because students typically have fewer encounters with these types of texts. The author of this chapter has used this three-phase approach in teaching the science report writing genre. The science report graphic organizer was posted on the board. A science report comprises three genres—a sequential, procedural genre of the steps in the experiment; a descriptive genre that reports the observed results of the experiment; and an explanatory genre that explains the cause–effect relationships occurring in the experiment. Students conducted three related experiments on a topic. Each experiment was slightly different, but all reinforced the same scientific principle. For example, when investigating water tension, students conducted three experiments.

- They filled two cups with water—one with pure water and one with water to which a small amount of detergent had been added. They then counted how many pennies they could put into each cup until the water overflowed.
- Using an eyedropper, students dropped pure water on one penny and water to which detergent had been added on a second penny. They counted how many drops of water they could put on each penny until the water overflowed
- Students made a small "bug" from an index card and glued tabs from soda cans to each foot of the bug. They placed the bug carefully on the surface of water in a tray and squirted a small amount of detergent behind the bug and watched what happened.

For the first experiment on a topic, the teacher modeled each component of the report (as shown in Figure 10.1). After students completed the second experiment on a topic, they jointly constructed the report as the teacher wrote it on an overhead. This jointly written report was Xeroxed and given to students in another class, who followed the procedures when they conducted the experiment. Consequently, the students and teacher carefully edited the report, making certain that their information was clear and explicit. After the third experiment on the topic, students wrote a report independently in their science journals.

Syntactic Structures

The writings of good authors can provide students with syntactic patterns. Students must know how to express their ideas clearly in coherent, cohesive, grammatically correct sentences. To write effectively, students must also be capable of a range of syntactic and cohesive strategies. By middle elementary school, children must be capable of producing a variety of independent and dependent clause structures (see examples in Chapter 9) linked by coordinating and subordinating conjunctions. Table 10.2 lists and defines these coordinating and subordinating conjunctions.

Although it would seem intuitive that explicitly teaching the grammatical structure of a language would result in better reading comprehension and writing, such is not the case (Hillocks & Smith, 2003). In fact, nearly all studies have found that the explicit teaching of grammar in traditional ways (identifying parts of speech, practicing grammatical forms and grammatical corrections

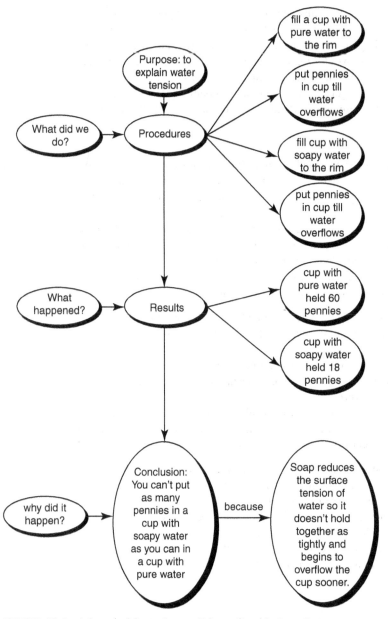

First, we filled the cups with pure water to the rim. Then we carefully dropped pennies into the cup one by one. We counted each penny we dropped into the cup. We watched until we saw a drop of water flow over the rim of the cup. We recorded the number of pennies we had put in the cup before the water overflowed. Next, we filled cups with water that had a little soap in it. We carefully dropped pennies into the cup one by one. We counted each penny we dropped into the cup. We watched until we saw the water overflow. We recorded the number of pennies we had put in the cup before the water overflowed.

The cup of pure water held 66 pennies before it overflowed. The meniscus of the water got higher and higher until a little water began to spill over the rim of the cup. The cup of water with detergent held only 18 pennies before the water overflowed. The meniscus of the water with detergent didn't get as high as the meniscus of the pure water.

Soap reduces the surface tension of water so the water molecules don't hold together as tightly. The cup with soapy water couldn't hold as many pennies as the cup of pure water because the soap reduced the water tension. Therefore, the soapy water overflowed sooner than the pure water.

FIGURE 10.1   A Sample Science Report Using a Graphic Organizer.

TABLE 10.2   Clausal Connecting Words

Connecting Words	Definition	Words with Similar Meaning
Coordinating connectors: Link independent clauses		
and	Plus Together with Occurring at the same time	In addition As well as
or	Tells us we have a choice	No true synonyms; in some contexts *optionally*, *alternatively*, or *on the other hand* may be substituted
but	Contrary to expectations	On the contrary However Yet, still Nevertheless Except that
hence	As a result From this time	Therefore As a result From now on
therefore	For that reason	Consequently Hence
yet	Means the same as *but*	But However Nevertheless Still Except that
Subordinating connectors: Link dependent clauses		
After	Following the time that	
Although/though	In spite of the fact	Even though Even if Supposing that
As	To the same degree that In the same way that	While Because
Because	For the reason that Since	For In view of the fact Inasmuch as
Taking into account that Before	In advance of the time when	Prior to
If	In the case that In the event that Whether	Granting that On condition that
Meanwhile	During or in the intervening time At the same time	

(continued)

TABLE 10.2 *(Continued)*		
Since	From the time that (preferred meaning) Continuously from the time when As a result of the fact that	Inasmuch Because for
Subordinating connectors: Link dependent clauses		
So that/in order that	For the purpose of	So With the wish that With the purpose that With the result that
Than	Compared to the degree that	
Unless	Except on the condition that	
Until	Up to the time that To the point or extent that	
When/whenever	At the time that	As soon as If While (although not synonymous)
Where/wherever	At what place In a place that To a place that	
While	During the time that At the same time that Although	As long as

on worksheets, and diagramming sentences) is negatively correlated with quality of writing (Hillocks & Smith, 2003; Saddler & Graham, 2005). The writing of students who had received traditional grammar instruction was worse than the writing of students who did not receive such instruction. In response to this research, many educators simply ceased all instruction in grammar and sentence structure. This research, however, should not be interpreted as indicating that students do not need explicit knowledge of grammar and sentence patterns. There are ways to explicitly teach grammar and sentence patterns that have been found to significantly improve children's writing and reading comprehension. The *Writing Next* report (Graham & Perin, 2007b) indicated that sentence combining activities, rather than traditional grammar teaching, positively affect the quality of students' writing.

By exploring extended passages written by authors, students can be taught grammar in context in meaningful ways. They can explore how and why authors use particular syntactic patterns to convey meaning. Dean (2008) calls such texts "mentor texts," rather than model texts. She notes that models are a likeness, pattern, or copy; in contrast, a mentor guides, advises, and supports. Dean suggests presenting students with high-quality published texts in which specific vocabulary or syntactic patterns are removed. The students read the passage and discuss the language and the mood that is established. Then the instructor replaces some components that were omitted, and students discuss how the added information clarifies the passage or makes it more interesting. Finally, all components are added back in. For example, the author of the 2009 Newbury award book *The Graveyard Book* (Gaiman, 2008) employs a variety of complex syntactic patterns. In this story, an 18-month-old baby is the sole survivor of an attack on his family. He escapes his house and toddles to a nearby graveyard. Quickly recognizing that the baby is orphaned, the graveyard's ghostly residents adopt him, name him Nobody ("Bod"), and allow him to live in their tomb. The syntactic patterns add to the eerie tone of the story. Consider these sentences without participial phrases:

> Now he got to his feet and walked forward more carefully, *startling an owl which rose on silent wings.* (Gaiman, p. 17)

> When he was satisfied he stepped out into the morning's dark, *his head churning with unpleasant possibilities,* and he returned to the graveyard, to the chapel spire where he slept and waited out the days. (Gaiman, p. 32)

The Accelerated Literacy program described in Chapter 7 is one framework for using high-quality texts to mentor students in literate syntactic patterns. Sentence combining is another approach that is effective in teaching children to construct more complex sentences (Saddler & Graham, 2005; Strong, 1986). The goal of sentence combining is to make sentence construction in writing more automatic and less labored and at the same time to make students more conscious of sentence options because text revision requires such awareness. One can begin by providing students with support for the combining. In the following examples, connecting words are put in parentheses following the sentences in which they appear; the word SOMETHING is a placeholder word for noun constructions; words or phrases that will be embedded (inserted) into a sentence are underlined; word-ending cues (e.g., [-ING], [-LY]) can be introduced after students get comfortable with the basic cues. One can generate novel sentences to provide practice on a particular type of combining, or one can take complex sentences from literature and textbooks, reduce them to simple sentences, have students recombine them, and then compare their combined sentences with the original texts. These examples are also from *The Graveyard Book.*

The man Jack was rattling the gates to the graveyard. The man wanted to get into the graveyard. (BECAUSE)	The man Jack was rattling the gates to the graveyard because he wanted to get in.
Mrs. Owens knew SOMETHING. The man shaking the gates wasn't the baby's family. (THAT)	Mrs. Owens knew that the man shaking the gates wasn't the baby's family.
The ghost woman said (SOMETHING). The man is trying to harm the baby. The man is <u>evil</u>.	The ghost woman said that the evil man is trying to harm the baby.
The Owens needed to figure out SOMETHING. Silas could bring food to the baby (HOW).	The Owens needed to figure out how Silas could bring food to the baby.
The Lady of Gray's horse was <u>ripping up</u> a clump of thick grass. The horse was <u>masticating</u> the clump of thick grass. The horse was content. (-LY)	The Lady of Gray's horse was contently ripping up and masticating a clump of thick grass.
There is a statue on the grave. (IF) The statue will be headless. The statue will be scabbed with fungus and lichen. (OR) The statue will look like fungus itself (AS TO)	If there is a statute on the grave, it will be headless or scabbed with fungus and lichen as to look like fungus itself.

Students can also be given a series of sentences and encouraged to work in groups to see how many different ways they can be combined, for example:

Titania was working hard on her test.

Kaylene slipped her a note.

Titania unfolded the paper carefully.

She didn't want her teacher to see.

Examples:

Titania was working hard on her test when Kaylene slipped her a note. Not wanting the teacher to see it, Titania unfolded the paper carefully.

Or

While Titania was working hard on her test, Kaylene slipped her a note, which Titania unfolded carefully because she didn't want the teacher to see.

Killgallon and Killgallon (2000, 2006) included sentence combining in a series of sequential strategies that employed the use of models to teach a variety of complex syntactic patterns to students from elementary school through college. In teaching each pattern, they select models of the patterns from a wide variety of the literature that students in each age range would be reading. Teaching of each syntactic structure begins with a definition and examples of the structure, followed by a series of systematic activities that begin with identifying the structure in sentences, combining sentences, unscrambling parts of sentences, expanding sentences, and producing novel sentences by imitating sentence types from books. Students then apply what they have learned in writing their own sentences and paragraphs.

The Killgallons use a series of worksheet activities to teach the various literate syntactic patterns. Educators can use the Killgallons' materials to introduce the particular syntactic patterns, but then develop activities using materials that the students are reading. For example, sentences from the book, *Harry Potter and the Chamber of Secrets* (Rowling, 2000) were used to develop adjective clauses following the Killgallons' protocol. Adjective clauses are defined as the part of a sentence that makes a statement about a person, place, or thing named in the sentences and that usually begins with words such as *who, which, that,* or *whose.* Adjective clauses can occur between a subject and verb (subject–verb split) (e.g., "Overhead, the bewitched ceiling, *which always mirrored the sky outside,* sparkled with stars"), or they can occur at the end of a sentence (e.g., "They said good-bye to the Grangers, *who were leaving the pub for the Muggle street on the other side*").

Practice 1: Identifying. First, students identify adjective clauses in sentences such as:

Dudley hitched up his up his trousers, <u>which were slipping down his fat bottom</u>.

Fred, <u>who had finished his own list</u>, peered over at Harry's.

They couldn't use the real Quidditch balls, <u>which would have been hard to explain if they had escaped and flown over the village</u>.

Practice 2: Combining. Next, students are given sentences to combine. They are told, "Combine the two sentences by making the underlined part of the second sentence an adjective clause to put at the ^. Write the new sentence and underline the adjective clause."

The red envelope ^ burst into flames and curled into ashes.

It was the red envelope <u>which had dropped from Ron's hand</u>.

The red envelope, <u>which had dropped from Ron's hand</u>, burst into flames and curled into ashes.

Practice 3: Unscrambling. Students are given a list of sentence parts to unscramble. They are to write out the sentence, underlining the adjective clause.

so that it resembled a park bench

She and Ginny got into the front seat

which had been stretched

She and Ginny got into the front seat, <u>which had been stretched so that it resembled a park bench</u>.

Practice 4: Expanding. Students are to create an adjective clause to complete a sentence.

They took turns riding Harry's Nimbus Two Thousand, which . . . (e.g., was easily the best broom).

The wizard who . . . kept winking cheekily up at them all. (e.g., Harry supposed was Gilderoy Lockart).

Practice 5: Combining to Imitate. Students are presented with a model sentence from a book. They are then given several novel, related sentences and asked to combine the sentences using the model sentence as a pattern, such as:

Not daring even to look at each other, Harry and Ron followed Snape up the steps into the vast, echoing entrance hall, which was lit with flaming torches.

Celia and Monica whispered softly to each other.

Celia and Monica crept along the cold, dripping cave.

The cave was filled with flying bats.

Whispering softly to each other, Celia and Monica crept along the cold, dripping cave, which was filled with flying bats.

After students have had experiences with this sequence of practice activities based on model sentences from high-quality children's literature, they are given activities to use the structures more independently. Sentence combining can be one activity that is part of exposing students to high-quality written models to imitate. Appendix 7.1 in Chapter 7 lists books that can be used to teach some syntactic structures.

To engage in sentence combining, students need to recognize the typical order of words, phrases, and clauses in sentences. Rog (2007) suggested giving students a graphic organizer to help them "stretch" their sentences. Table 10.3 shows sentence examples using a variant of Rog's graphic. The "where" column typically uses adverbial prepositional phrases. The "when" column can use an adverbial preposition phrase ("at noon") or a dependent adverbial clause (all the other examples). The "why" column can use an infinitive phrase ("to make everyone laugh") or a dependent adverbial clause ("so no one else would get hurt"). One should be cautious in using this sentence graphic organizer. This organizer does not incorporate all aspects of sentence structure. Relative clauses, adjectival prepositional phrases, and participial phrases are not included, although one could include them after the second column to describe the "who" or "what." Also, sentence elements do not always conform to the order shown in the graphic organizer. In many instances the

TABLE 10.3	Sentence Stretching Graphic Organizer					
What kind?	Who or what?	Did what?	How	Where?	When?	Why?
large, green	turtle	crawled	slowly	up the hill	at noon	to have lunch with his friend
ancient, wise	wizard	flicked his wand	deftly	toward the evil dementor	as soon as it appeared	because he did not want to see another child harmed
angry, teenage	boy	chased the dog	hurriedly	off the playground	after it bit the child	so no one else would get hurt

"when" and "why" elements can be placed at the beginning of a sentence. Once students are able to produce sentences using the graphic organizer, show them how sentence structures can vary.

Books can also be used to demonstrate punctuation. In *Punctuation Takes a Vacation*, Pulver (2003) shows what happens if there were no punctuation:

> THIS IS WEIRD THE PUNCTUATION IS MISSING UH OH WHERE COULD IT BE YIKES MAYBE PUNCTUATION TOOK A VACATION WE ARE IN BIG TROUBLE NOW.

Each vacationing punctuation mark writes a postcard to Mr. Wright's classroom, demonstrating their use. For example, the question marks write:

> Do you miss us?
>
> How much?
>
> Why couldn't we take a vacation sooner?
>
> Guess who?

The bestselling adult book on punctuation, *Eats, Shoots & Leaves: The Zero Tolerance Approach to Punctuation* (Truss, 2003), drew attention to the important role that punctuation plays in creating meaning in texts. A children's version with a similar title, *Eats, Shoots & Leaves: Why, Commas Really DO make a Difference!* (Truss, 2006), provides humorous examples of how punctuation can change meaning. To prove her point, the author provides contrasting examples of the same sentence, punctuated in different ways. For example,

> "Go, get him doctors!" shows a child who has fallen from a playground climber. An adult is shouting to children, telling them to get a doctor for the child.

In contrast,

> "Go get him, doctors!" shows a person with a mask running out of a hospital with a child.

An adult seeing this yells to nearby doctors to go get the fleeing person.

The book *Twenty-Odd Ducks: Why, Every Punctuation Mark Counts!* (Truss, 2008) emphasizes the importance of punctuation in general. In one example, a child gazes at a tower of presents obscuring a Christmas tree, and Truss writes, "'Do you know who came last night?

Santa Claus,' said my mom." On the facing page, Santa addresses his elves: "'Do you know who came last night?' Santa Claus said. 'My mom.'" (Needless to say, no pile of presents accompanies the arrival of Santa's mom.) The roles of apostrophes are explained in *The Girl's Like Spaghetti: Why, You Can't Manage without Apostrophes* (Truss, 2007). In each example in the books, the pertinent punctuation marks are printed in red, and an afterword provides additional explanations for each pair of examples.

Summarizing

Teaching students to summarize improves not only the quality of their writing, but also their reading comprehension (Graham & Hebert, 2010; Graham & Perin, 2007b). Ideally, students should be asked to summarize texts that are well structured at both microstructure and macrostructure levels (Kintsch, 1990). Well-structured microstructures (sentences and connective words) make the relationships among concepts and ideas in text more explicit and obvious, and well-structured macrostructures highlight the primary ideas in texts. Thus, it is easier for students to recognize what should be included in the summary, and the structure of the text provides a framework for the summary the student is writing. Writing summaries is a complex task; students must identify the most important information in a text, condense the information into a very brief form, and then restate the information in their own words. Educational researchers (Brown, Campione, & Day, 1981; Brown & Day, 1983; Kintsch & van Dijk, 1978) have suggested teaching students a rule-based summary strategy that operates on the text macrostructure. The macrorules for summarization include

- Delete material that is trivial.
- Delete material that although important, is redundant.
- Substitute a superordinate term or event for a list of items or actions; if a text lists cats, dogs, goldfish, gerbils, and parrots, one can substitute the word *pets*; or integrate events or concepts by substituting a superordinate action for a list of subcomponents of that action, for example, "Michael went on vacation" for "Michael packed his bag, took a cab to the airport, boarded a plane for Cancun. . . ."
- Select a topic sentence, or
- If there is no topic sentence, then invent your own.

The task of summarizing taxes working memory. To use these summarization strategies, students must analyze information at a fairly deep level while simultaneously manipulating the text and generating sentences to express the relationships in the texts concisely. Being aware of the explicit structure of the text can be an aid to summarizing information. The more students are aware of this explicit structure and the more fluent they are in sentence generation the better they able to summarize (Armbruster, Anderson, & Ostertag, 1987).

Summarization skills develop from late elementary school through the college years. By sixth grade, students have a good understanding of what summarizing means, but they have difficulty with identifying the important ideas and especially trying to formulate main point statements of their own (Kintsch, 1990). To facilitate students' summarizing skills, it is helpful to know the micro- and macrostructures of the texts that students are to summarize, and then to employ backward design to develop the specific skills students need to summarize particular texts. Rather than beginning with a list of skills to teach and then combining the skills to achieve some product, one looks at a product, determines what students need to produce that product, and then teaches the specific skills.

Summarization requires that students integrate their microstructure knowledge and skills with their macrostructure knowledge and skills. When producing expository macrostructures, students must clearly identify the relationships between propositions in the texts and the relationship of the propositions to the overall theme of the texts. Consequently, there is an interaction between students' syntactic microstructure skills and their presentation of ideas in macrostructures. In addition, summarizing expository texts requires the ability to make inferences. Students must employ several types of inferences when they summarize. They make *generalizations,* which are inferences that reduce the number of text propositions or ideas. These are inferences about the overall gist or meaning of the text. Students make *elaborations,* which are inferences that are not directly implied by the text; they originate from the reader's own knowledge about the content or related information. They make *reorderings,* which are inferences that rearrange text content in an order that is different from the original text. And finally, they use *connective* words that express bridging inferences and that function to provide coherence between expressed ideas. Sixth-grade students are able to relate the details of what they read to a global topic, whereas older students are able to differentiate more levels of importance in the information they read.

Sixth-grade students produce few generalizations, elaborations, reorderings, and bridging inferences in the form of connectives. By 10th grade, students are producing all these types of inferences, and college students produce significantly more generalizations, elaborations, and reorderings than the 10th-grade students. The limited use of inferred information in summaries of the younger students indicates that they were composed largely of information selected sequentially from the original text. In contrast, older students, particularly college students, used inferences to formulate their summaries and reorder the information to highlight the main points of the passage. With age, there was a significant decrease in the importance of text details and an increase in macropropositions. This indicates that older students are more aware of the major ideas in the text and in the overall organization of the text.

In a program to train teachers in strategies to improve the comprehension of students in fourth and fifth grades (Westby, Culatta, Lawrence, & Hall-Kenyon, 2010), teachers were trained to work with students to identify text structures and to use graphic organizers to identify the main and supporting ideas. Students read expository texts and with teachers developed graphic organizers that highlighted the overall macrostructure of the texts. Initially, teachers partially completed the graphic organizers and then encouraged students to complete the organizer. On the graphic organizers, teachers also showed the relationships among ideas in the texts and explicitly taught the specific connectives that were needed to express the relationships among the ideas in the texts.

Students' summaries of texts provided information about how students integrated microstructure and macrostructure skills. Figure 10.2 shows a partially completed graphic organizer for a compare–contrast passage about bears. The compare–contrast bears passage and a couse–effect wildfires passage are in Appendix 10.2. A holistic rubric was developed to evaluate students' summaries. The rubric was based on Scardamalia's concept of working memory (1981), which was based on number of elements of working memory used in the production of the summary. Expository texts and summaries require coordination of at least four content units: (1) Statements must link to a central topic/theme; (2) Statements must be linked to one another; (3) The nature of the link between statements can be explicit (*because, as a result, if–then*) rather than general (*and, then, so*); and (4) Statements are simultaneously linked to the central topic and to each other according to the discourse genre. In the rubric, the primary defining characteristics of each level in terms of working memory were as follows:

- *Level 0:* Students wrote statements or ideas that may have been triggered by the topic but that were not presented in the passage. The sentences did not link to the central topic or to one another, for example, in response to the wildfire passage, a student wrote:
  - If you're trieing to start a fir by prepared to bring sum water.

And in response to the bears passage a student wrote:
  - Polar bears diggin there to look for babi sils

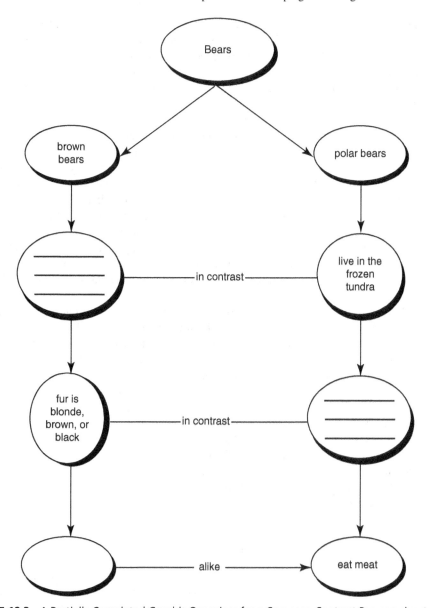

FIGURE 10.2   A Partially Completed Graphic Organizer for a Compare–Contrast Passage about Bears

- *Level 1:* Students relied on their short-term memories to retell information in the texts. They were not employing working memory—they did not evidence awareness of the overall gist or theme of the passage. They reported details of the passage, but did not indicate the relationships among the details, or the summary was too brief to indicate relationships. For example,
  - People can start wildfires with campfires. Wildfires harm people, plants and animals. Wildfires can be started by lightning.
- *Level 2:* Students held or manipulated two concepts in working memory—they either related ideas to the central topic, or they chained one idea in temporal or causal relationship

to the next. They did not, however, both simultaneously chain and center ideas. In chaining, statements (ideas) are related in a temporal or causal relationship to one another. In centering, statements are related to a central topic, but not necessarily to one another. For example,

- Brown Bears live in mountains and forests. There fur is blonde, brown, or black. They eat meat. Polar Bears live in the frozen tundra. There fur is black or white. They eat meat like the Brown Bears.

- *Level 3:* Students held and manipulated three concepts in working memory—they simultaneously chained ideas to one another and linked (or centered) each idea to the overall topic. Their summaries conveyed the overall gist of the text and indicated that they had a clear sense of the text structure. They may not use a topic sentence and may not be consistent in the way they use the organization structure. They use some connectors to express relationships between ideas, but they may use a limited variety of earlier developed connectives (*but, when, then, so, because*). (I have bolded the connective words and italicized the dependent clauses to highlight the increasing syntactic complexity.)

  - Polar Bears and Brown bears are both alike in some ways **but** they are also both different in some ways. Brown bears live in the mountains and desserts. Polar bears live in the frozen tundra. Brown bears fur is blond, brown, or black. Polar bears fur is white. **But** brown bears and Polar bears both eat meat.

- *Level 4:* This level requires manipulation of four concepts in working memory. The text structure is obvious; it is often introduced with a topic sentence. There is simultaneous chaining and centering of ideas with use of explicit connectives in clauses that make the relationships between ideas explicit with a variety of connectives and later developing connectives and conjunctives (e.g., *before, because, consequently, when, if–then, but, in contrast, similarly*). The summary captures the main ideas and primary supporting details and presents the information in a particular discourse genre.

  - Brown Bears and Polar Bears are dislike and alike in these ways. Brown bears live in mountains and forests, ***however,*** Polar Bears live in the frozen tundra. Brown bears fur is blonde, brown, or black. **But** Polar Bears fur looks white **but** is really clear. ***Although*** *they are different in these ways* they are alike **because** *they both eat meat.*

  - Wildfires are dangerous **because** *there hard to put out.* A wildfire may be started by people **when** *they start campfires* and a spark spreads to dry grass catching it on fire. Another way is **when** *people lighting fireworks* and a spark also catches it on fire. A natural way is **if** *lightning strikes a tree or dry grass.* Any way it starts, ***if*** *it's not taken care of* it may turn into a wildfire **which** *may hurt people, plants, and animals.*

At levels 0 and 1, students produce very brief summaries with few ideas. There can be considerable variation in the length of summaries that score as level 2. To achieve a level 3, the summaries need to be long enough if students are to show the relationships among ideas and to the overall gist of the text.

DEVELOPING WRITING PROCESSES

If children are to be effective writers, they must understand the writing process as well as have the writing foundations. They must have something to write about; they must know how to gather information, plan their writing, organize it, review it, and revise it; and they must be able to regulate their behavior in the process. Teaching students strategies to carry out the writing process is highly effective in improving their writing and reading comprehension (Graham & Hebert, 2010; Graham & Perin, 2007a, b).

Each aspect of the writing process requires metacognitive strategies:

- *Prewriting planning strategies:* Students must consider the purpose of writing (the why), the audience (the who), and the knowledge they have or need to have.
- *Organizational strategies:* Students must have strategies for considering the genre structure, putting ideas into related groups, and labeling groups of ideas.
- *Drafting strategies:* Students must have strategies for ordering ideas, translating ideas into syntactic units and print, and expanding/supporting ideas.
- *Editing/revising strategies:* Monitoring if the plan was met; monitoring organization and meaningfulness.

Strategy instruction should address the phases of the writing process. The phases should be viewed as recursive, not linear. That is, one plans before one begins to write, but one may adjust plans as one translates and revises. Similarly, revision may occur in all phases; it need not be limited to the final phase. One can revise as one plans and as one is producing the text. In the last 15 years, the Self-Regulated Strategy Development (SRSD) writing program (Graham & Harris, 2005; Harris, Graham, Mason, & Friedlander, 2008) has been extensively studied. With SRSD, students learn specific strategies for accomplishing tasks along with strategies for regulating their use and undesirable behaviors (such as impulsivity) that impede performance. As with strategies for effective reading comprehension, strategies for effective writing must consider *declarative, procedural,* and *conditional* knowledge. Students must know what is expected at each stage of the writing process (declarative knowledge), they must have strategies for how to perform each stage (procedural knowledge), and they must know when and where to employ particular strategies (conditional knowledge). For example, one must know that narratives have particular elements (story grammar components) and that one can use knowledge of these elements to generate a story. One must also realize that these elements cannot be used to generate a comparison/contrast text.

High-quality children's literature can provide a model for the writing process as well as for the foundational skills. *What Do Authors Do?* (Christelow, 1995) and *From Pictures to Words: A Book about Making a Book* (Stevens, 1995) describe the process that writers go through. In *What Authors Do?* Christelow introduces neighboring authors who are watching their pets, a cat and a dog, chase each other into a pond. The authors decide to write a story about their pets. They take notes, make outlines, read, and do research. The male author writes a chapter book about a dog and cat who travel around the country on a freight train; the female author writes and illustrates a picture book about a dog-chasing cat that saves its family from a fire. The authors deal with rejection, revision, working with editors, and publishing. In *From Pictures to Words*, the author also goes through all stages of the writing process, but her story characters assist her in the process by offering suggestions for how the story should begin and develop—what is the setting, what is the plot, what problems arise for the characters in the story, and how are the problems resolved.

Strategies for Generative Ideas and Planning

The first step in the writing process is developing an idea. Graham and Perrin's meta-analysis (2007a, b) indicated that prewriting activities that help students generate ideas and inquiry activities that engage children in finding content information for a task are both effective in improving the students' written products. When asked to write, many students are quick to respond that they have nothing to write about. They are told to "write what you know." They are, however, unaware of what they do know and may require assistance in discovering ideas for their writing. *Nothing Ever Happens on 90th Street* (Schotter, 1997) encourages students to develop stories based on what they see around themselves. In this story, Eva's homework assignment is to write what she knows. She sits on her stoop thinking that observing the neighborhood happenings will be boring. At first it is, but she encounters neighbors with a variety of problems—being unemployed, having difficulty making a tasty mousse, one who doesn't smile. All of them have suggestions for Eva's writing, though. They advise her to not neglect the details, use her imagination, stretch the truth, add action as if it were seasoning, and most of all, when the story bogs down, ask, "What if . . .?" and try to figure out what happens next. That's just what Eva does, and with imaginative ideas she develops a story in which neighbors fall in love, open restaurants, and add mocha to mousse.

Once students have their ideas, they must struggle with finding the words that will truly "show" the reader their ideas. In *Show; Don't Tell: Secrets of Writing* (Nobisso, 2004), the author offers insight into authors' decisions regarding their choices of nouns and adjectives. A lion explains to his friends (a hippo, a duck, a penguin, and a cow) that they need to use their five senses and their intuition when writing. The animals try out the lion's suggestions. The book has some interactive materials to encourage using language of the senses—a mesh grid to feel, a scratch and sniff page to smell, and a sound module (of breaking glass) to listen to. For each of these, the characters (and readers) are encouraged to find the right words to "show" what they are sensing; and in a variety of illustrations, they are shown what happens when the chosen words are not specific enough. Both Cleary and Heller have a series of books that demonstrate the effective use of the parts of speech in vivid, colorful ways. (See children's books reference list at the end of this chapter.)

Writing what you know works for personal narratives and some imaginative stories, but works less well for assignments requiring students to produce expository texts because students do not have the background knowledge required for writing tasks. The Writing for Understanding approach (Hawkins, Ginty, Kurzman, Leddy, & Miller, 2008) recognizes that most students require explicit instruction in gathering information and employing the appropriate organizational structures to convey that information. The Writing for Understanding approach makes extensive use of text models and modeling of the writing process as well as a backward design approach to curriculum design. When employing backward design, educators note the knowledge and skills required to complete a particular task, for example, what content knowledge students must possess, what genre or genres students must use, whether they know the macrostructure organization of the genre, and whether they have the necessary microstructure skills (vocabulary and syntactic skills) to complete the task. Rather than teaching a general hierarchy of skills, when employing a backward design approach to the curriculum, the skills that are taught are based on what skills and knowledge the students require for the task. Educators must ensure that students engage in prewriting and inquiry skills to gain knowledge about their topics. In today's world, this necessitates that educators develop students' multiliteracy skills, that is, the ability to access information through a variety of multimedia sources in addition to books and magazines (Westby, 2010). Students must be able to effectively search Internet hypertext and use video and graphic media to gather and organize information.

Many students, at all age levels, do no planning when they write. When given a topic, they employ *knowledge telling,* simply writing down anything that comes to mind (Bereiter & Scardamalia, 1987). To plan, students must have adequate background information on a topic, and they must have declarative knowledge about the structural components of the genre. A planning strategy can be as simple as having a student outline the components of a text, as described in the use of the story wheel for developing narratives. The CSIW employs "think-sheets" that function like the story wheel. They are designed to make the strategies for each of the text structures explicit (Englert & Mariage, 1991). In a generic plan-think sheet, the students indicate:

Topic

Who: Who am I writing for?

Why: Why am I writing?

What: What do I know? (Brainstorm a list of what is known about the topic)

How: How can I group my ideas?

A think-plan sheet for an explanatory text may include

What is being explained?

     Materials/things you need?

     Setting?

What are the steps?

     First,

     Next,

     Third,

     Then,

     Last

Harris, Graham and Mason (2003) presented students with a general three-step mnemonic for writing, POW (**P**ick my idea, **O**rganize my notes, **W**rite and say more), then followed this with specific mneumonics for particular genres. For example, W-W-W What = 2 How = 2 is used to help children remember parts to include in a story:

Who is the main character?

When does the story take place?

Where does the story take place?

What does the main character do or want to do; what do others characters do?

What happens then? What happens with the other characters?

How does the story end?

How does the main character feel; how do the other characters feel?

The mnemonic TREE is used with elementary school children to plan an opinion or persuasive essay (Harris & Graham, 1996b):

• Note **T**opic sentence
• Note **R**easons
• **E**xamine reasons—will my reader by this?
• Note **E**nding

Older students use the STOP strategy. When using this strategy, students first think about their audience and their purpose for writing, then they:

• **S**uspend judgment
• **T**ake a side

- **O**rganize ideas
- **P**lan more as you write

In the first step, students generate all the ideas they can that support each side of an issue. In the second step, they evaluate the ideas and take a side. In the third step, they organize their ideas by putting a star next to ideas they want to use, an X next to arguments they want to dispute, and then number the ideas in the order they will use them.

The final step is a reminder to continue to plan throughout the writing process. During the writing process, students consult a cue card with the acronym DARE that reminds them to check that they are including all the structural components of the argument:

Develop your topic sentence

Add supporting ideas

Reject possible arguments for the other side

End with a conclusion

Strategies for Production

During the translating or actual writing, students are encouraged to use self-verbalizations to make certain they are following their plans and self-regulating their performance. For example,

- Focusing attention and planning: I've got to come up with a topic sentence. Maybe I could say, "The world cannot exist without rain forests."
- Self-evaluating and error correcting: I've given two reasons. But I haven't really said why they are important; this isn't long enough—I've got to write some more.
- Coping and self-control: I'm not going to crumple the paper and start over.
- Self-reinforcement: I know a lot about rainforests. This last sentence is good.

For elementary school children, Harris and Graham (1996a) recommend working with them to develop self-regulatory statements in categories such as: things to get me started (problem definition and focusing/planning); things to say while I work (focusing/planning, strategy, self-evaluating/error correcting, coping, and self-reinforcement), and things to say when I'm done.

Strategies for Revising

Students frequently resist revising, and when they do revise, they tend to confine their revisions to proofreading for spelling errors rather than revising to improve meaning and organization. Revising is a difficult, complex activity that taxes working memory. Students must be able to compare what they have written with their goals, evaluate the degree to which they have achieved their goals, and when the text does not meet the goals, modify the text.

Bereiter and Scardamalia (1987) proposed a compare–diagnose–operate (C–D–O) strategy that reduces the working memory or executive demands on students. Students are given cards with the following evaluative statements:

1. People won't see why this is important.
2. People may not believe this.
3. People won't be very interested in this part.
4. People may not understand what I mean here.
5. People will be interested in this part.
6. This is good.

7. This is a useful sentence.
8. I think this could be said more clearly.
9. I'm getting away from the main point.
10. Even I'm confused about what I'm trying to say.
11. This doesn't sound quite right.

Students read a sentence in their drafts, then choose one of these evaluative statements. If students select an evaluative statement such as, "This is a useful sentence," they go on to the next sentence and choose another evaluative card. If they choose a statement such as, "Even I'm confused about what I'm trying to say," they then choose a directive statement to facilitate tactical choice:

1. I think I'll leave it this way.
2. I'd better give an example.
3. I'd better leave this part out.
4. I'd better cross this sentence out and say it a different way.
5. I'd better say more.
6. I'd better change the wording.

If they chose a statement such as "I'd better change the wording," they make a wording change and then go on to the next sentence.

The C–D–O strategy may be a good way to get students to begin to think about revision; however, because it focuses on sentence-level revision, it may not influence higher text-level issues related to content and organizational structure. One may want to add another series of statements that students use for the overall text:

1. Too few ideas.
2. Part of the essay doesn't belong with the rest.
3. Incomplete idea.
4. I've ignored the obvious point someone would bring up against what I'm saying.
5. Weak reason.
6. Choppy—ideas are not connected to each other very well.
7. Hard to tell what the main point is.
8. Doesn't give the reader reason to take the idea seriously.
9. Too much space given to an unimportant point.

Harris and Graham (1996b) use a very simplified version of this procedure, which they term SCAN:

- **SCAN** each sentence:
  Does it make **S**ense?
  Is it **C**onnected to my central idea?
  Can I **A**dd more detail?
  Note errors.

Writing process classrooms often use peer revising strategies. Students may come to an author's chair, where they read their papers to a small group of other children. The children:

1. Listen to the text.
2. Comment on something they like about the text and why they like it.
3. Comment on something they think could be done better and how the text could be revised.

Effective use of the author's chair and peer revision requires modeling by adults of types of statements that can be helpful. Otherwise, students give vague responses such as, "I liked it cause it's a story," or "make it look neater."

Summary

Expert writers are made not born. Some current process approaches to the teaching of writing assume that students learn to write simply by writing a lot; they do not need explicit teaching of form and style. Although it may be true that some students do learn to write simply by writing, many students require more specific teaching or mentoring. Such assistance is particularly important for students such as those with language learning disabilities who have difficulty acquiring the written language code or those from culturally/linguistically diverse backgrounds who have less exposure to the English written language code. More explicit teaching and careful scaffolding of teacher–student interactions around writing would probably be beneficial for all students. Coe (1994) suggested,

> People learned to swim for millennia before coaches explicitly articulated our knowledge of how to swim, but kids today learn to swim better (and in less time) on the basis of that explicit knowledge. The same can be said about most athletic and craft skills. Might it be true for writing as well? (p. 159)

If teachers and speech-language pathologists are to provide explicit teaching to develop students' writing, they must know how writing develops in a variety of genres. They must be able to assess students' present writing abilities, provide meaningful activities for writing, and provide both scaffolded support and direct instruction in the components of writing (handwriting, keyboarding, punctuation, spelling, sentence construction, genre organization). Finally, they must ensure that students acquire cognitive strategies and the motivation and ability to use these strategies to become independent writers.

References

Armbruster, B. B., Anderson, T. H., & Ostertag, J. (1987). Does text structure/summarization instruction facilitate learning of expository text? *Reading Research Quarterly, 22*, 331–346.

Bereiter, C., & Scardamalia, M. (1987). *The psychology of written communication.* Hillsdale, NJ: Erlbaum.

Berninger, V. W., & Amtmann, D. (2003). Preventing written expression disabilities through early and continuing assessment and intervention for handwriting and/or spelling problems: Research into practice. In H. L. Swanson, K. R. Harris, & S. Graham (Eds.), *Handbook of learning disabilities* (pp. 345–363). New York: Guilford.

Brown, A. L., Campione, J. C., & Day, J. D. (1981). Learning to learn: On training students to learn from texts. *Educational Researchers, 10*, 14–21.

Brown, A. L., & Day, J. D. (1983). Macrorules for summarizing texts: The development of expertise. *Journal of Verbal Learning and Verbal Behavior, 22*, 1–14.

Coe, R. M. (1994). Teaching genre as process. In A. Freedman & P. Medway (Eds.), *Learning and teaching genre* (pp. 157–169). Portsmouth, NH: Heinemann.

Dean, D. (2008). *Bringing grammar to life.* Newark, DE: International Reading Association.

Dorfman, L. R., & Cappelli, R. (2007). *Mentor texts: Teaching writing through children's literature, K–6.* Portland, ME: Stenhouse Publishers.

Dorfman, L. R., & Cappelli, R. (2009). *Nonfiction mentor texts: Teaching informational writing through children's literature, K–8.* Portland, ME: Stenhouse Publishers

Emig, J. (1971). *The composing processes of twelfth graders.* Urbana, IL: National Council of Teachers of English.

Englert, C. S., & Mariage, T. V. (1991). Shared understandings: Structuring the writing experience through full text available. *Journal of Learning Disabilities, 24*, 330–342.

Esterreicher, C. A. (1994). *Scamper strategies.* Eau Claire, WI: Thinking Publications.

Graham, S. (1992). Issues in handwriting instruction. *Focus on Exceptional Children, 25*, 1–16.

Graham, S., Berninger, V., Abbott, R., Abbott, S., & Whitaker, D. (1997). The role of mechanics in composing of elementary school students: A new methodological approach. *Journal of Educational Psychology, 89,* 170–182.

Graham, S., & Harris, K. R. (2005). *Writing better: Effective strategies for teaching students with learning difficulties.* Baltimore: Brookes.

Graham, S., & Hebert, M. (2010). *Writing to read: Evidence for how writing can improve reading.* Washington, DC: Alliance for Excellent Education.

Graham, S., & Perin, D. (2007a). A meta-analysis of writing instruction for adolescent students. *Journal of Educational Psychology, 99,* 445–476.

Graham, S., & Perin, D. (2007b). *Writing next: Effective strategies to improve writing of adolescents in middle and high school.* Washington, DC: Alliance for Excellence in Education.

Graves, D. H. (1983). *Writing: Teachers and children at work.* Portsmouth, NH: Heinemann.

Halliday, M. A. K. (1985). An introduction to functional grammar. London: Edward Arnold.

Harris, K. R., & Graham, S. (1996a). Constructivism and students with special needs: Issues in the classroom. *Learning Disabilities: Research and Practice, 11,* 133–137.

Harris, K. R., & Graham, S. (1996b). *Making the writing process work: Strategies for composition and self-regulation.* Cambridge, MA: Brookline Books.

Harris, K. R., Graham, S., & Mason, L. H. (2003). Self-regulated strategy development in the classroom: Part of a balanced approach to writing instruction for students with disabilities. *Focus on Exceptional Education, 35*(7), 1–16.

Harris, K. R., Graham, S., Mason, L. H., & Friedlander, B. (2008). *Powerful writing strategies for all students.* Baltimore: Brookes.

Hawkins, J., Ginty, E., Kurzman, K. L., Leddy, D., & Miller, J. (2008). *Writing for understanding: Using backward design to help all students write effectively.* Hopewell, NJ: Authentic Education.

Hillocks, G., & Smith, M. W. (2003). Grammars and literacy learning. In J. Flood, J. Jensen, D. Lapp, & J. Squire (Eds.), *Handbook of research on teaching the English language arts* (2nd ed., pp. 721–737). Mahwah, NJ: Erlbaum.

Killgallon, D., & Killgallon, J. (2000). *Sentence composing for elementary school.* Portsmouth, NH: Heinemann.

Killgallon, D., & Killgallon, J. (2006). *Grammar for middle school: A sentence composing approach.* Portsmouth, NH: Heinemann.

Kintsch, E. (1990). Macroprocesses and microprocesses in the development of summarization skill. *Cognition and instruction, 7,* 161–195.

Kintsch, W., & van Dijk, T. A. (1978). Toward a model of text comprehension and production. *Psychological Review, 85,* 363–394.

Moreau, M. R., & Fidrych-Puzzo, H. (1994). *The story grammar marker.* Easthampton, MA: Discourse Skills Productions.

Nelson, N. W., Roth, F. P., & Van Meter, A. M. (2009). Written composition instruction and intervention for students with language impairment. In G. A. Troia (Ed.), *Instruction and assessment for struggling writers* (pp. 187–212). New York: Guilford.

Olsen, J. (1998). *Handwriting without tears.* Cabin John, MD: Author.

Rog, L. J. (2007). *Marvelous minilessons for teaching beginning writing, K–3.* Newark, DE: International Reading Association.

Saddler, B., & Graham, S. (2005). The effects of peer-assisted sentence combining instruction on the writing performance of more and less skill young writers. *Journal of Educational Psychology, 97,* 43–54.

Scanlon, D., Deshler, D. D., & Schumaker, J. B. (1996). Can a strategy be taught and learned in secondary inclusive classrooms? *Learning Disabilities: Research & Practice, 11,* 41–57.

Scardamalia, M. (1981). How children cope with the cognitive demands of writing. In C. H. Frederiksen & J. F. Dominic (Eds.), *Writing: The nature, development, and teaching of written communication* (pp. 81–103). Hillsdale, NJ: Erlbaum.

Singer, B. D., & Bashir, A. S. (2004). Developmental variations in writing composition skills. In C. A. Stone, E. R. Silliman, B. J. Ehren, & K. Apel (Eds.), *Handbook of language and literacy* (pp. 559–582). New York: Guilford.

Strong, W. (1986). *Creative approaches to sentence combining.* Urbana, IL: National Council of Teachers of English.

Truss, L. (2003). *Eats, shoots & leaves: The zero tolerance approach to punctuation.* New York: Gotham Books.

Westby, C. E. (2010). Multiliteracies: The changing world of communication. *Topics in Language Disorders, 30,* 64–71.

Westby, C. E., Culatta, B., Lawrence, B., & Hall-Kenyon, K. (2010). Summarizing expository texts. *Topics in Language Disorders, 30*(4), 275–287.

Westby, C. E., Moore, C., & Roman, R. (2002). Reinventing the enemy's language: Developing narratives in Native American children. *Language and Linguistics, 13*(2), 235–269.

Children's Books

Christelow, E. (1995). *What do authors do?* New York: Clarion House.

Cleary, B. P. (2000). *Hairy, scary, ordinary: What is an adjective?* New York: Scholastic.

Cleary, B. P. (2001). *To root to toot to parachute: What is a verb?* Minneapolis, MN: Lerner.

Cleary, B. P. (2002). *Under, over, by the clover: What is a preposition?* Minneapolis, MN: Lerner.

Cleary, B. P. (1999). *A rink, a fink, a skating rink. What is a noun?* Minneapolis, MN: Lerner.

Cleary, B. P. (2005). *Dearly, nearly, insincerely: What is an adverb?* Minneapolis, MN: Lerner.

Cleary, B. P. (2006). *I and you and don't forget who. What is a pronoun?* Minneapolis, MN: Lerner.

Cleary, B. P. (2009). *Slide and slurp, scratch and burp: More above verbs.* Minneapolis, MN: Lerner.

Cleary, B. P. (2009). *Quirky, jerky, extra perky: More about adjectives.* Minneapolis, MN: Lerner.

Cleary, B. P. (2008). *A lime, a mime, a pool of slime: More about nouns.* Minneapolis, MN: First Avenue Editions.

Cleary, B. P. (2010). *Lazily, crazily, just about nasally: More about adverbs.* Minneapolis, MN: First Avenue Editions.

Cleary, B. P. (2010). *But and for, yet and nor: What is a conjunction?* Minneapolis: Lerner.

Cleary, B. P. (2010). *Punctuation station.* Minneapolis, MN: Lerner.

Duke, K. (1992). *Aunt Isabel tells a good one.* New York: Dutton.

Gaiman, N. (2008). *The graveyard book.* New York: HarperCollins.

Heller, R. (1988). *Kites sail high: A book about verbs.* New York: Putnam.

Heller, R. (1998). *Many luscious lollipops: A book about adjectives.* New York: Putnam.

Heller, R. (1998). *Behind the mask: A book about prepositions.* New York: Putnam.

Heller, R. (1998). *Up, up and away: A book about adjectives.* New York: Putnam.

Heller, R. (1998). *Merry-go-round: A book about nouns.* New York: Putnam.

Heller, R. (1999). *Mine, all mine: A book about pronouns.* New York: Putnam.

Lyon, G. E. (1999). *Where I'm from.* Spring, TX: Absey & Co.

Nobisso, J. (2004). *Show, don't tell: Secrets of writing.* New York: Gingerbread House.

Orloff, K. K. (2004). *I wanna iguana.* New York: Putnam.

Pulver, R. (2003). *Punctuation takes a vacation.* New York: Holiday House.

Rowling, J. K. (2000). *Harry Potter and the chamber of secrets.* New York: Scholastic.

Schotter, R. (1997). *Nothing ever happens on 90th street.* New York: Scholastic.

Stevens, J. (1995). *From pictures to words: A book about making a book.* New York: Holiday House.

Spiegelman, A. (1997). *Open me . . . I'm a dog!* New York: HarperCollins.

Teague, M. (1996). *The secret shortcut.* New York: Scholastic.

Truss, L. (2006). *Eats, shoots & leaves: Why, commas really DO make a difference.* New York: G.P. Putnam.

Truss, L. (2007). *The girl's like spaghetti: Why, you can't manage without apostrophes.* New York: G.P. Putnam.

Truss, L. (2008). *Twenty-odd ducks: Why, every punctuation mark counts.* New York: G.P. Putnam.

Appendix *10.1*

Students' Postmodern Stories

Read Me, I'm a Baseball

It all started when a boy named Babe, who loved baseball, walked into a baseball shop. He walked to the front desk and asked for a decent bat. It was then he saw me. He said, "Never mind about that bat. I want that baseball!" He brought me to every baseball game he ever had. Even when he was in the major leagues. On the big night of his life he made it to the world series. The announcer said The one the only Babe Ruth!" Bottom of the 9th . . . down by 3 . . . bases loaded. . . . What! I go flying . . . Through the air and over the back wall! Babe Ruth has hit a grand slam with me. The Yankees has won!!!!!!!!!!! Babe is so happy that it was his ball, me, that won the world series.

Open Me, I'm a Penguin

What's that? You think I smell of paper and lead?" You think I look like a book? Well I can assure you I'm not a book. See I can waddle and can squeak "squeak squeak." See I can be your cute Arctic pet. We will go skiing together and slide down slides together on our bellies. Let me be your penguin and I will tell you my story. It all started when I went hunting for fish and I started getting chased by a killer whale. Then the killer whale king saw me and turned me into a . . . high flyer! But not like this one, a balloon flyer . . . high in the sky! Over the icy landscape I saw an alba-tross! I went down to saw hi but I accidentally bumped into him. He got really mad and turned me into a . . . fish! But not like this one. I was big, fat and juicy. And I fell the albatross was right behind me. Suddenly, I landed on a human wizard that was walking over a frozen plateau. He got sup mad and turned me into this book. That's my story. But I can still squeak "squeak, squeak" and cuddle in your lap. If you let me be your Arctic pet, I'll tell you my story anytime you like.

Appendix 10.2

Wildfires Passage

Wildfires are fires that are large and out of control. People should do everything they can to prevent wildfires. People need to be careful when using fire. If people start a campfire then a spark may spread and catch dry grass on fire. People also need to be careful when lighting fireworks because the sparks from the fireworks can also catch the nearby grass on fire. Sparks from campfires or fireworks can cause a wildfire. Not all wildfires happen because of people. A thunderstorm may cause lightning to strike the dry ground or a nearby tree. As a result, a wildfire can start. Whether a wildfire is started by people or a storm, it can be very dangerous and may result in harm to people, plants, and animals.

Bears Passage

Bears are found throughout the world. Two main types are brown bears and polar bears.

Brown bears live in mountains and forests. Their fur is blonde, brown, or black. The tips of their fur are gray, giving them a grizzled look. This is why they are sometimes called grizzly bears. It also helps them hide in the shrubs and trees where they live. Polar bears live on frozen tundra by the ocean. It is difficult to live there. It is mostly cold and dark and there are very few plants and animals. In order to survive, the polar bear has adapted in special ways. The skin of the bear is black. This draws every bit of possible heat from the sunlight. The bear's hairs appear to be white, but they are actually clear. Below these hairs are orange or yellow, "underhairs".

Brown bears are omnivores. They eat some meat, but mostly they eat plants. This includes grasses, bulbs, seeds, berries, and roots. They will also eat insects, fish, and small mammals. Some bears eat large animals, including moose, caribou, and elk. Polar bears are also omnivores. They eat some plants, but of all bears, the polar bear eats the most meat. Polar bears hunt seals. Seals must make holes in the ice so they can come up to breathe. The bears will sit near these holes for hours waiting to capture the seals.

INDEX